RETURN

Judy Thompson

SOFT-TISSUE MANIPULATION

An authoritative textbook dealing with Neuro-Muscular Technique,
Muscle Energy Technique and Strain-Counterstrain — diagnostic and
therapeutic methods which restore the structural, functional
and postural integrity of the body, removing pain,
muscular tension, stress and restrictions to health.

SOFT~TISSUE MANIPULATION

A Practitioner's Guide to the Diagnosis and Treatment of
Soft Tissue Dysfunction and Reflex Activity

by
LEON CHAITOW
N.D., D.O., M.B.N.O.A.

Illustrated by Bevil Roberts

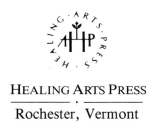

HEALING ARTS PRESS

Rochester, Vermont

Healing Arts Press
One Park Street
Rochester, Vermont 05767

ISBN 0-89281-276-1

Printed and bound in the United Kingdom.

3   5   7   9   10   8   6   4   2

Healing Arts Press is a division of Inner Traditions International Ltd.

Distributed to the book trade in the United States by Harper and Row Publishers, Inc.
Distributed to the book trade in Canada by Book Center, Inc., Montreal, Quebec
Distributed to the health food trade in Canada by Alive Books,
Toronto and Vancouver

Contents

	Page
Acknowledgements	7
Introduction	9

Chapter

1. Somatic Dysfunction — The Soft Tissue Component	15
2. Reflex Areas and Somatic Dysfunction	41
3. Diagnostic Methods	75
4. Postural and Emotional Considerations	97
5. Techniques and Index of Neurolymphatic Reflexes	121
6. Basic Spinal Neuro-muscular Techniques	173
7. Basic Abdominal Techniques	187
8. NMT in Clinical Use	195
9. Muscle Energy Techniques	201
10. Strain-Counterstrain (Tender Point) Technique	241
11. On Energy	257
Bibliography	265
Index	267

To my wife, Alkmini and our
daughter, Sasha.

Acknowledgements

My grateful thanks go to Dr Boris Chaitow for the notes, photographs and guidance which greatly aided me in the preparation of the chapter on abdominal technique in particular and the whole book in general. I also wish to express my thanks to Peter Lief D.O. for his permission to quote from his written and spoken comments on his and his late father's contribution to manipulative therapy. My thanks go, too, to Brian Youngs B.Sc., D.O. for his generous permission to quote from his authoritative articles on the theoretical and practical aspects of Neuro-muscular Technique. Also, my special thanks to Terry G. Moule N.D., D.O. for his contribution to Chapter 8 'NMT in Clinical Use'.

I acknowledge with gratitude Michael M. Patterson Ph.D., Associate Professor of Osteopathic medicine at The College of Osteopathic Medicine, Ohio University, for his assistance in giving permission to quote from his writings. My thanks, also, to Churchill Livingstone for permission to quote from the book *Connective Tissue Massage* by Maria Ebner (a book now sadly out of print).

Thanks are also due to the Rolf Institute's Executive Director, Richard Stenstadvold, for permission to quote from the writings of the late founder of the Institute, Ida Rolf; to The Japan Publishing Company for their permission to quote from *Tsubo—Vital Points for Oriental Therapy* by Katsusuke Serizawa M.D.; to Randolph Stone D.C. for the quotations from his work on Polarity Therapy—there is a lot of common ground between his methods and those of Stanley Lief; and to Williams & Wilkins Co. for muscle tests quoted from *Posture and Pain* by Kendall, Kendall and Boynton.

My sincere thanks go to all the writers, medical, osteopathic, chiropractic and others, whose work I have alluded to or quoted from; and especially Bevil Roberts for his dedicated work in illustrating this book.

On a more personal level I wish to thank my father, Max Chaitow, for providing the information regarding the early family history of his cousin Stanley Lief; and to thank most sincerely my wife, Alkmini, without whose patient help this book would not have been written.

Finally, and most importantly, I wish to express my thanks and deep respect to the memory of that giant among men, the late Stanley Lief. His work goes on, and the spread of the knowledge of Neuro-muscular Technique serves to underline yet further his contribution to natural healing. I hope I have done him justice.

Introduction

The role of the soft tissue of the body in terms of health and dysfunction deserves re-emphasis, as does the relationship of the muscle, fascia and connective tissue in general to the overall economy of the body and to its ability to function efficiently. The ways in which dysfunction in the soft tissue mirrors deeper pathology of both mind and body, and the ways in which it influences such pathology, directly or reflexly, are profoundly important.

A factor common to the various reflex systems (such as acupuncture points, Chapman's neurolymphatic reflexes, myofascial trigger points etc.) seems to be their siting in fascial tissue. The stresses and strains produced in this ubiquitous tissue produce definite patterns, many of which are related to lines of postural stress, which are fairly uniform in man. Andrew Taylor Still, the founder of osteopathic medicine, was clearly prophetic when he stated that the fascia is the place to look for the cause of disease, and the place to begin the action of remedies. Palpable tender areas of dysfunction, which often display measurable changes of cutaneous electrical potential, may be regarded as common to all these systems.

This aspect of soft tissue manipulation will form a major part of this book. It is the intention to introduce a variety of systems, which have in common the use of distinct, palpable, usually sensitive, areas of the soft tissues which may be contracted, in either a diagnostic or a therapeutic manner, or both. The classification of such points into particular types, with their own characteristics, in terms of the effects they have on local or general function and pain, is a practical necessity. It has been suggested, however, with some seriousness, that there are in fact so many points and areas charted that the entire body surface is potentially of diagnostic or therapeutic value. This will be discussed further in Chapter 2, when we examine some of the more developed classifications of reflex points, as well as acupuncture points with which they are often interchangeable.

The designation of some of these points as being 'neurovascular', or 'neurolymphatic' points, does not indicate that these are necessarily accurate descriptions of their nature. What is clear is that they are not mere figments of the imagination.

The noted chiropractic researcher, and developer of a system of treatment of the musculo-skeletal system known as Receptor-Tonus technique, Raymond Nimmo D.C., stated in 1971 (*The Receptor*, Vol. 2, No. 1, pp. 47): 'There is no such thing as a neurolymphatic reflex, and the osteopathic profession discredited the Chapman system years ago.'

This is far from the truth, as evidenced by the employment of neurolymphatic reflexes in clinical trials. In Chapter 2, for example, details are given of one clinical trial, conducted under hospital conditions in 1979, in which stimulation of the Chapman's neurolymphatic adrenal point was shown to produce significant alterations in serum aldosterone levels, over a three-day period, whilst a 'dummy' point nearby, produced no alteration on stimulation. These points may not be related neurologically to the lymphatics, in a direct sense. Clinically, however, they have been shown to beneficially influence lymphatic stasis. The neurovascular points, described by Bennett (Chapter 2), may also have no proven neural connection with vascular structures, but improvement in circulatory function follows their employment. Bennett's points have a close resemblance to some of the reflex abdominal areas, described by McKenzie, and both sets of points have many resemblances to traditional acupuncture points. Their description in this book relates to the designations given them by the practitioners who noted their importance, and who rightly or wrongly, named them in these ways, Frank Chapman and Terence Bennett.

The methods of treatment of these reflex areas vary, and these will be discussed. We will also present variations in the use of soft-tissue manipulation, which are applicable to such areas. The use of other modalities, such as local anaesthetic injections of trigger points, will not be discussed, as such information is available in appropriate texts. Apart from the various systems, involving reflex points, and the discussion of the significance and methods of treating trigger points, the three methods of soft-tissue manipulation which will be presented are Neuro-muscular Technique, Muscle Energy Technique, and the functional technique known as Strain Counterstrain.

There are a number of additional individual techniques, specifically related to particular areas, such as the psoas, piriformis and tensor fascia lata, which will be included in the text but what will not be presented in detail are those techniques which form the major part of traditional massage therapy. These are available for study in appropriate texts, and it is not considered necessary to do more than briefly review these. Soft-tissue manipulation is capable of being used as part of any physical form of treatment, and may be combined with osteopathic, chiropractice, physiotherapeutic and gymnastic therapy, to great advantage. It may also be used on its own, in a paliative or corrective manner, as we shall discover.

All dysfunction of the musculo-skeletal system requires that an overall appreciation be made as to causative factors. The treatment of symptoms is never more than of short-term value, without attention to the correction of those factors from which these symptoms derive, whether these be postural, occupational, habitual, emotional or any other form of misuse of the primary machinery of life, the musculo-skeletal system. The accusation may be that by paying undue attention to the soft-tissue component of the musculo-skeletal system other vital aspects are being ignored. If the advice of this book were that correction of joint problems, and overall postural and functional re-education, as appropriate, were to be ignored, then this would be a valid criticism. This is not the viewpoint expressed in this book. We are stressing the vital need for attention to be paid to the soft-tissue component, but not to the exclusion of attention to the joints and skeletal structures, and certainly not with any thought of avoiding the correction of those contributory factors, which are identifiable and correctable.

Manipulation has, to a large extent, minimized the importance of the soft-tissues in general, and the muscles and fascia in particular. There has, to be sure, been a great deal written, regarding these structures, and a number of osteopathic and chiropractic practitioners and authors have made major contributions to our knowledge in these areas. However, the majority of practitioners involved in physical therapy, of all sorts, do not exploit the diagnostic and therapeutic potential of the soft tissues fully. This is a tendency which is changing, as the newer, less stressful, methods of manipulation, such as functional technique, and muscle energy methods, are being adopted. It is to be hoped then, that it is quite clear that the methods presented in this work are designed to contribute towards the understanding and treatment of somatic dysfunction, and that this is seen to be but a part of the overall rehabilitation and re-education of the total structure.

There are many conditions in which the use of soft tissue manipulation, as presented in this book, can obviate the requirement for any other form of physical therapy or manipulation, but this is not, by any means, always the case, and in most situations these methods should be seen as part of an overall treatment plan, which among other benefits, offers access to diagnostic information which cannot be obtained, other than from the soft tissues.

The objectives, if not the methods, outlined herein, are not new. Carl McConnel D.O., a major force in early osteopathic history, discussed the soft tissues thus: 'A pathological point of prime importance, for example, is that osseous malalignment is sustained by ligamentous rigidity. This rigidity is incepted by way of muscular fascial and tendinous tensions and stresses. Every case portrays a uniqueness in accordance with location, architectural plan and laws, tissue texture, regional and strength ratios, resident properties, environmental settings, resolution of forces etc. Remember I am speaking of the solid biological background of individual pathogenesis, the veritable soil of prediseased conditions.' He continues, 'The lack of either sufficient, or efficient, soft-tissue work, is one reason for mediocre technique and recurrence of lesions. The same is evident in the correction of postural defects.' (*1962 Year Book*, Osteopathic Institute of Applied Technique.)

These views will be found echoed in the words of more recent practitioners and researchers into the correction of musculo-skeletal dysfunction. The methods outlined in this book aid in the correction of the fundamental problems of this structure.

Neuro-muscular Technique (NMT) is a method of diagnostic and therapeutic value, which is simple in its application yet has enormous potential. The developer of this technique was Stanley Lief who was born in Lutzen in the Baltic state of Latvia in the early 1890s. He was one of the five children of Isaac and Riva Lief (Riva was the author's grandfather's eldest sister). The family emigrated to South Africa in the early 1900s where Stanley was given a basic primary school education before starting work in his father's trading store in Roodeport, Transvaal.

His health was poor and this led to an interest in physical culture, one source of inspiration for which was in the form of magazines from America. Eventually he worked his passage to the U.S.A. in order to train under the legendary Bernarr Macfadden. He qualified in chiropractic and naturopathy before the First World War, and was in Britain at the outbreak of war. After serving in the army during the war he returned to England and worked in institutional Nature Cure resorts until 1925 when he established his own Hydro, Champneys, at Tring in Hertfordshire.

At this world-famous healing resort he established his reputation as a daring and pioneering healer. By using the dietetic, fasting, hydrotherapeutic and physical methods, by which means naturopathy aims to restore normality to the sick body, he developed a huge following. During his most successful years before the Second World War he evolved the technique which this book attempts to describe.

Stanley Lief and his cousin Boris Chaitow, who worked as his assistant at Champneys before and during the Second World War, developed and refined the uses of NMT. Boris Chaitow was also born in Latvia and as a child went to live in South Africa. He was qualified as a lawyer and was in practice with my father when he became inspired by Stanley Lief's example and, with Lief's help, trained in America before joining him at Champneys in 1937. Boris Chaitow is still in practice at his superb health resort in the Cape, South Africa.

In this book the basic application, together with some specialized soft tissue manipulation techniques, will be presented, as will various reflex systems which fall within the scope of soft tissue treatment in general and NMT in particular. Detailed reference to and illustrations of the neurolymphatic reflexes of Chapman, together with illustrations of other reflex patterns such as myofascial trigger points, have therefore been included.

NMT, as a modality, may be incorporated into any system of physical medicine. It may (and indeed often should) be used as a treatment on its own, or it may accompany (preceding for preference) manipulative and other physical modalities. Its main use up to the present has been in the hands (literally) of the osteopathic profession. However, those physiotherapists, chiropractors and doctors of physical medicine who have studied and used NMT have found it complementary to their own methods of practice.

I firmly believe that this method, if comprehended and used as Stanley Lief and Boris Chaitow intended, can substantially aid practitioners in resolving the problems of many of their patients. Since it offers a simultaneous diagnostic and therapeutic capability NMT is time saving, energy saving and, above all, efficient.

The specialized soft tissue manipulative methods described, as well as muscle energy technique (MET), may be used independently or as part of NMT treatment. Practice is required in all these methods, and the key to the successful use of NMT is the ability to sense accurately what it is that the hands are feeling, together with having a clear picture of what the particular movement of technique being employed is aimed at achieving. If the practitioner can learn to 'see' with his hands, and by using them let the patient's body 'tell its own tale', then the intelligent application of the methods described here will provide a major step towards the recovery of health.

Holistic methods of healing demand that in order to create the situation for the maintenance or the restoration of health the individual must be seen as a totality. It is necessary, therefore, to recognize all the various factors affecting both the internal and external environment of the individual as being part of the complex interacting totality which can influence the individual for good or ill. In the end the body is self-healing, self-repairing and self-maintaining, if the prerequisites for health are present. Emotional stability, nutritional balance, hygienic considerations all play their parts, as does the structural and mechanical integrity of the body.

No method that is worthy of consideration as part of the therapeutic resources of practitioners conscious of the holistic approach should have undesirable side-effects. Nothing that is done to the body in the name of therapeutic endeavour should detract from the body's ability to function normally and efficiently. NMT and MET which aim at restoring structural and functional integrity to the musculo-skeletal component of the body is safe and efficient and produces no adverse reactions or effects if used correctly.

NMT takes its place as part of the armamentary of all those who seek to aid the healing capacity of the body. In setting down the methods employed in NMT the author is acutely aware of the limitations of the written word in conveying the essence of such techniques. The illustrations provide a further aid, but nothing can take the place of individual instruction. It is to be hoped that courses and seminars will continue to provide the opportunity for practitioners to learn, at first hand, the scope of these methods. This book should aid such study as it provides the practitioners or student with the raw material with which to begin the study of an invaluable technique.

Chapter 1

Somatic Dysfunction—
the Soft Tissue Component

The soft tissues of the body are the source of a great deal of pain and dysfunction. This pain can be localized or general and it can also be referred or reflex in nature. Terminology applied to soft tissue lesions and problems is not always accurate. Such terms as 'fibrositis' and 'muscular rheumatism' do not necessarily indicate anything at all in a clinical sense. Such expressions as 'stringy', 'nodular', 'indurated' etc. are also inexact.

They do, however, describe what the practitioner's hands feel and, as such, have a subjective value. But, for the purpose of accuracy, a comprehensive term can be applied to all lesions of the musculo-skeletal system. This term is 'somatic dysfunction' and it can be defined as impaired or altered function of related components of the somatic (body framework) system, i.e. skeletal, arthrodial, and myofascial structures and related vascular, lymphatic, and neural elements.

This general expression (somatic dysfunction) obviously requires specific definition in any given case and this should include identification of the particular structure, tissue or area involved. The soft tissues of the body have specific interrelated functions to perform. A variety of factors can contribute to local or general dysfunction of traumatic, postural, pathological or psychological origin. Such dysfunction might itself become the source of referred pain and other symptoms.

Some of the various components which might contribute towards somatic dysfunction and the ramifications thereof will be considered, as will several therapeutic techniques which aim at normalizing the soft tissues and the reflex end-products of somatic dysfunction. A number of researchers in this field have examined different aspects of the causes of soft tissue dysfunction and it will be advantageous to examine some of the findings and theories which have resulted, as well as their solutions.

Sixty per cent of the mass of the body comprises the musculo-skeletal system. There is structural and functional continuity between all the hard and soft tissues which make up this mechanical component of the human machine. The tendency to think of a local lesion as existing in isolation should be discouraged and an awareness should be cultivated of the interrelated nature of this assortment of tissues. The musculo-skeletal system consists of muscles, ligaments, tendons, bones and fascia (connective tissue) and is the main consumer of body energy. Apart from its obvious role in the support and motion of the body it is involved in biochemical and biomechanical activities.

The Fascia   The fascia is of great significance in its role of supporting and providing cohesion to the body structures. Its functions are varied and complex and include the following:

1. Connective tissue provides a supporting matrix for more highly organized structures.

2. Because it contains mesenchymal cells of an embryonic type, connective tissue provides a generalized tissue capable of giving rise, under certain circumstances, to more specialized elements.

3. It provides, by its fascial planes, pathways for nerves, and lymphatic vessels.

4. It supplies restraining mechanisms by the differentiation of retention bands, fibrous pulleys, check ligaments, etc.

5. Where connective tissue is loose in texture it allows movement between adjacent structures and, by the formation of bursal sacs, it reduces the effects of pressure and friction.

6. Deep fascia ensheaths and preserves the characteristic contour of the limbs, and promotes the circulation in the veins and lymphatic vessels.

7. The superficial fascia, which forms the panniculus adiposus, allows for the storage of fat and also provides a surface covering which aids in the conservation of body heat.

8. By virtue of its fibroplastic activity, connective tissue aids in the repair of injuries by the deposition of collagenous fibres (scar tissue).

9. The ensheathing layer of deep fascia, as well as intermuscular septa and interosseous membranes, provides additional surface areas for muscular attachment.

10. The meshes of loose connective tissue contain the 'tissue fluid'; they provide an essential medium through which the cellular elements of other tissues are brought into functional relation with blood and lymph. Connective tissue has a nutritive function.

11. The histiocytes of connective tissue comprise part of an important defence mechanism against bacterial invasion by their phagocytic activity. They also play a part as scavengers in removing cell debris and foreign material.

12. Connective tissue represents an important 'neutralizer' or detoxicator to both endogenous toxins (those produced under physiological conditions), and exogenous toxins (those which are introduced from outside the organism). Much of this neutralizing or detoxicating function appears to be associated with reactions at the surface of the numerous fibres.

These, then, represent the major functions of this ubiquitous, tenacious connective tissue which is a living tissue deeply involved in the fundamental processes of the body's metabolism.·

Modern techniques of electron and phase microscopy have been used to study myofascial biochemistry activity. Much of the fascia and connective tissue is made of tubular structures. Erlinghauser[1] has shown that lymph and cerebrospinal fluid spreads throughout the body via these channels. The implications of this knowledge have not yet been fully realized or investigated by physiologists.

GAS and LAS   Selye[2] called stress the non-specific element in disease production. In describing the relationship between the General Adaptation Syndrome (GAS)—i.e. alarm reaction, resistance phase, exhaustion—and the Local Adaptation Syndrome (LAS), Selye emphasized the importance of connective tissue. He indicated that stress results in a pattern of adaptation, individual to each organism.

In assessing the patient the neuro-muscular-skeletal changes represent a record of the attempts on the part of the body to adapt and adjust to the stresses imposed upon it. The repeated postural and traumatic insults of a lifetime, combined with the tensions of emotional and psychological origin, will often present a confusing pattern of tense, contracted, bunched, fatigued fibrous tissue.

The minutiae of the process are not for the moment at issue. What is important is the realization that, due to prolonged stress of a postural, psychic or mechanical type, a discrete area of the body will become so altered by its efforts to compensate and adapt to this stress, that structural and, eventually, pathological changes will become apparent. Other researchers have shown that the type of stress involved can be entirely physical in nature (e.g. repetitive postural strain such as that adopted by a dentist or hairdresser), or purely psychic in nature (e.g. chronic repressed anger).

More often than not a combination of mental and physical stresses will so alter neuro-muscular-skeletal structures as to create an identifiable physical change, which will itself be a generator of further stress, such as pain, joint restriction, general discomfort and fatigue. Such changes can also be the result of traumatic episodes and one could have either chronic or acute lesions which in all respects duplicate each other, apart from the long-term tissue changes which would be manifest in the chronic lesion.

When an individual is conscious of being in danger, real or imagined, the total organism is involved and the homeostatic mechanism is activated to protect itself from danger. The chronic stress pattern that can result in the total organism will produce long-term muscular contraction. This in turn, if prolonged, will have profound effects on, for example, the cardio-vascular system. Even simple muscular contraction of the arm, if sustained, will elevate blood pressure by 10mm to 20mm Hg[3] Jacobson[4] stated:

> Physiological studies indicate beyond reasonable doubt that, with or without attendant emotion, neuro-muscular hyperkinesis is characteristic of over-energetic living and, in consequence, the heart overworks protractedly with resultant wear and tear, manifested in diversified cardiac pathology.

The ramifications of neuro-muscular stress are therefore more widespread than the simple pain and discomfort level. Energy loss, mechanical inefficiency, pain, cardio-vascular pathology, hypertension etc., all are a possible result of neuro-muscular dysfunction and are therefore amenable to correction by whatever means will normalize this dysfunction.

The tissues which we are concerned with and some of the changes that occur in them will be considered later in the book. At this stage, however, it is necessary to establish beyond reasonable doubt that soft tissues of the musculoskeletal system, when subjected to acute or chronic embarrassment, will change and adapt themselves in a predictable manner. This adaptation will be seen almost always to be at the expense of optimum functional ability. Such changes will also be seen to be the on-going source of further physiological embarrassment. Finally it will be seen that removal of such changes or lesions or dysfunction is frequently possible.

Our concern in this work is with the soft tissue component of such processes. As such there is a large degree of overlapping of interest with the practitioner whose prime interest in restoring structural integrity focuses more on the bony structures of the body. Manipulative therapists, physiotherapists, chiropractors and osteopaths all use techniques to attempt to normalize positional and motional disturbances within the body framework. To some extent all take into account the soft tissues when assessing and correcting such problems. The aim of this book is to emphasize the importance of the soft tissue component. From the therapeutic viewpoint a specific technique for the alleviation of the soft tissue aspect of such problems will be seen at times to obviate the necessity for joint manipulation.

Stress Responses

Stress responses[5] on the part of the body have been divided into four general areas of consideration. All or some of these factors can be present in any given case.

Physiological. This might involve general overall muscle tension of a postural nature or specific localized tension resulting from particular over-use of a part (typists, dentists, tailors, etc.).

Emotional. All emotional changes are mirrored in muscular changes. Emotional attitudes, such as anger or fear, as well as moods such as excitement or depression, all produce muscular postures and patterns. There is a close relationship between habitual tension patterns and postures, and psychological attitudes and conflicts.

Behavioural. All movement requires muscular activity. Certain patterns of use establish themselves. Often individual awareness of the pattern of use is diminished and habitually repetitive actions take place with resultant muscular hypertension.

Structural. Muscle tissue will change in texture, chemistry, tone etc. and will also modify and alter the framework of the body, warping and cramping its potential for normal use. The body will be bent and distorted to meet the stresses imposed from without and within.

Barlow, whose work follows that of Alexander,[6] suggests that there exists a self-regulating tendency in muscular behaviour. The term 'postural homeostasis' implies a return to a balanced resting state after activity. Such regulation is usually at an unconscious level. He gives the example of a patient with persistent low back pain who, in the resting position, demonstrates a particular set of muscular distortions such as tense erector spina on the left and a tense trapezius on the right, together with a pelvic twist to the right. On activity all these spasms become accentuated.

This demonstrates a residual tension pattern which has never been resolved. This, Barlow suggests, can be normalized by restoring a 'balanced resting state'. It might be, however, only partially released through treatment which only deals with part of the causative components. In such a case activity or stress would reactivate the whole pattern of imbalance. In this suggested restoration of homoeostatic equilibrium Barlow would, of course, employ postural re-education of the individual. I would contend that greater success would be achieved by the use of soft tissue normalization, through neuro-muscular treatment and possibly manipulation, combined with such re-education.

Source of Pain

Where pain exists in tense musculature, Barlow suggests that in the absence of other pathology such pain results from:

1. The muscle itself through some noxious metabolic product (this has been called 'Factor P'[7]) or an interference in blood circulation due to spasm, resulting in relative ischaemia.

2. The muscular insertion into the periosteum, such as that caused by an actual lifting of the periosteal tissue by marked, or repetitive, muscular tension (e.g. 'tennis elbow').

3. The joint involved, which can become restricted and over-approximated. In advanced cases osteo-arthritic changes can result from the repeated microtrauma of repeated muscular misuse. Many chronic joint conditions are preventable if early muscular stress patterns are spotted and normalized prior to such damage taking place.

4. Nerve irritation, which can be produced spinally or along the course of the nerve as a result of chronic muscular contractions. These can produce disc and general spinal mechanical faults, with all that that can lead to.

5. Variations in pain threshold will make all these factors more or less significant and obvious.

Where pain has been produced by repetitive habits, postural and otherwise, with emotional and psychological overtones, the task of the therapist is complex indeed. It is certainly true that tension can be partially released or relaxed without resolving the underlying pattern. This must be avoided if repeated recurrence of painful episodes is to be minimized. What must be aimed at is a state of relative equilibrium of body structure and function.

Reich[8] outlined an understanding of the postures and defensive tensions produced by neurotic patients. He showed that such individuals often behaved as though they were 'half-dead'. Their normal functioning, on all levels, was diminished and restricted. 'They were disturbed sexually, they were disturbed in their work function, their bodily processes lacked rhythm, their breathing was unco-ordinated'.[9]

Reich and his followers have demonstrated the capability of emotions to mobilize or paralyse the body. Continued and repeated stress is shown to produce 'blockages' and restrictions in the musculoskeletal system which, if unreleased become self-perpetuating and are themselves the source of pain and further stress. The ability to relax is lost and the drain on nervous energy is profound.

Neurosis would seem to be the disease of modern times. The bioenergetic answer to this problem is to aid in the release of these tensions by a complex set of exercises, including facial expressions and body positions, accompanied by breathing techniques. These methods are doubtless successful in many cases, but do not concern our present study. What is important is the realization that neuro-muscular restriction, as evidenced by stiff body use, may often be a manifestation of deep psychological and emotional stress. Its release, by whatever means, can be seen to be a desirable step in the restoration of normality.

Tissue Changes

Taylor[10] has postulated that the tissue changes, apparent to the trained palpating hand, often result from changes in the thermo-dynamic equilibrium. He states that the body is a thermo-dynamic system and, as such, the alterations in the extracellular fluids, viscosity, pH, electrophoretic changes, colloidal osmotic pressure, etc. are subject to thermo-dynamic laws. One of these states that the total energy of such a system and its surroundings must remain constant, though the energy may be changed from one form to another due to alterations of the stresses imposed. Through postural misuse and gravitational effects, particular changes would result in energy loss and therefore stasis and stagnation in the fascia involved. One of the phenomena of thermo-dynamics is that of thixotropy in which gels become more solid with energy loss and more fluid with energy input. Such changes are certainly palpable in soft tissues before and after neuro-muscular treatment.

Taylor has stated that manipulative pressure and stretching are the most effective ways of modifying energy potentials of abnormal soft tissues. Little[11] believes that an additional beneficial effect results from the interaction of the bio-energy mechanism of the practitioner and the bio-energy field of the patient.

Eeman[12] has shown that after each simple movement that we perform we retain a degree of unconscious contractive muscular activity. This unconscious continuation of objective contraction is not only wasteful of energy but productive of long-term changes within the tissues involved.

He has further shown that unless, and until, neuro-muscular relaxation is achieved there cannot be a total resting state of the mind. Over and above the important factors of posture, functional ability and pain the musculoskeletal element is seen to play a vital role in the conservation, or otherwise, of energy and in the attainment, or otherwise, of a truly relaxed mind. Whilst the origins of musculo-skeletal tensions can be either psychic or physical their continuity ensures a constant degree of psychic stress as a feedback from this tension.

Rolfing   Rolf[13] suggests that the human organism as an energy mass is subject to gravitational law. As a plastic medium, capable of change, Rolfing attempts to reorganize and balance the body in relation to gravitational forces. This is done by using pressure and stretch techniques on the fascial tissues in a precise sequence of body areas. The beneficial effects are claimed to be physical, emotional, postural and behavioural.

Rolf states:

Our ignorance of the role and significance of fascia is profound. Therefore even in theory it is easy to overlook the possibility that far-reaching changes may be made not only in structural contour, but also in functional manifestation, through better organization of the layer of superficial fascia which enwraps the body. Experiment demonstrates that drastic changes may be made in the body, solely by stretching, separating and relaxing superficial fascia in an appropriate manner.

Osteopathic manipulators have observed and recorded the extent to which all degenerative change in the body, be it muscular, nervous, circulatory or organic, reflects in superficial fascia. Any degree of degeneration, however minor, changes the bulk of the fascia, modifies its thickness and draws it into ridges in areas overlying deeper tensions and rigidities. Conversely, as this elastic envelope is stretched, manipulative mechanical energy is added to it, and the fascial colloid becomes more 'sol' and less 'gel'. The biophysics of this process has been discussed in a classical paper by R. B. Taylor.[14]

As a result of the added energy, as well as of a directional contribution in applying it, the underlying structures, including the muscles which determine the placement of the body parts in space, and also their relations to each other, have come a little closer to the normal. ('Normal' as used there must be differentiated from 'average'.) The patient feels 'so much better'.

Gutstein[15] seeks to denote localized functional sensory and/or motor abnormalities of musculoskeletal tissue (comprising muscle, fascia, tendon, bone and joint) as myodysneuria. He sees the causes of such changes as multiple and among these are:

(a) Acute and chronic infections which it is postulated stimulate sympathetic nerve activity via their toxins.

(b) Excessive heat or cold, changes in atmospheric pressure and draughts.

(c) Mechanical injuries, both major and repeated minor micro-traumas. Postural strain, unaccustomed exercises etc., which may predispose towards future changes by lowering the threshold for future stimuli.

(d) Allergic and endocrine factors which can cause imbalance in the autonomic nervous system.

(e) Inherited factors making adjustment to environmental factors difficult.

(f) Arthritic changes: since muscles are the active components of the musculoskeletal system it is logical to assume that their circulatory state has influence over bones and joints. Spasm in muscle may contribute towards osteoarthritic changes and such changes may produce further neuro-muscular changes which themselves produce symptoms.

(g) Visceral diseases may intensify and precipitate somatic symptoms in the distribution of their spinal and adjacent segments.

Diagnosis of myodysneuria is made according to some of the following criteria:

(a) A varying degree of muscular tension and contraction is usually present although sometimes adjacent, non-indurated tissue is more painful.

(b) Sensitivity to pressure or palpation of affected muscles and their adjuncts.

Marked contraction may require the application of deep pressure to demonstrate tenderness.

Pathophysiology

The changes which occur in tissue involved in the onset of myodysneuria, according to Gutstein, are thought to be initiated by localized sympathetic predominance, associated with changes in the hydrogen ion concentration and calcium and sodium balance in the tissue fluids.[16] This is associated with vasoconstriction and hypoxia. Pain results, it is thought, by these alterations affecting the pain sensors and proprioceptors. Muscle spasm and hard nodular localized tetanic contractions of muscle bundles[17] together with vasomotor and musculomotor stimulation intensify each other, creating a vicious cycle of self-perpetuating impulses. There are varied and complex patterns of referred symptoms which may result from such 'trigger' areas as well as local pain and minor disturbances.

Such sensations as aching, soreness, tenderness, heaviness and tiredness may all be manifest as may modification of muscular activity due to contraction resulting in tightness, stiffness, swelling etc.

Cathie[18] maintains that the contractive phase of fascial activity supercedes all other qualities of fascia. The attachments of fascia he states have a tendency to shorten after periods of marked activity which are followed by periods of inactivity and the ligaments become tighter and thicker with advancing age. The properties of fascia (connective tissue) that he regards as being important to therapeutic consideration are listed as being that:

1. It is richly endowed with nerve endings.
2. It has the ability to contract and to stretch elastically.
3. It gives extensive muscular attachment.
4. It supports and stabilizes, thus enhancing the postural balance of the body.
5. It is vitally involved in all aspects of motion.
6. It aids in circulatory economy, especially of venous and lymphatic fluids.
7. Fascial change will precede many of the chronic degenerative diseases.
8. Fascial changes predispose towards chronic tissue congestion.
9. Such chronic passive congestion precedes the formation of fibrous tissue which then proceeds to an increase in hydrogen ion concentration of articular and periarticular structures.
10. Fascial specializations produce definite stress bands.
11. Sudden stress (trauma) on fascial tissue will often result in a burning type of pain.
12. Fascia is a major arena of inflammatory processes.
13. Fluids and infectious processes often travel along fascial planes.
14. The CNS is surrounded by fascial tissue (dura mater) which in the skull attaches to bone. Dysfunction in these tissues can have profound and widespread effects.

Changes which occur in connective tissue, and which result in such alterations as thickening, shortening, calcification and erosion, may be a result of sudden or sustained tension or traction. Cathie points out that many 'trigger spots' correspond to points where nerves pierce fascial investments. The causes of derangement may therefore be seen to result from faulty muscular activity, alteration in bony relationships, visceral positional change (e.g. visceroptosis) and the use of unnatural positions. All these can be sustained, repetitive causes or single, violently induced changes. Chemical (nutritional) factors must also be considered. As Pauling[19] points out:

> Many of the results of deprivation of ascorbic acid involve a deficiency in connective tissue. Connective tissue is largely responsible for the strength of bones, teeth, skin, of the body. It consists of the fibrous protein collagen.

He goes on to point out that in deficiency of Vitamin C this binding material becomes less efficient and more fluid. Pauling concludes that the effectiveness of Vitamin C in helping the body contain virus particles may to some extent be a result of its strengthening action on connective tissue, which would impede the motion of virus particles through tissue. This illustrates again the unbiquitous nature of the musculoskeletal tissues in general and fascia in particular and the profound effect on the body economy of dysfunction in any of its myriad components.

Fibrositis   Cyriax[20] believes that all primary 'fibrositic' conditions are a result of articular lesions (dysfunctions). A secondary fibrositic change may result, he states, from traumatic injury to soft tissues (e.g. capsular adhesion at the shoulder after injury) which should be called fibrosis, not fibrositis. This he sees as scar tissue formation. Other secondary fibrositic conditions can result from rheumatoid disease, infection (such as epidemic myalgia) and parasitic infection (*triclina spiralis*). All other muscular and soft tissue dysfunctions Cyriax regards as a result of joint dysfunction which can then produce muscular protective spasm, muscular wasting, pain etc., and which can only be normalized, he maintains, by correction of the joint lesion. Neuro-muscular theory and practice show that appropriate normalization of the soft tissues can often achieve joint normalization without active manipulative treatment of such a joint.

Cyriax does point out that fibrous tissue is capable of maintaining inflammation, originally traumatic, almost as a matter of habit. In such cases he opts for hydrocortisone injections as the appropriate measure to 'break' this habit. Such treatment can work, but all too often fails as underlying mechanical dysfunction has not been normalized.

Stoddard,[21] in discussing contracted musculature, describes its 'stringy' feel resulting from the continuous contraction of some muscle fibres and, like Cyriax ascribes the cause to the underlying joint dysfunctions. The resulting ache and pain is usually a result of circulatory embarrassment as metabolic wastes build-up due to sustained muscular contraction. Muscular guarding is always seen to indicate deeper pathological changes (e.g. T.B. spine, osteomyelitis, disc herniation etc.).

Stoddard sees the metabolic wastes, which may result from a degree of stasis, as causing a vicious cycle in perpetuating muscular contraction, leading eventually to fibrous changes occuring. There is no indication that Stoddard considers such changes to be of primary importance in his treatment programme. He does stress the importance of exercises to strengthen muscle groups and of correct posture, but does not indicate any great interest in treatment of the soft tissue themselves.

Connective Tissue Massage

A system which does concentrate on the soft tissues is Connective Tissue Massage. This is a soft tissue system of German origin which has marked similarities to Neuro-muscular Technique. Maria Ebner[22] describes its principles as follows:

Principles of application. The autonomic nervous system serves to co-ordinate the various structures of the human body. The structures under autonomic control continue to function as long as the body is alive, and are independent of voluntary control. The severance of a somatic spinal nerve will absolish the function of the organ which it supplies. The severance of an autonomic nerve will not interfere with the function of the supplied organ during the resting state. The heart with all autonomic connections severed will continue to beat, provided its nourishment is maintained. The impulse for its basic function arises in the organ itself. The function of the autonomic nervous system is to co-ordinate the various structures and make them adaptable to varying and changing stimuli arising from changes in the environment. The autonomic centres serve to modify the reaction to peripheral stimuli of somatic and autonomic origin, and establish harmonious interaction of structures under somatic and autonomic control, e.g., thermal stimuli registered by the terminal somatic nerves will cause adaptive constriction or dilatation of peripheral blood vessels. The close interrelation between the somatic, autonomic and endocrine systems makes it impossible for pathological changes to take place in any one structure without causing adaptive changes in other structures. Surface changes relating to sensibility and contour in organic pathological disturbances have already been reported by Head in 1898.

Capillary changes in skin segments within the dermatome supply of a pathologically affected organ have been investigated microscopically by Dittmar (1943) and by Rouanet (1946).

Changes in muscular tension and pain senisbility have been discussed by Mackenzie (1917) and others. The most universally known example is the circumscribed abdominal tension in appendicitis.

The pathway responsible for peripheral changes in pathological organic disturbances may also be responsible for changes in the opposite direction. Hartman (1928) describes changes in connective tissue within the dermatomes of the heart, causing heart symptoms and clearing up after treatment of the peripheral connective tissue.

Nonnenbruch and Gross (1952) describe similar phenomena which they investigated. These observations should prove that body surface, organs and connective tissue within the segmental nerve supply are connected by reflex pathways. Changes in one part of the segment may be responsible for alteration in other parts of the segmental supply. The previously described distribution of autonomic cell stations and fibres will have made it clear that tissue changes due to alteration in blood supply will not remain confined to one particular segment. Treatment of peripheral changes should therefore be continued until the circulation over the whole body surface is normalized to the greatest possible extent. Hypersensitive zones must disappear before terminating the treatment.

Pathways concerned may be as follows, choosing stomach pathology as an example. The stomach is supplied by the great splanchnic nerve which derives its fibres from the segments T.5 to 9. Ascending sympathetic branches pass to cervical ganglia from the same segments. Maximal points for stomach pathology lie in the dermatomes of C.3 to T.5 to 9.

Viscero-cutaneous. Afferent from stomach—Posterior Root Ganglion (PRG)—lateral horn cell white ramus—sympathetic ganglion—grey ramus—somatic nerve carrying fibres to blood vessels.

Result. Vasoconstriction in the periphery and hyperaesthesia. Changes in subcutaneous tissue.

Cutaneo-visceral. Altered tension in the periphery registered by posterior afferent—PRG—lateral horn—sympathetic ganglion—postganglionic fibre to stomach.

Result. Interference with stomach blood supply and new flare-up. The peripheral changes are invariably present but usually clear up within two to three weeks. For unknown reasons they sometimes do not clear up and cause new flare-up.

Viscero-motor. This is a variation of the viscero-cutaneous effect, except that the connector fibre establishes a relay into the anterior horn. The new fibre carries excitatory impulses to muscles within the segmental supply.

Result. Alteration in muscle tension.

The treatment itself employs pulling and stretching of the various soft tissues of the body in a precise manner. Such 'strokes' are both diagnostic and therapeutic, having both local and distal reflex effects. This is in common with Neuro-muscular Technique.

R. L. Nimmo[23] described his system for normalizing body structures as one which detected and eliminated noxious 'points' which generate reflex effects; eliminated hypertonia and hypotonia in muscles to enable restoration of bony normality; and corrected abnormalities in ligaments and tendons. The sensitive points generating noxious stimuli result, according to Nimmo, from repetitive irritation resulting from facilitation. Travell, Mennell and others have worked in this field and some of their therapeutic ideas will be discussed later. At this point it would be advantageous to examine that aspect of body function which has been so closely investigated by Korr, the great osteopathic researcher and theoretician.

Korr[24] states:

> The spinal cord is the keyboard on which the brain plays when it calls for activity or for change in activity. But each 'key' in the console sounds, not an individual 'tone', such as the contraction of a particular group of muscle fibres, but a whole 'melody' of activity, even a 'symphony' of motion. In other words, built into the cord is a large repertoire of patterns of activity, each involving the complex, harmonious, delicately balanced orchestration of the contractions and relaxations of many muscles. The brain 'thinks' in terms of whole motions, not individual muscles. It calls selectively, for the preprogrammed patterns in the cord and brain stem, modifying them in countless ways and combining them in an infinite variety of still more complex patterns. Each activity is also subject to further modulation, refinement, and adjustment by the afferent feedback continually streaming in from the participating muscles, tendons, and joints.

Reporting Stations

In order to understand the problems affecting any particular joint or soft-tissue area it is necessary to have an awareness of the various reporting organs which lie with them. There is a constant feedback of information from all tissues as to their state of tone, tension, movement etc. The sensory information is added to by changes in blood chemistry, to which the sympathetic nervous system is sensitive. Depending upon the environmental demands, and the requirements dictated by the conscious and unconscious mind, the tissues will be 'tuned' accordingly.

The reporting mechanisms in and around joints may be thought of as providing answers to a number of basic questions. These are posed by Keith Buzzell D.O. as follows (*The Physiological Basis of Osteopathic Medicine*, Postgraduate Institute of Osteopathic Medicine and Surgery, New York, 1970): 'What is happening in the peripheral machinery with respect to three questions? What is the present position? If there is motion, where is it taking us? And, third, how fast is it taking us there?' A variety of inputs of information will give the answer to these important questions, so that the body can provide an appropriate response. Some important structures involved in this are:

Ruffini End-Organs: These are found within the joint capsule, around the joint, so that each is responsible for an angle of approximately 15 degrees, with a degree of overlap with that of the adjacent end-organ. These are not easily fatigued organs, and are progressively recruited as the joint moves, so that movement is smooth and not jerky. The prime concern of Ruffini end-organs is a steady position. It is also to some extent concerned with the direction of movement.

Golgi End-organs: These, too, adapt slowly, and continue to discharge over a lengthy period. They are found in the ligaments associated with the joint. Unlike the Ruffini end-organs, which respond to muscular contraction which alters tension in the joint capsule, Golgi end-organs are not thus affected, and can deliver information independently of the state of muscular contraction. This helps the body to know just where the joint is at any given moment, irrespective of muscular activity.

The Pacinian Corpuscle: This is found in peri-articular connective tissue, and

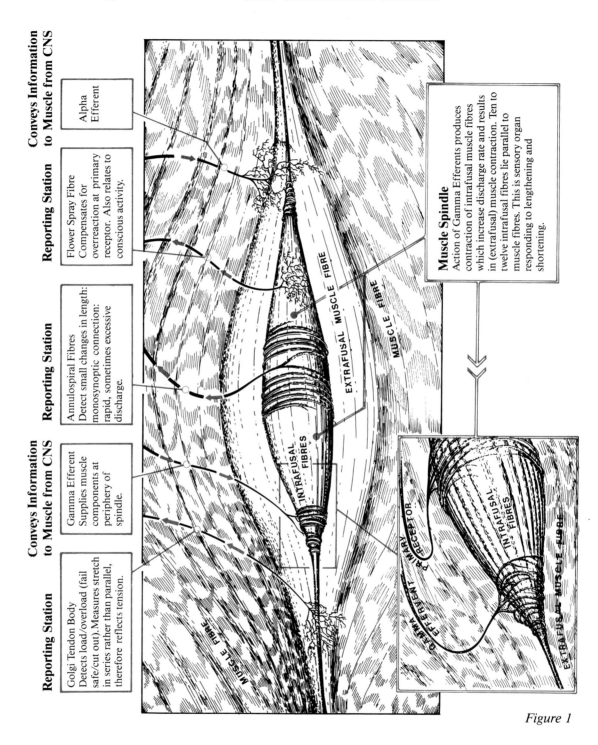

Conveys Information to Muscle from CNS

Alpha Efferent

Reporting Station

Flower Spray Fibre Compensates for overreaction at primary receptor. Also relates to conscious activity.

Reporting Station

Annulospiral Fibres Detect small changes in length: monosynoptic connection: rapid, sometimes excessive discharge.

Conveys Information to Muscle from CNS

Gamma Efferent Supplies muscle components at periphery of spindle.

Reporting Station

Golgi Tendon Body Detects load/overload (fail safe/cut out). Measures stretch in series rather than parallel, therefore reflects tension.

Muscle Spindle
Action of Gamma Efferents produces contraction of intrafusal muscle fibres which increase discharge rate and results in (extrafusal) muscle contraction. Ten to twelve intrafusal fibres lie parallel to muscle fibres. This is sensory organ responding to lengthening and shortening.

EXTRAFUSAL MUSCLE FIBRE

MUSCLE FIBRE

INTRAFUSAL FIBRES

MUSCLE FIBRE

PRIMARY RECEPTOR

INTRAFUSAL FIBRES

GAMMA EFFERENT

EXTRAFUSAL MUSCLE FIBRE

Figure 1

Illustration of Muscle spindle, Golgi tendon organ, and nerve supply to and from these reporting stations.

adapts rapidly. It triggers discharges, and then ceases reporting in a very short space of time. These messages occur successively, during motion, and the CNS can therefore be aware of the rate of acceleration of movement taking place in the area. It is sometimes called an acceleration receptor.

There are other end-organs, but these three can be seen to provide information as to present position, direction and rate of movement of any joint.

Muscle Spindle: This receptor is sensitive and complex. It detects, evaluates, reports and adjusts the length of the muscle in which it lies, setting its tone. Acting with the Golgi tendon body, most of the information as to muscle tone and movement is reported. The spindles lie parallel to the muscle fibres, and are attached to either skeletal muscle, or the tendinous portion of the muscle. Inside the spindle are fibres which may be one of two types. One is described as a 'nuclear bag' fibre, and the other as a chain fibre. In different muscles the ratio of these internal spindle fibres differ. In the centre of the spindle is a receptor called the annulospiral receptor (or primary ending) and on each side of this lies a 'flower spray receptor' (secondary ending). The primary ending discharges rapidly, and this occurs in response to even small changes in muscle length. The secondary ending compensates for this, because it fires messages only when larger changes in muscle length have occurred.

The spindle is a 'length comparator', and it may discharge for long periods at a time. Within the spindle there are fine, intra-fusal, fibres which alter the sensitivity of the spindle. These can be altered without any actual change taking place in the length of the muscle itself, via an independent gamma efferent supply to the intrafusal fibres. This has implications in a variety of acute and chronic problems. Buzzell describes the neural connections with the CNS thus: 'The central connections of the spindle receptors are important. The annulospiral fibre has the only known monosynaptic relationship in the body. As the fibre passes to the cord, and through the dorsal horn, it goes without synapse, directly to the anterior horn cells that serve the muscle fibres in the vicinity of the spindle. This is the basis of the so called 'tendon reflex', which actually is not a tendon reflex, but simply a spindle response to a sudden elongation of the muscle.' In contrast the secondary fibres have various synapses in their central connection which can be traced to higher cortical centres. Conscious activity may involve a modifying influence, via these structures, on muscle tone. The activities of the spindle appear to provide information as to length, velocity of contraction and changes in velocity. (*Gray's Anatomy*, 35th Edition, 1977).

Golgi Tendon Receptors: These structures indicate how hard the muscle is working since they reflect the tension of the muscle, rather than its length, as does the spindle. If the tendon organ detects excessive overload it may cause cessation of function of the muscle, to prevent damage. This produces relaxation.

Let us again recall Korr's words regarding the nature of the information which these, and other, reporting stations are providing to the CNS. These represent 'the complex, harmonious, delicately balanced orchestration of the contraction and relaxation of many muscles.' The pattern of information fed back to the CNS and brain, reflects, at any given time, the steady state of joints, the direction and speed of alteration in position of joints, together with data on the length of muscle fibres, the degree of load that is being borne, as well as the tension this involves. This total input is what occurs, rather than the individual pieces of information, as outlined above, from particular reporting stations. Should any of the information

Effect of Contradictory Information

be contradictory, to actually conflict with other information being received, what then? Buzzell states it this way: 'It is possible, for example, for the excessive force exerted by external trauma to induce such hyperactivity of the joint and muscle receptors that the reports from that area become gibberish.' Should conflicting reports reach the cord from a variety of sources simultaneously, no discernable pattern may be recognized by the CNS. In such a case no adequate reponse would be forthcoming, and it is probable that activity would be stopped. Spasm or splinting could therefore result. It is in such situations that the techniques of muscle energy (MET), which will be fully described in Chapter 9, have their major influence, for they allow, in many cases, for the 'resetting' of the reporting stations, which allows them to again 'march in step, one with the other', and to provide usable information. NMT, MET and Strain-counterstrain are the tools which we may employ in attempting to assess the nature of soft-tissue dysfunction, and to normalize this.

Korr discusses a variety of insults which may result in increased neural excitability; the triggering of a barrage of supernumary impulses, to and from the cord, and also what he terms 'cross-talk', in which axons may overload and pass impulses to one another directly; muscle contraction disturbances, vasomotion, pain impulses, reflex mechanisms, disturbances in sympathetic activity, all may result from such activity, due to what might be relatively slight tissue changes in the intervertebral foramena, for example. He adds the concept that when any tissue is disturbed, whether bone, joint, ligament or muscle, the local stresses feed constant information to the cord, and effectively jam normal patterned transmission from the periphery. These factors, combined with any mechanical alterations in the tissues, are the background to much somatic dysfunction. He summarizes thus: 'These are the somatic insults, the sources of incoherent, and meaningless feedback, that causes the spinal cord to halt normal operations and to freeze the status quo in the offending and offended tissues. It is these phenomena that are detectable at the body surface, and are reflected in disorders of muscle tension, tissue texture, visceral and circulatory function, and even secretory function; the elements that are so much a part of osteopathic diagnosis.'

Our task in assessing and dealing with this complex of somatic dysfunction is aided by the diagnostic and therapeutic ability of neuro-muscular technique, as well as by the more recent development of muscle energy techniques. The addition of the gentle functional techniques of Lawrence Jones (Chapter 10) which utilize 'tender points' as diagnostic and monitoring aids, are a further weapon which can be employed in the normalization of the soft tissues and joints of the body, thus affected. Mediating much somatic dysfunction is the process of segmental facilitation.

Theory of Facilitation   Professor Michael Patterson[25] explains the theory of facilitation as follows:

> The concept of the facilitated segment states that because of abnormal afferent or sensory inputs to a particular area of the spinal cord, that area is kept in a state of constant increased excitation. This facilitation allows normally ineffectual or subliminal stimuli to become effective in producing efferent output from the facilitated segment, causing both skeletal and visceral organs innervated by the affected segment to be maintained in a state of overactivity. It is probable that the 'osteopathic lesion', or somatic

dysfunction with which a facilitated segment is associated, is the direct result of the abnormal segmental acitivity as well as being partially responsible for the facilitation.

Although the effects of the facilitated segment on various skeletal and visceral functions are well documented, little is understood about the genesis and maintenance of spinal facilitation. Even the question of why some traumas cause facilitation and others do not remain unanswered.

The concept of the facilitated segment is essentially that abnormal or altered inputs from a source of irritation impinging on the spinal cord will keep the interneurons or motoneurons of that spinal segment in a constant state of excitement, thus allowing normally ineffectual inputs to produce outputs to all organs receiving innervation from the excited area. This concept implies that the spinal cord is a relatively passive mediator of the influences imposed on it and that the neural paths act as communicators of that activity.

The recent research on spinal functions seems to indicate, however, that the spinal cord, besides being the determiner of where abnormal activity is sent by virtue of predetermined pathways, may participate actively in either controlling abnormal or unusually intense inputs or amplifying and retaining such inputs in certain circumstances.

Initially, only intensities of afferent input above a certain level would result in increased sensitivity of the spinal pathway. Inputs of lower intensity either would cause no alterations or would cause an actual decrease in sensitivity as a protective mechanism against undue changes in homoeostatic mechanisms. It is apparent that the potential for sensitization by different types of afferent inputs may differ widely. Thus, inputs from pain receptors may sensitize the pathway at low levels because of the properties of the initial synapses between pain afferent fibres and interneurons. In this event an initially protective increase in response might occur, but a detrimental facilitation of a segment would follow. On the other hand, inputs from joint receptors have a less dramatic effect at similar input levels.

The model also permits the prediction that emotional arousal would affect the susceptibility of the pathways to sensitization. The increase in descending influences from the emotionally aroused subject would result in an increase in toxic excitement in the pathways and allow all additional inputs to produce sensitization at low intensities. Thus, highly emotional persons or those in a highly emotional situation would be expected to show a higher incidence of facilitation of spinal pathways. Since the higher brain centres do influence the tonic level of the spinal paths, it might be expected also that physical training and mental attitudes would tend to alter the tonic excitability as well, reducing the person's susceptibility to sensitization from everyday stress. Thus the athlete would be expected to withstand a comparatively high level of afferent input prior to experiencing the self-perpetuating results of sensitization.

A further corollary of the hypothesis is that slowly developing conditions or slowly increasing inputs would result in less sensitization at high levels than sudden inputs. The slow developing of chronic source of increased sensory input initially would cause habituation, resulting in resistance to sensitization until the input level was abnormally high. On the other hand, sudden increases in input, such as a sudden postural stress, would be expected to produce sensitization of the neural pathways most rapidly.

The hypothesis presented here explains a phenomenon observed in clinical practice and described by Jones in 1964. He termed it 'spontaneous release by positioning'. Jones outlined a procedure developed to reduce somatic dysfunction in several apparently severe cases. He noted that a patient with a severe lesion which was interfering with normal movement and function gained considerable relief from the lesion if he was positioned in such a way that the discomfort was stopped. Although placing the patient in such a position of comfort apparently required heroic positioning at times, holding the patient in the exaggerated position for at least 90 seconds often allowed a return to normal posture and activity with no recurrence of the symptoms. It would be assumed from the model that the sensitization caused by the constant pain inputs from the affected area would drop below a critical level during the period of pain cessation. A corollary to the decrease in sensitization over time would be that for a time following the aforementioned treatment, the patient would be highly liable to recurrence of the problems as a result of residual sensitization and the long-lasting effects of conditioning of the abnormal activity. This liability would be gradually reversed by normal inputs and responses. It would also be expected that highly nervous persons might require a longer period in a position of comfort to achieve relief and that such persons would remain vulnerable for longer periods to reacquisition of sensitization or facilitation than would less emotional patients. A closely allied aspect of the sensitization concept is that a relatively minor increase in sensitization which might be caused during daily activity could be corrected during sleep as a result of the decrease in descending activity and the accompanying muscular relaxation. Thus, besides the damping effects of habituation, normal relaxation should tend to relieve minor segmental problems which otherwise might become increasingly acute. However, it will also be expected that drugs often used to relieve somatic dysfunction, such as muscle relaxants or central nervous system depressants would be successful only if a sufficient degree of relaxation or decrease in the overactive sensory input could be achieved. It is possible that often such drugs do not work because of increased inputs from visceral and non-muscular tissues which remain a source of high afferent bombardment.

The application of high-velocity and muscle energy manipulative techniques to the somatic dysfunction remains the most effective means of treating these disorders. In a brilliant recent article, Korr proposed a mechanism involving the gamma motor system and muscle proprioceptors as one of the common causes of sustained muscle contraction associated with the somatic dysfunction. He proposed that manipulative procedures involving high-velocity, short-amplitude forces as well as muscle energy techniques would act to force the central nervous system to correct abnormally high excitation of the muscle spindles and allow the muscle to return to its normal length and the joint to its normal motion. Similar reasoning with regard to decreasing the spindle activity would apply to functional techniques, which, instead of forcing a contracted muscle against its contraction, would allow it to continue to shorten until relaxed normally. In any of these procedures afferent input to the cord would be reduced for a sufficient time to allow the sensitization to decrease below the critical level. That is, afferent input would be reduced either directly or via central brain influences, to a level below that required to sustain sensitization.

The Muscle's Role in Low Back Pain Problems

If we examine the role of the muscular component of the musculo-skeletal structures we find strong evidence as to its involvement in many acute and chronic conditions. Jokl ('Muscle and low back pain' *The Journal of the American Osteopathic Association*, Vol 84, No. 1, pp 64-65) tells us that disuse muscular atrophy, following back injury, is a major factor in the progression from an acute back problem to a chronic one. Changes take place which are observable, histologically and biochemically, in the muscle fibres, and which are translated into functional changes. The effects of these changes involves decreased endurance and weakened muscles, as well as spasm. We should remind ourselves of the basic anatomy of the low back, which includes the division of the musculature into *deep muscles*, connecting the adjacent spinous processes (interspinales), adjacent transverse processes (intertransversari) and the rotatores, connecting the transverse process below to the laminae above. The *intermediate muscles* include multifidus, which connects the transverse processes to the spinous processes of the vertebra above.

The *superficial group* includes iliocostalis, longissimus and spinalis (erector spinae). The origin of this is on the ischium, and the insertion the 6th and 12th ribs. Together with the psoas major and minor, and the quadratus, these greatly influence spinal stability.

The *prevertebral muscles*, which further stabilize and support the spine are those which encircle the abdomen, such as the internal and external oblique, and rectus abdominus muscles.

Any, or all, of these can have a major influence of the onset of low back problems and pain. The division of muscles into different types is of some importance. Muscle fibres may be differentiated into types by virtue of their role, as well as their main energy source. For example, those muscles which are mainly involved in activities of a nature which require stamina, rather than speed of action, derive their energy via oxidative phosphorylation. This is in contrast to those muscles which produce power and speed, and which derive energy from carbohydrate sources via glycolytic breakdown. The muscles which support the spine are mainly type 1, endurance and stamina muscles; their activities are in the main related to static, anti-gravity efforts, which require prolonged contraction. These are far more susceptible to disuse atrophy and shortening. The strength of such muscles may not indicate much change, even after a period of disuse, but the endurance factor could be greatly affected. This makes for a certain degree of caution being required in interpreting muscle strength tests, involving the paravertebral musculature.

Muscle Types

Jokl points out that EMG studies indicate that paraspinal muscles show marked fatigue in individuals with low back pains. This fatigue factor may be a major part in worsening, or accentuating, an already demonstrable degree of dysfunction in such a region. When such a situation is in existence (pain and easy fatigue of supporting musculature) it may be assumed that an increased number of muscle fibres have been recruited in order to maintain spinal stability. This results in increased muscular pressure. Jokl tells us that normal muscle can work for long periods without any EMG evidence of fatigue. As muscles become weaker, they work at an increased percentage of their maximum voluntary contraction. Ultimately this leads to muscle spasm, which allows ischemia to develop, and pain to result. The cycle of increased effort, local spasm and ischemia, leading to pain, ultimately may result in paraspinal spasm and splinting.

The use of both neuro-muscular technique and muscle energy technique, is indicated in such a situation, as a means of breaking the cycle and, initially, relaxing the contracted muscles. NMT methods have a combined effect in both relaxing the tissues as well as increasing the vascularity and mobility of these structures. They become more 'extensible', to use Grieve's phrase (*Mobilisation of the Spine*, Churchill Livingstone). He enlarges on this aspect thus:

There is new evidence to support the view that suppleness and flexibility of muscle and connective tissue, are of prime importance. Long and continued occupational and postural stress, asymmetrically imposed upon the soft tissues, tends to cause fibroblasts to multiply more rapidly and produce more collagen. Besides occupying more space within the connective tissue element of the muscle, the extra fibres encroach on the space normally occupied by nerves and vessels. Because of this trespass, the tissue loses elasticity, and may become painful when the muscle is required to do work in co-ordination with others. In the long term collagen would begin to replace the active fibres of the muscle, and since collagen is fairly resistant to enzyme breakdown, these changes tend to be irreversible.

We can see that an understanding of the mechanisms involved , as described by Jokl, Korr, Patterson and Grieve, helps us to picture the neurological and structural changes involved in much joint and spinal dysfunction.

In 1948 Korr stated that:

1. The body is a unit; all parts function in the context of the entire organism.

2. Disease is a reaction of the organism as a whole. Abnormal structure or function in one part exerts abnormal influence on other parts and, therefore, on the total body economy.

3. The organism has the inherent capacity to defend itself, to repair itself, and to resist serious upsets in equilibria.

4. The nervous system plays a dominant organizing role in the disease processes.

5. There is a somatic component to every disease which is not only a manifestation of the disease, *but an important contributing factor*.

6. Appropriate treatment of the somatic component has important therapeutic value in that it leads to improvement in the other components.

The consensus of opinion would seem to indicate that the neuro-muscular component of joint dysfunction is of importance in both the production and maintenance of the problems. Its normalization can remove a major contributory factor to be affected joint and can further be of value by removing the site of trigger points whose ramifications can affect the body adversely in numerous ways. Postural integrity and a reasonable level of relaxation are also dependent upon neuro-muscular tonus being normal. The correction of joint dysfunction by manipulation or exercise may be speeded up by soft-tissue correction as can maintenance of the affected area in an improved state of functional integrity.

Stanley Lief Neuro-muscular Technique (NMT) is a system that has evolved over the past forty years from the original work of the late Stanley Lief. Lief was a pioneering and gifted practitioner of manipulative therapy. As a trained chiropractor and osteopath he was aware of the need for a means by which soft-tissue structures could be prepared for subsequent manipulation. In the 1930s he studied the work of Rabagliatti whose work *Initis* influenced his work towards dealing with connective tissue problems. He also studied the work of a practitioner of Hindu manipulation Dewanchand Varma who was practising in Paris. Varma used a system called 'Pranotherapy' and in his book *The Human Machine and its Forces* (London, 1938) he states:

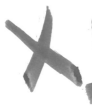

We have discovered that the circulation of the nervous currents, slows down occasionally because of the obstruction caused by adhesions; the muscular fibres harden and the nervous currents can no longer pass through them. We have demonstrated effective and positive methods designed to restore nervous equilibrium which promotes the healthy circulation of blood, so that new tissues begin to be built up, again. Our method of treatment, by the removal of all obstacles to the flow of nervous current, allows energy to proceed unimpeded.

Lief found various techniques of Varma useful and out of these ideas and methods developed his own soft tissue method—NMT. His cousin Boris Chaitow D.C., who worked with Lief during this period, describes the early development of NMT as follows: [26]

In the middle of the 1930s Stanley Lief realized that the integrity of a joint was to a great extent related to the character of the tissues surrounding the joint, related to muscle, tendons, ligaments, blood and nerve supply etc. He felt that in order the better to achieve effective mobility and integrity of function of joints—particularly in the spine but also in *all* bony articular relationships—it was advisable to normalize, as best one could, the adjacent soft tissues by removing any function-interfering factors, such as tensions, contractions, adhesions, spasms, fibrositic contractures etc., with appropriate use of fingers and hands to those tissues. To this end the neuro-muscular technique was evolved to cover *every* possible type of lesion in *whatever* part of the body (articular, soft tissue, abdominal, glandular, nervous, vascular etc.).

It so happened that at that particular time Stanley Lief had heard of a well-known Indian practitioner named Varma operating in Paris, who was applying an unusual but very effective soft-tissue technique on patients with remarkable benefits. Lief decided to arrange to have a series of treatments on himself from Varma, and finally persuaded the latter to teach him this specialized technique. Much as he appreciated the method used by Varma, he felt it could be improved, and began to develop and subsequently practised the method for which he devised the name of 'Neuro-muscular Technique'. This name was an accurate definition of the purpose of the method he evolved from the rather crude technique used by Varma. This involved an application of hands and fingers to the appropriate areas of soft tissue related to the affected bony articulations, as well as all other areas of soft tissue which his sensitive fingers found to be abnormal in texture. This enables adverse factors in such tissue to be corrected to allow the full function of *muscles* and nerves to be re-established. In doing so the double benefits are achieved in improving nerve and blood circulation, improving texture of muscle tissue and in being better able to get effective results in manipulating the bony articulations involved, and assuring lasting integrity of their normal function.

Stanley Lief also maintained that bony joint lesions were not the only factors in the interference in nerve force integrity, but that tensions contractions, adhesions, muscle spasms and fibrositic contractures in soft tissues could in themselves constitute primary factors in disease causation by reducing effective nerve and blood circulation. To this end he developed his diagnostic sensitivity with his fingers so that in a few seconds of palpation over any area of the body, he was able to assess abnormalities present in relation to tensions, adhesions, spasms etc.

The body's integrity of prime health and its functional efficiency at a high level, depends not only on its chemistry influenced by the nature of the food and drink we ingest, but also on the effective nerve and blood circulation free of mechanical and functional obstructions. To this second vital purpose there is no formula devised by the osteopathic or chiropractic professions that will more effectively achieve the optimum result than the philosophy and technique devised by Stanley Lief. There is no single part of the body that he was not able to apply his method to to achieve remarkable physiological responses.

Stanley Lief's son, Peter, has described [27] the 'neuro-muscular' lesion as being associated with:

1. Congestion of the local connective tissues.
2. Disturbance of the acid-base balance of the connective tissues.

3. Fibrous infiltration (adhesions).
4. Chronic muscular contractions or hyper- or hypotrophic (tone) changes.

Etiology of the neuro-muscular lesion, according to Lief, include a number of causative factors, giving rise to neuro-muscular lesions, which may include:

1. Fatigue, exhaustion, bad posture.
2. Local trauma.
3. Systemic toxaemia (lack of exercise and oxygen).
4. Dietetic deficiencies.
5. Psychosomatic causes bringing about muscular tensions.

The presence of a lesion is always revealed by an area of hypersensitivity to pressure.

Tissues Involved in NMT

Boris Chaitow and Peter Lief have both evolved the theory and application of NMT as first described by Stanley Lief. Brian Youngs[28] has given the following general explanation of the tissues involved in NMT:

Site of Application
As the technique operates primarily on connective tissue it will be concentrated at those areas where such tissue is most dense, e.g. muscular origins and insertions, especially the broad aponeurotic insertions. The most frequent sites are the superior curved line of the occiput, the numerous insertions and origins of the large, medium and small muscles which attach to the vertebral column; the iliac-crest insertions; the intercostal insertions and abdominal-muscle insertions. Nevertheless, the technique can of course be applied to any area which requires it—head, face, wrists, etc. Connective tissue is, after all, ubiquitous.

To understand the therapeutic effect of the technique one must have some knowledge of the pathophysiology of the tissue upon which it operates. Connective tissue consists of a matrix containing cells and fibres. It was largely ignored until recently, but has now been made the subject of close study—and even international conferences—in regard to its structure and functions. Dr Rabagliatti, forty-five years ago, was so interested and far-seeing that his book, *Initis*, contained concepts the general truth of which is being proved today. He was, however, a lone voice and because he held unorthodox ideas he was, typically, ignored.

The ubiquity of connective tissue caused Dr Rabagliatti to analogize it to the ether—as the medium for, as he termed it, 'the zoodynamic life force'.

Through the connective tissues' planes run the trunks and plexuses of veins, arteries, nerves, and lymphatics. Connective tissue is the support for the structural and, therefore, functional relationships of these systems.

Chemical Structure
Briefly, the matrix consists of a jelly-like ground substance in which the fibres, cells, vessels, etc., lie. This ground substance is the 'physical expression of the *milieu intérieure* intervening everywhere between the blood and lymph vessels and the metabolizing cells; it plays a major role in the transport, storage and exchange of water and electrolytes. The chemical structure is essentially polysaccharide, hyaluronic acid, chondroitin sulphuric acid, chondroitin sulphate and chondroitin itself, together with proteins which contain a considerable amount of the amino acid tyrosine, which forms the majority of the thyroxin molecule.

The fibres are white fibrous (collagen), yellow (elastin), and reticulin. The collagen fibres are also protein and polysaccharide in composition and are stabilized chemically by the presence of the ground substance constituents. The presence of chondroitin sulphate, for example, renders the enzymatic breakdown of collagen much more difficult. The importance of this point will become more clear later. The formation of fibres appears to be due to a precipitation of fibre constituents by serum glycoproteins under the influence of adrenocorticotrophic hormone.

Reticulin contains more polysaccharide than collagen, and some lipid also. Elastin is also protein and polysaccharide in composition. Sulphur is a constituent of all three. Cells include fibroblasts, mast cells, macrophages and others.

A Function of Circulation
The nature and composition of connective tissue is a function of circulation. Circulatory efficiency in any area will determine (1) the influx of materials to the area, and (2) the drainage of the area.

Incoming blood leads to the production of lymph and this fluid permeates the ground substance, bringing all the constituents of the blood except the proteins to the connective tissue. Some of these constituents are hormones. Thyroxin, adrenoglucocorticoids and adrenomineralocorticoids are only three of these. Oestrogen and androgens are two more. All these have known effects upon the structure of connective tissue. Thus, a diminution of thyroxin leads to an increase of water retention in most cells and an increase in the quantity of ground substance. The sex hormones also do this, but of most interest to us, here are the opposing groups of the adrenocortical hormones. Selye divides these into anti- and pro-inflammatory hormones (A-Cs and P-Cs). These are produced in response to stress situations and they exert both a general and a local effect. By regulating the balance between these two the body can control the ability of the tissues to produce an inflammatory response. But when the A-Cs and the P-Cs are both present in the blood the A-Cs always win the contest, i.e., there is an anti-inflammatory response.

Stressor Stimulus
The A-Cs are produced in response to a stimulus—the stressor. The stressor in neuro-muscular technique is pain. Effective technique appears to be accompanied by pain in all (I generalize here deliberately) such conditions (and also in the condition without treatment). Pain is probably due to two factors. A much reduced threshold in the area due to circulatory inhibition enabling a build up to just below the threshold level of Lewis pain substance or, alternatively, a disturbance of electrolyte level (e.g., increase of hydrogen ions or disturbance in the calcium/sodium/potassium balance due to the same circumstances). Consequently pain will be produced by even slight stimulus, let alone the heavier movements of neuro-muscular technique. Also, pressure and tension proprioceptors may be overstimulated and pain can result from an over-application of any ordinary stimulus.

The A-Cs liberated will produce both general effects (General Adaptation Syndrome) and local effects (Local Adaptation Syndrome) and their effect is anti-inflammatory, both generally and locally, at the area of application of the stressor, i.e., at the areas of technique application. Consequently, there is a break-down of collagen fibres and a general decrease in water retention in the ground substance; the congested area is decongested.

Different Muscle Types

We have noted previously that different muscle types (type 1 and 2) have different roles to play, as well as having different sources of energy. They are also prone to different observable forms of dysfunction, one from the other, in response to pathological states.

Thus type 1 muscles are mainly concerned with supportive static activities and derive their energy primarily from oxidative phosphorylation. They are prone to loss of endurance capabilities, when disused or subject to pathological influences. These muscles become shortened or tighter, when this occurs. Those muscles which play a more active role in terms of strength and speed of action, are known as type 2, and are predominantly phasic, in that they are seldom called upon to maintain effort for long periods. These muscles derive energy primarily from glycogen breakdown, and when disused, or pathologically influenced, become weak.

Among the more important postural muscles which tighten and shorten (become hyperactive) in response to dysfunction, are trapezius (superior aspects), sternocleidomastoid, levator scapulae and upper aspects of pectoralis major, in the upper trunk. Quadratus lumborum, erecta spinae oblique abdominals and iliopsoas, in the lower trunk. Tensor fascia latae, rectus femoris, biceps femoris, adductors (longus brevis and magnus) piriformis, hamstrings, semitendinosus, in the pelvic and lower extremity region; and the flexors of the arms.

Phasic muscles, which weaken in response to dysfunction (i.e. are inhibited), include the paravertebral muscles and scaleni, the extensors of the upper extremity (flexors are primarily postural) the abdominal aspects of pectoralis major; middle and inferior aspects of trapezius; the rhomboids, serratus anterior, rectus abdominus; the internal and external obliques the gluteals, the peroneal muscles, and the extensors of the arms. (Identification of these variations is via tests for strength and tightness.)

Note: Lewit[29] does not subscribe to the theory that phasic and postural muscles can be differentiated by virtue of their fibre type, as do Grieve[30] and Jokl.[31]

The logical approach to correction of dysfunction, involving shortened tight musculature, is to lengthen and stretch these tissues. NMT and Muscles Energy Technique (which will be described in Chapter 9) are useful in achieving this. Such an approach may involve any combination of these technique, and could include deep NMT, followed by isometric methods, which employ post isometric relaxation, as well as reciprocal inhibition, and also isotonic methods which contribute towards breaking down fibrocytic contractions.

Correct Sequence Therapy Those muscles which have become weak will respond to initial attention to them, via isotonic concentric MET methods, as well as exercises specific to the area. General postural and body-toning exercises should follow. In the early stages, however, it is important to allow the beneficial effects of the attention to the shortened muscles to proceed without confusing the issue by attention to the weakened antagonists. If, after several weeks of treatment of the shortened, contracted, postural muscles, there is not an observable and measurable improvement in the weak antagonists, then MET and exercise should be introduced.

The use of gentle functional techniques, such as those of Lawrence Jones, (which are described in detail in Chapter 10) are suitable for combining with NMT and MET methods. By using muscle energy techniques, to help to lengthen shortened structures, and NMT to aid in this, as well as in identifying localized areas of soft-tissue dysfunction (myofascial trigger points, Jones' tender points or other forms of soft-tissue dysfunction) the operator has a wide array of diagnostic and therapeutic methods, literally at his finger tips.

We should not lose sight of the tried and tested effects of massage on the soft tissues. The degree of that effect will vary with the type of soft-tissue manipulation employed, and the nature of the patient and the problem.

Soft-tissue techniques, apart from those specifically associated with NMT, may include *Stroking* (to include relaxation and reduce fluid congestion) *stretching* (along or across the belly of muscles. Heel of hand, thumb or fingers are involved in slow movements, rhythmically applied). *Inhibition* via pressure (directly applied to the belly of contracted muscles or to local soft-tissue dysfunction, for a minute or more, or in a make and break manner, to reduce hypertonic contraction or for reflex effect) *kneading* (to improve fluid exchange and to achieve relaxation of tissues). *Vibration* and friction (used near origins and insertions, and near bony attachments, for relaxing effects on the mucle as a whole). Other methods which we would associate with the above techniques of traditional massage (soft tissues manipulation) would include the various applications of NMT, as described in this text, and the connective tissue massage methods which are primarily used for reflex effects (see Chapter 4).

How are the various effects of massage and soft-tissue manipulation explained? It seems that a combination of effects occur. Pressure, as applied in deep kneading or stroking along the length of a muscle, tends to displace its fluid content. Venous, lymphatic and tissue drainage is thereby encouraged. The replacement of this with fresh oxygenated blood, aids in normalization, and reduces the effects of pain-inducing substances which may be present. These observations are not mere conjecture but have been demonstrated in animal experiments to involve the opening of capillaries, which would otherwise be closed, resulting in increased capillary filtration, and reduction in oedema. Venous capillary pressure is also increased by massage in this manner. Massage also causes a decrease in the sensitivity of the gamma efferent control of the muscle spindles, and thereby reduces any shortening tendency of the muscles. Pressure techniques, such as are used in NMT, and the methods employed in MET, have a direct effect on the Golgi tendon organs, which detect the load applied to the tendon or muscle. These have an inhibitory capability, which can cause the entire muscle to relax. The Golgi tendon organs are set in series in the muscle, and are affected by both active and passive contraction of the tissues. The effect of any system which applies longitudinal pressure or stretch to the muscle, will be to evoke this reflex relaxation. The degree of stretch has, however, to be great, as there is little response from a small degree of stretch. The effect of MET, articulation techniques, and various functional balance techniques depends to a large extent on these tendon reflexes. ('The Physiology of Soft Tissue Massage', Sandler, S., *British Osteopathic Journal*, 1983 15:1-6).

We are in the midst of a change in the concepts of manipulative therapy which has far-reaching implications. One of the major changes is the restoration of the soft-tissue component to centre stage, rather than the peripheral role to which it has been assigned in the past. Lewit discusses aspects of this in his book *Manipulative Therapy in Rehabilitation of the Motor System* (Butterworth, 1985):

**Effects
Explained**

'It soon became clear that treatment of restricted joint movement has its limits, and that passive mobility itself involves not only joints but also muscles. This close relationship between joints and muscles became the starting point for further advances.' He discusses the 'no-man's land', which lies between neurology, orthopaedics and rheumatology which, he says, is the home of the vast majority of patients with pain derived from the locomotor system, and in whom no definite pathomorphological changes are found. He makes the suggestion that these be termed cases of 'functional pathology of the locomotor system'. These include most of the patients attending osteopathic, chiropractic and physiotherapy practitioners.

The most frequent symptom of individuals involved in this area of dysfunction is pain, which may be reflected clinically by reflex changes such as muscle spasm, myofascial trigger points, hyperalgesic skin zones, periostial pain points, or a wide variety of other sensitive areas which have no obvious pathological origin.

It is a major part of the role of NMT to help in both identifying such areas, as well as offering some help in differential diagnosis. NMT and muscle energy methods are then capable of normalizing many of the causative aspects of these myriad, mysterious, sources of pain and disability. Lewit makes great claims for those aspects of MET which are related to post isometric relaxation (see Chapter 9) in this regard. He says: 'By involving muscular physiology we have increasingly engaged the patient's own activity; originally passive manipulative techniques became semi-active, until finally the patient began to learn self-treatment, independent of the therapist. Since these techniques are very effective in producing muscular relaxation, they can also be used to treat muscular spasm, trigger points and even referred pain.'

It is the intention in this book to explore a variety of aspects of the dysfunction which lie in these grey areas, of which Lewit speaks. By learning how to use NMT diagnostically and therapeutically, a good deal of information is obtained as to the patterns of dysfunction operating. It is important to stress, at the outset, that NMT may be used in both a diagnostic mode and a therapeutic mode, and that to some extent these overlap, and may be carried out simultaneously. Once having identified those structures and tissues which required greater attention, NMT is available as a tool with which to make contact and give direct localized treatment to areas which are contracted or tightened. Specific techniques are also available to deal with reflex activity, such as is noted in trigger points, Muscle energy methods, as described by Lewit, and elaborations on this, derived from a variety of sources, provide a further array of methods which can then be brought into operation, depending upon the particular indications. Soft tissue manipulation is capable of normalizing a great many joint problems, without recourse to active manipulative effort. In many cases, as will be seen in Chapter 9, MET also offers the opportunity to make subsequent manipulation a much easier task by reducing the muscular restrictions, as well as preparing the specific tissues involved for manipulation. MET and NMT are symbiotic, and it is possible to achieve more by combining their repertoire of useful techniques, than either can achieve individually. By adding the knowledge of suitable techniques by which to influence reflex activity, demonstrated by the presence of localized areas of soft-tissue dysfunction (trigger points, Chapman's points, etc.) as well as using the tender points described by Lawrence Jones (Chapter 10) in gentle functional techniques of joint restoration, the scope of the application of soft-tissue manipulation becomes apparent. This does not necessarily preclude active joint manipulation in correcting structural dysfunction, but should make for a lesser need to utilize such methods as thrust or long-lever techniques, and to make their employment simpler, and less likely to traumatize the local tissues or the patient.

We have now looked at the soft tissues through a variety of eyes. What emerges is the certainty that therapeutic effort is well aimed if directed at normalizing the neuro-muscular component (to include connective tissue) of any dysfunction. Whether the object is to improve local or general function or to prepare for active manipulation or to remove reflex pain patterns, the objects of attention are the soft-tissue structures with their altered feel and sensitivity to pressure. Various workers have described the same changes using different terminology and advising a variety of therapeutic methods. NMT offers a simple system of diagnosis and treatment based on over fifty years of use and development. In skilled hands it can remove pain, improve function, obviate manipulation or prepare for it, enhance the body's economy, relieve stress, induce relaxation and well-being and greatly aid in the restoration of health—without side effects.

Before considering the technique itself it will be necessary to examine reflex symptoms and trigger areas which originate in the soft tissues.

[1] Erlinghauser, R. F., 'Circulation of C.S.F. Through Connective Tissues,' *Academy of Applied Osteopathy Yearbook* (1959).

[2] Selye, H., *The Street of Life*, (McGraw Hill, 1956).

[3] Humphreys, P. W. and Lind, A. R., *Journal of Physiology* (1963), pp. 120-135.

[4] Jacobson, E., 'Principles Underlying Coronary Heart Disease,' *Cardiologia* (1955), pp. 26-83.

[5] Barlow, W., 'Anxiety and Muscle Tension Pain', *British Journal of Clinical Practice*, Vol. 3, No. 5.

[6] Alexander, F. M, *The Use of the Self*, (Educational Publications, 1957).

[7] Lewis, Sir Thomas, *Pain*, (New York, 1942).

[8] Reich, Wilhelm, *Character Analysis*, (Vision Press, 1949).

[9] Boadella, David, 'The Language of the Body in Bio-energetic Therapy', *Journal of the Research Society for Natural Therapeutics* (1978).

[10] Taylor, R. B., 'Bio-energetics of Man', *Academy of Applied Osteopathy Yearbook* (1958).

[11] Little, K. E., 'Toward More Effective Manipulative Management of Chronic Myofascial Strain and Stress Syndromes', *Journal of the American Osteopathic Association*, Vol. 68 (March, 1969).

[12] Eeman, L., *Co-operative Healing*, (Frederick Muller, 1947).

[13] Rolf, Ida, 'Structural Dynamics', *British Academy of Applied Osteopathy Yearbook* (1962).

[14] Taylor, R. B., *op. cit.*

[15] Gutstein, R., 'A Review of Myodysneuria (Fibrositis)', *American Practitioner and Digest of Treatments,* Vol. 6, No. 4.

[16] Petersen, W., *The Patient and the Weather: Autonomic Disintegration*, (Edward Bros., Ann Arbor, 1934).

[17] Bayer, H., Pathophysiology of Muscular Rheumatism, *Ztschr. Raeumaforsch 9:210* (1950).

[18] Cathie, Dr A., 'Selected Writings', *Academy of Applied Osteopathy Yearbook* (1974).

[19] Pauling, Linus, *The Common Cold and 'Flu*, (W. H. Freeman and Company, 1976).

[20] Cyriax, J., *Textbook of Orthopaedic Medicine*, (Cassell, 1962).

[21] Stoddard, Dr Alan, *Manual of Osteopathic Practice*, (Hutchinson, 1969).

[22] Ebner, M., *Connective Tissue Massage*, (Churchill Livingstone, 1962).

[23] Lecture to Research Society for Natural Therapeutics, 1969.

[24] Korr, I., 'Spinal Cord as Organiser of Disease Process', *Academy of Applied Osteopathy Yearbook* (1976).

[25] Patterson, M., 'Model Mechanism for Spinal Segmental Facilitation', *Academy of Applied Osteopathy Yearbook* (1976).

[26] Personal communication to the author.

[27] Lief, P., *British Naturopathic Journal*, Vol. 5, No. 10.
[28] Youngs, B., 'Physiological Background of NM Technique', *British Naturopathic Journal*, Vol. 5, No. 6.
[29] Lewit, K., *Manipulative Therapy in Rehabilitation of the Motor System* (Butterworth 1985).
[30] Grieve, G., *Mobilisation of the Spine* (Churchill Livingstone 1985).
[31] Jokl, Peter., 'Muscle and low back pain' (JAOA, Sept 1984, p64).

Chapter 2

Reflex Areas and
Somatic Dysfunction

Much work has been done in recent years in the field of myofascial trigger points. Janet Travell[1] M.D. has stated that if a pain is severe enough to cause a patient to seek professional advice it is usually a referred pain and therefore a trigger area is involved (if there is no evidence of organic or metabolic disease). She maintains that patterns of referred pain are constant in distribution in all people, only intensity will vary. Among the effects of an active trigger point there may be numbness, tingling, weakness, lack of normal range of movement as well as pain. The etiological myofascial trigger point for a particular pain pattern is always located in a particular part of a particular muscle.[2] Eradication of the trigger, by whatever means, will remove all symptoms. Treatment of the target or reference area is useless.

There is some disagreement about the role of bony or joint.lesions in the maintenance of such pain patterns. One school of thought maintains that such 'lesions' should be corrected manipulatively, prior to dealing with the myofascial trigger. The importance of the fourth dorsal segment and the lumbo-dorsal junction is emphasized in this regard. Others, notably Travell, suggest such manipulative procedures should be performed after the myofascial pain pattern has been normalized.

Trigger Areas

The trigger areas, in so far as they concern our present study, are localized areas of deep tenderness and increased resistance. Pressure on such a trigger will often produce twitching and fasiculation. Pressure maintained on such a point will produce referred pain in a predictable area. If there are a number of active trigger points the reference areas may overlap. Any physical or psychic stress factor can result in alterations in normal tone in muscles, fascia and other soft tissues. This can affect changes in joint play, breathing, posture etc. and result in abnormal and constant tension. This in turn can lead to swelling, myositis and spasm which is the predisposing condition in the production of trigger points and their referred pain and dysfunction. Trauma or chilling may also be part of the etiology.

A number of methods exist for the obliteration of such trigger points, ranging from pharmacological agents such as novocaine or xylocain, to coolant sprays and acupuncture techniques. It is noteworthy that direct pressure techniques can also effectively reduce and ultimately remove such trigger areas. In so far as such a course of action would fit into neuro-muscular treatment it is of value to this study. Individual preference for one or other technique will allow scope for the effective removal of these pain sources. It is important to remember that a trigger point is self-perpetuating unless it is correctly treated.

Once symptoms have been relieved the muscle containing the trigger must be gently stretched to its longest resting length. Failing this, symptoms will return, irrespective of the technique used (chilling, pressure, injection, acupuncture etc.). Such stretching should be gradual and gentle.

Dr J. Mennell[3] states that a muscle that can attain and maintain its normal resting length is a pain-free muscle. One that cannot (a muscle in spasm) is usually a source of pain, regardless of whether the source of the spasm is in that muscle or not. Whatever the means used to 'block' the trigger activity and whatever the neuropathological routes involved, the critical factor in the restoration of pain-free normality is that during any relief from the state of spasm or contraction, the affected muscle should have its normal resting length restored by stretching. Mennell defines trigger points as localized palpable spots of deep hypersensitivity from which noxious impulses bombard the CNS to give rise to referred pain. Mennell favours chilling the trigger area by vapo-coolant or ice-massage. Details of his recommended method will be given in the treatment section.

Muscle Energy Techniques will be found to play a large part in achieving the desired resting length of muscles, and to be particularly useful in dealing with trigger points.

It is not always easy to determine whether a soft tissue pain is referred, or whether it is arising locally. Kellgren, in Copeman's *Textbook of Rheumatic Diseases* (Churchill Livingstone, 1978, pp. 62-77) tells us that there are two methods of doing so. The first is by applying pressure to a tender area, and noting whether the pain increases out of all proportion to the degree of pressure applied. If so, the pain is of local origin. With referred pain this does not happen, and the pain noted on pressure is directly proportional to the pressure being employed.

The other method is to use a local anaesthetic. This will provide little relief if the area relates to referred pain (and may even exacerbate it) whereas pain arising locally, and thus anaesthetized, will show dramatic relief from pain.

It should be kept in mind that pain is not the only symptom likely to derive from trigger points. Travell ('Temperomandibular Joint Pain, Referred from Muscles of Head and Neck', *Jnl. Prosth. Dent.*, Vol. 10, 1960, pp. 745-763) found that, on occasion, trigger points within the neck muscles could cause the teeth to become hypersensitive to hot and cold. Triggers in the temporalis muscle could increase lacrimation in the adjacent eye, and triggers in the midportion of the temporalis could increase salivation. She suggested a strong relationship between trigger points and the autonomic nervous system.

Similar trigger involvement in other symptomatology involves gastric disturbances and sudomotor activity (Kellgran, K., 'Somatic Structure Simulating Visceral Pain', *Clin. Science*, 1939-42, pp. 303-309).

Gutstein There are many factors involved in the role of reflexes in both pathological and physiological activity. Neuro-muscular Technique provides the opportunity to both seek out reflex trigger areas and to treat them manually. It further allows for the application of other reflex effects. Gutstein[4] has shown that conditions such as ametropia may result from changes in the neuro-muscular component of the craniocervical area as well as more distant conditions involving the pelvis or shoulder girdle. He states:

> Myopia is the long-term effect of pressure of extraocular muscles in the convergence effort of accommodation and by spasm of the ciliary muscles, with resultant elongation of the eyeball. A sequential relationship has been shown between such a condition and muscular spasm of the neck.

Normalization of these muscles by manipulation relieves eye symptoms as well as facial, dorsolumbar and abdominal tenderness. Gutstein terms these reflexes 'myodysneuria' and suggests that the reference phenomena of such spots or triggers would include pain, modifications of pain, itching, hypersensitivity to physiological stimuli, spasm, twitching, weakness and trembling of striated muscles; hyper- or hypo-tonus of smooth muscle of blood vessels, and of internal organs; hyper- or hypo-secretion of visceral, sebaceous and sudatory glands. Somatic manifestations may also occur in response to visceral stimuli of corresponding spinal levels.

Many such trigger areas are dormant and asymptomatic. Gutstein's method of treatment is the injection of an anaesthetic solution into the trigger area. He indicates however that where accessible (e.g. muscular insertions in the cervical area) the chilling of these areas combined with pressure will yield good results. This is in line with Mennell's work and fits into the field of Neuro-muscular Technique. Amongst the patterns of vasomotor, sebaceous, sudatory and gastro-intestinal dysfunction quoted by Gutstein are the following, all of which relate to reflex trigger points or 'myodysneuria'.

1. Various patterns of vasomotor abnormality such as coldness, pallor, redness, cyanosis etc. The variations in response to stimulation relates to the fact that most organs respond to weak stimuli by an increase in activity and to very strong stimuli by inhibiting activity. Menopausal hot flushes are one example and these seem often to be linked with musculoskeletal pain. Gutstein found that obliteration of overt and silent triggers in the occipital, cervical, interscapular, sternal and epigastric regions was accompanied by years of alleviation of premenopausal, menopausal and late menopausal symptoms. NMT has long emphasized the importance of normalizing these very structures.

2. Gutstein maintains that normalization of skin secretion and therefore of hair and skin texture and appearance may be altered for the better by the removal of active trigger areas in the cervical and interscapular areas.

3. The conditions of hyper- and hypo- and an-hidrosis accompany vasomotor and sebaceous dysfunction. The trigger areas were similar and it was often found that abolition of excessive perspiration as well as anhidrosis followed adequate treatment.

4. Gutstein quotes a number of practitioners who have achieved success in treating gastro-intestinal dysfunctions by treating trigger areas. Some of these were treated by procainization, others by pressure techniques and massage. The abdominal wall lends itself to this latter procedure as evidenced by the work of Cornelius[5] whose treatment was not dissimilar to that of Lief's NMT.

Among the conditions that have responded to such treatment are the following:

Pylorospasm, bad breadth, heartburn, regurgitation, nausea, abdominal distension, constipation, nervous diarrhoea etc.

Obviously other causes, notably of a dietary nature, might be involved. However, in a number of instances the 'trigger' points might well be the major factor.

The main area of these triggers, relating to gastro-intestinal dysfunction, were found to be in the upper, mid and lower portions of the rectus muscles, over the lower portion of the sternum, the epigastrium, including the xiphoid process and the parasternal regions. The latter correspond with the insertions of the three portions of the rectus muscle into the cartilages of the fifth, sixth and seventh ribs. These triggers are found by careful palpation and pressure (*see illustration on page 188*).

Travell and Bigelow[6] have produced evidence that supports much of what Gutstein has reported. They indicate that high intensity stimuli from active trigger areas produce, by reflex, prolonged vaso-constriction with partial ischaemia in localized areas of the brain, spinal cord, or peripheral nerve structures. There might result a wide pattern of dysfunction affecting almost any organ of the body. The phenomenon of hysteria with symptoms as varied as disordered vision, respiration, motor power and cutaneous sensation, were often mediated by afferent neural impulses from trigger areas in skeletal muscle. These triggers when similarly located, produced the same pattern of clinical effects, whether activated in one patient by psychogenic factors or in another by other factors (e.g. mechanical or traumatic).

The Variety of Reflex Points

A number of respected researchers and clinicians are frequently in error when they describe as trigger points localized soft tissue areas which palpate as sensitive. It must be clear that with a variety of different types of discrete, palpable, soft tissue changes, we must be extremely careful as to what description we apply. A trigger point will always be palpable, and always be sensitive to pressure, but then so will most other 'points', whether these be Chapman's reflexes, Gutstein's myodysneuria points, or acupuncture alarm points. What is distinctive about active trigger points (myofascial trigger points) is that they also refer sensation or symptoms to a distinct target area, and that this target area is more or less reproducible in other individuals, when trigger points are located in similar positions. No other soft-tissue dysfunction has this particular attribute.

Travell's definition of a trigger point is that, 'it lies in skeletal muscle, and is identified by localized deep tenderness, in a palpable firm band of muscle (muscle hardening); and at the point of maximum deep hyperalgesia, by a positive "jump sign", a visible shortening of the part of the muscle which contains the band. To elicit the jump sign most effectively, one must place the relaxed muscle under moderate passive tension, and snap the band briskly with the palpating finger.'

The trigger point must also refer symptoms or sensations to a target area. Otherwise, rather than being active it may a latent trigger point, which could be activated by stress or strain on the tissues in which it lies. The difference between most other areas of discrete palpable soft tissue dysfunction, and an active trigger, is this quality of referring symptoms. All other points may be prospective triggers, but are not active.

Chapman's reflexes, as we will see later in this chapter, are also sensitive to pressure, and are characterized by having an altered texture (stringy, amorphous shotty plaques, pellet like, etc.). They also occur in pairs, one anterior and one posterior. Unless both are found in the predicted area, and unless both are palpable and sensitive (though without the referred sensitivity, pain or other symptoms noted with trigger points) they are not Chapman's (neurolymphatic) reflex points. Jones (see Chapter 10) describes tender points associated with joint dysfunction. These he equates with trigger points, and some may indeed be so described. However, the vast majority are not, are are merely localized areas of soft-tissue dysfunction, which palpate as tender, and which in most cases may be equated with the Ah Shi points in traditional acupuncture terminology. These have been described for many hundreds of years as 'spontaneously arising tender points' associated with joint dysfunction, or pathology. In acupuncture these are thought to be amenable to pressure or needling techniques. Jones uses them as a guide to the correct positioning of the joint, for when this is achieved the tenderness vanishes, or reduces markedly.

These are found singly, and not in pairs, as are the neurolymphatic points described above. Thus, we have the ability to distinguish one sort of soft-tissue dysfunction from another. We also have the ability to locate them precisely, via the methods used in NMT, which combs the soft tissues for just such aberrations.

There also exists a range of sensitive points which lies on the periostium (see list) and which is related to disturbances of function of the locomotor system. These points are, in some degree, interchangeable with Jones' points and Ah Shi points. Many of these points are at the site of tendon or ligament attachment, and the tenderness appears to relate to acute or chronic tension in the associated muscles. This can apply to spinal and all their attachments.

This is not an exhaustive list of all possible 'points', but is hopefully indicative of some of the variations of which we should be aware. Morphological examination of acupuncture points, overlying periosteal structures, shows that the fatty and connective tissues are the determining factor in the looked for 'acupuncture sensation'. These structures are equally amenable to pressure techniques.

List of Important Periosteal Pain Points (PPP)

(Adapted from Karel Lewit's *Manipulative Therapy in Rehabilitation of Motor System*). These will usually related to acute or chronic contraction of associated muscles.

Site	Muscular or Joint Implication
Pain on head of metatarsals.	Dropped arch; flat foot.
Spur or calcaneum (pain on pressure).	Tight plantar aponeurosis.
Pain of tubercle of tibia.	Tight long adductors. Perhaps hip dysfunction.
Pain at head of fibula.	Biceps femoris tightness.

Site	Muscular or Joint Implication
Posterior superior iliac spine tenderness.	Various possible implications, involving low back, gluteal and sacro-iliac region.
Lateral aspects of symphysis pubis.	Adductors tight. Hip or sacro-iliac dysfunction.
Pain on coccyx.	Gluteus maximus tightness, possibly piriformis or levator ani involvement.
Crest of Ilium — pain.	Tight quadratus lumborum/gluteus medius and/or lumbodorsal dysfunction.
Pain on greater trochanter.	Tight abductors. Hip dysfunction.
Pain on lumbar spinous processes. (especially L5)	Tight paraspinal muscles.
Pain mid-dorsal spinous processes.	Lower cervical dysfunction.
Pain spinous process of C2.	Levator scapular tight: C1-2, 2-3, dysfunction.
Pain on xyphoid process.	Rectus abdominus tight. 6-8 rib dysfunction.
Pain on ribs, on mammary or axillary line.	Pectoralis tightness. Visceral dysfunction referred to here.
Pain at sternocostal junction - upper Ribs.	Scalenus tightness.
Pain on clavicle, medial aspect.	Tight sternocleidomastoid.
Pain transverse process of atlas.	Tight sternocleidomastoid and/or recti capitis lateral. Atlanto-occipital dysfunction.
Pain on occiput.	Upper cervical or atlas dysfunction.
Pain on styloid process of radius.	Elbow dysfunction.
Pain on epicondyles.	Local muscular or elbow dysfunction.
Pain at deltoid attachment.	Scapulohumeral dysfunction.
Mandibular condyles painful.	TMJ dysfunction. Tight masticators.

Felix Mann MB, pioneer acupuncture researcher and author, describes periosteal acupuncture as being more effective than ordinary acupuncture in a number of conditions. He lists the following as being amongst the common sites:

1. Appropriate transverse cervical process.	Associated with headache, migraine, inter scapular pain and cervical spondylosis.
2. Area of sacro-iliac joint.	Associated with low back pain sciatica without neurological deficit, testicular pain, etc.
3. Coracoid process	Associated with painful shoulder joint.
4. Medial condyle tibia.	Knee pain, without advanced pathology.
5. Neck of femur.	Hip pain, without major changes evident on X-ray.
6. Lateral aspect of posterior spine of lower lumbar vertebrae.	If sacro-iliac joint, as above, does not yield benefit, then these areas may be used.

Note that pressure techniques, and Muscle energy methods, are as likely to achieve results in treating these points as is traditional needling.

Evans[7] in discussing reflex pain describes the mechanism as follows: **Reflex Pain**

> A prolonged bombardment of pain impulses sets up a vicious circle of reflexes spreading through a pool of many neuron connections upward, downward and even across the spinal cord and perhaps reaching as high as the thalamus itself. Depending upon the extent of the pool (internuncial pool), we detect the phenomena of pain and sympathetic disturbances a long distance from the injured (trigger) area of the body and occasionally even spread to the contra-lateral side.

Dittrich[8] has shown a constant pattern of fibrosis of subfascial tissue, with adhesions between this and the overlying muscle fascia, in a number of distinctive and common pain patterns. In what he calls the 'mid-sacral syndrome' which develops from sacral lesions, referred pain is almost always present in the buttock and sometimes in the thigh, leg or foot. Referred tenderness is elicited in the lower part of the buttock. The fibrous adhesions (trigger area) are found at the level of the *third sacral vertebra near the spine..*

In the 'mid-lumbar syndrome' there is referred pain and tenderness in the lower lumbar, upper sacral and sacro-iliac regions. The trigger point is found over the lateral third of the sacro-spinalis muscle at the level of the *upper margin of the iliac crest*.

The 'latissimus-dorsi syndrome' may result from irritation of the *aponeurosis of this muscle* at either of the sites of injury, sacral or lumbar mentioned above.

Referred pain would develop in the sclerotonic distributions of the sixth, seventh, and eighth cervical nerves.

He points out that pathological changes at the two sites have been discovered by operative findings. His technique is to surgically remove these triggers or to obliterate the triggers by injection of local anaesthetic. No concern is expressed for the mechanical, postural or other reasons that may have produced them, nor is any mention made of more conservative manipulative methods of normalization. The presence of 'fibrosed subfascial tissue' supports the theories of Stanley Lief and Boris Chaitow. The locale of these, close to bony insertions, further supports the rationale behind Neuro-muscular Technique.

It seems that soft tissue lesions, characterized by fibrosis of subfascial tissue (fat etc.) with fibrous connections between the structure and the overlying fascia can initiate sensory irritation which produce referred pain and tenderness. In addition, autonomic nervous involvement may be activated to produce vasomotor, trophic, viseral or metabolic changes. Symptoms will disappear when the offending lesion is normalized by whatever method. However, a system that both corrects the offending trigger and attempts to prevent its recurrence would seem to have a greater scientific basis.

Viscerosomatic Reflexes

Many of the various points described in this book as belonging to one or another system or category (Chapman's reflexes, Bennet's reflexes, trigger points etc.) are examples of viscerosomatic reflex activity (otherwise called 'referred' pain or dysfunction). Myron Beal D.O. ('Viscerosomatic Reflexes: A review, *The Journal of the American Osteopathic Association*, Vol. 85, No. 12, December 1985, pp786-801) has described this phenomenon and its vast background of research documentation.

He points out that a viscerosomatic reflex is the result of afferent stimuli, arising from dysfunction of a visceral nature. The reflex is initiated by afferent impulses arising from visceral receptors, which are transmitted to the dorsal horn of the spinal cord, where they synapse with interconnecting neurons. The stimuli are then conveyed to sympathetic and motor efferents, resulting in changes in the somatic tissues, such as skeletal muscle, skin and blood vessels. Abnormal stimulation of the visceral efferent neurons may result in hyperasthesia of the skin, and associated vasomotor, pilomotor and sudomotor changes. Similar stimuli of the ventral horn cells may result in reflex rigidity of the somatic musculature. Pain may be associated with such changes. The degree of stimulus required, in any given case, will differ. Factors such as prior facilitation of the particular segment, as well as the response of higher centres, will differ from person to person. In many cases, it is suggested, by Korr and others, that viscerosomatic reflex activity may be noted prior to any symptoms of visceral change, and that this is of diagnostic and prognostic value.

The first signs of viscerosomatic change, in response to such reflex activity, are vasomotor reactions (increased skin temperature), sudomotor (increased moisture of the skin), skin textural changes (e.g. thickening), increased subcutaneous fluid, and increased contraction of muscle. These signs disappear if the visceral cause improves. When such changes become chronic, trophic alterations are noted, with increased thickening of the skin and subcutaneous tissue, and localized muscular contraction. Deep musculature may become hard, tense and hypersensitive. This may involve deep splinting contractions, involving two or more segments of the spine, with associated retriction of spinal motion. The costotransverse articulations may be significantly involved in such changes.

Patterns of somatic response will be found to differ from person to person, and to be unique, in terms of location, the number of segments involved, and whether or not the pattern is uni- or bi-lateral. The degree of intensity will also differ, and is related to the degree of acuteness of the visceral condition.

Research, involving animals, as well as observations in humans, using regional nerve blocks, has helped to define site locations of response, in various forms of visceral dysfunction. Beal notes that three distinct groups of visceral involvement are found in respect of particular sites. These are:

T1-T5: heart and lungs; T5-T10 oephagus, stomach, small intestine, liver, gall bladder, spleen, pancreas and adrenal cortex. T10-L2 large bowel, appendix, kidney, ureter, adrenal medulla, testes, ovaries, urinary bladder, prostate gland, uterus.

There appears to be a concensus as to sidedness being apparent, in reflexes of unpaired organs. Thus, left-sidedness is noted in conditions involving small intestine and the heart; right-sidedness for gall bladder disease and appendix. The stomach may produce reflex activity on either, or both sides.

A number of studies have been concerned with the identification of such reflexes. One five year study involved over 5,000 hospitalized patients (*The Journal of the American Osteopathic Association*, 70:570-92, Feb 1971). This concluded that most visceral disease appeared to have more than one region with increased frequency of segmental findings, and that the number of spinal segments involved was related to the duration of the disease. It was noted in this study, by Kelso, that there were an increased number of palpatory findings in the cervical region, related to patients with sinusitis, tonsillitis, diseases of the oesophagus and liver complaints. Somatic dysfunction was noted in patients with gastritis, duodenal ulceration, pyelonephritis, chronic appendicitis and cholycytitis, in the region of T5-T12. Other studies have confirmed this, as well as noting other patterns of reflex activity.

Somatic dysfunction is assessed most easily by use of palpatory investigation. Beal insists that investigation should pay attention to the various soft-tissue layers: 'The skin for changes in texture, temperature and moisture; the subcutaneous tissue for changes in consistency and fluid; the superficial and deep musculature for tone, irritability, consistency, visco-elastic properties, and fluid content; and the deep fascial layers for textural changes'. He advises: 'Special attention be given to the examination of the costotransverse area, where it is felt that autonomic nerve effects are predominant'. He notes that tests for the quality and range of joints have not been found to differentiate between visceral reflexes and somatic changes. This confirms the importance of the soft-tissue assessment in order to elicit such information.

He notes that the supine position is ideal for assessment of paraspinal tissues. The hand being gently inserted under the region, and pressure, or springing, techniques applied. He has not investigated the use of patient examination in the prone position, as he suggests that this position is precluded in acutely ill patients. Nevertheless, since Beal notes the difficulty of applying diagnostic measures with the patient supine, when the mid to lower thoracic area is under review, a prone position is suggested, unless the patient cannot manage this. The availability of a couch with a split head-piece would make this more comfortable. As we will see, the methods employed by those using connective tissue massage involve the patient being seated. This helps in assessing skin and superficial tissue status, but is not really suitable for deeper penetration.

Beal suggests that the diagnosis of a viscerosomatic reflex is based upon two or more adjacent spinal segments showing evidence of somatic dysfunction, and being located within the specific autonomic reflex area. There should be deep confluent spinal muscle splinting, and resistance to segmental joint motion. Skin and subcutaneous tissue changes, which are consistent with the acuteness or chronicity of the reflex, should be noted.

Specific identification of the origin of the reflex is, he suggests, difficult. When, however, a localized dysfunction fails to respond to treatment, suspicions should be alerted as to possible visceral activity maintaining the dysfunction.

It is noted that psychological stress often manifests as a bilateral contraction of the superficial spinal musculature in the cervical or thoracic regions. Other historic and physical evidence is required to support such findings.

Treatment of such reflex areas has been suggested to be of value. By interrupting the reflex arcs, and influencing the viscus through stimulation of the somaticovisceral reflex, and also by reducing potential preconditioning effects of somatic dysfunction to body stressors, this may be achieved. Response may be limited because of continued afferent stimulation from the diseased viscus. When this improves the reflex activity should diminish, and a better response be obtained from treatment of the reflex areas. A variety of improvements have been noted in this regard, with an overall feeling that symptomatic improvements are frequently observed and that such treatment, in a long-term programme, results in decreased incidence of recurrence of acute manifestations of disease, less somatic pain, less disability and a decrease in the potential stress effects, mediated through segmental facilitation.

Treatment itself, of such areas, according to Beal, is as follows:

> Treatment of the acute stage of somatic dysfunction, associated with visceral disease, is designed primarily to break into the reflex arc. In cases of serious illness the treatment may consist of gentle digital pressure, of short duration, to affect a local change in superficial tissues. When relaxation has been accomplished in the subcutaneous and superficial paraspinal musculature, the deep muscle contraction can be addressed. The duration of treatment is dependent upon the patient's condition and perceived energy level.

Beal suggests that acute conditions that are not life threatening may be addressed in a more aggressive manner (asthma is given as an example). It is suggested that NMT is an ideal method of addressing all aspects of such reflex activity. Offering as it does a diagnostic as well as a therapeutic opportunity to address both superficial and deep tissues.

Viscerosomatic reflex changes are just one of the many reasons for altered tissue findings, which may be noted in the general NMT assessment, described in Chapter 6. Awareness of the possibility of this adds to the potential for accurate diagnosis.

M. Blashey M.D.,[9] dealing with limb rehabilitation, describes the research of Julius **Fuchs' System** Fuchs, a Germany orthopaedist who died in 1953. Fuchs' system used supporting structures of a part elastic material and part non-elastic material which was arranged so that antagonistic muscle groups were supported in such a way as to produce 'kinetic fields'. These fields were kinetically facilitating where elastic tissue was used and kinetically impeding where inelastic tissue was used. However, where sensory nerve damage had occurred in the skin overlying these muscles no kinetic effect was obtained. Only light pressure on the muscular structures involved was found to be required to produce what Fuchs termed the 'orthokinetic' effect.

From this research we learn a good deal about the reflex effect on muscle groups which light manipulation of the overlying tissue of affected muscles can produce. Does there exist a specific function of structure or both, connecting skin surface with underlying muscle, in a direct and specific manner? It would seem so.

Hagbarth[10] has shown that both flexor and extensor responses can be elicited in a definite structural pattern. In the knee, for example, the flexors can be stimulated from the skin of the entire limb *apart* from the skin overlying the extensors. (In his experiments he was using the cat as a model but later work has shown it to valid for humans). The skin overlying the extensors is exitatory for the extensors. The converse applies, so that all skin covering the flexors is inhibitory for the extensors. This is summarized below:

Table 1. Areas of Inhibition and Excitation with Flexor and Extensor Responses in the Knee

Motion of Knee	Area of Inhibition	Area of Excitation
Flexion	over extensors only	over rest of limb
Extension	over flexors only	over rest of limb

These effects were obtained thermally, electrically and by tactile stimulation which did not need to be heavy. The 'skin motor areas' or 'orthokinetic fields' do not correspond in distribution to the skin fields of cutaneous nerves or with segmental arrangements.

I do not intend to become involved in the theoretical hypothetical neurological arguments that support these clinical facts. For the purposes of the study of neuro-muscular treatment the existence of a particular effect is in itself adequate. Physiologists, anatomists, biologists and zoologists will eventually produce profound definitive answers to all such conundrums. In the meantime, as in the case of acupuncture, the ethical practitioner can use knowledge gained by clinical means with equanimity as long as it is demonstrated that no harm can stem from the procedures involved. Such is the case in the present example.

To summarize this finding: there is a definite functional connection between a muscle and the portion of skin that covers it. They are integrated so that muscle is excited by stimuli within its own skin area. This area will be inhibitory to the antagonist of the underlying muscle.

Connective Tissue Massage

A system which incorporates a great deal of reflex effects is connective tissue massage (CTM). CTM involves the use of 'rolling' the tissues in order to achieve reflex and local effects. The strokes pull and stretch the tissues and it is suggested [11] that its effectiveness is based on a viscerocutaneous reflex. Bischof and Elmiger explain it thus:

> The specific mechanical stimulation of the pull on connective tissue seems to be the adequate stimulus to elicit the nervous reflex. Connective tissue massage acts first on the sympathetic terminal reticulum in the skin. The smallest branches of the autonomic nervous system contact the impulses activated by the pulling strokes to the sympathetic trunk and the spinal cord. The impulses travel from the skin either through a somatosensory spinal nerve via a posterior root ganglion to the grey matter or over the vascular plexus to the same segmental sympathetic ganglion or to the ganglion of the neighbouring segment, through the ramus communicans albus to the posterior root and grey matter of the spinal cord. They terminate either directly or by means of the internuncial neurons at the efferent autonomic root cells.
>
> In the efferent pathway the impulses travel from the autonomic lateral horn, or the intermediolateral column, over the anterior root, ramus communicans albus, to the segmental sympathetic ganglion or to the ganglion of the neighbouring segment and finally to the diseased organ. The origin of the connective tissue reflex zones and the influence of the CTM depend on the relationship between the function of the internal organs, vessels, and nerves as well as the tissues of the locomotor apparatus, which descend from the same metamere.
>
> Clara reminds us that the human embryo is composed of many homogeneous primitive segments (metameres) that are arranged serially. This arrangement is concerned with the mesoderm and the tissue regions derived from it—sclerotomes, myotomes, dermatomes, (ectoderm), angiotomes and nephrotomes, Secondly, the ectoderm participates in the segmentation (metamerism) since in each of the primitive segments or metameres one corresponding spinal nerve enters. The skin over the segment is also innervated, and in this way the segmentation is projected to the skin. This embryonal connection between the primitive segment and the spinal nerve (dermatome) develops early and remains unchanged postembryonically. Head was the first to point out that the internal organs that develop from the entoderm correspond to certain spinal cord segments, although the entoderm does not participate in the segmentation. The relationship between tissues and their spinal root innervation is the scientific foundation for CTM and other forms of segmental therapy. Most investigators differ little in their reports concerning the segmental connections of the internal organs. Different schemes have been proposed by Hansen, Keegan, Dejerine and others to relate skin topography with the internal organs.

During and after Connective Tissue Massage there are a number of reflex reactions including vaso-dilatation and diffuse or localized sweating. Some of these reflexes do not seem to be segmental in nature. For example, dilatation of the upper extremity blood vessels occurs when the pelvis is treated by CTM. The maximal skin temperature increase occurs about half an hour after CTM is discontinued and persists for an hour or so. It is of interest that the vaso-dilatory effect of CTM is as pronounced, or even more pronounced, after lumbar sympathectomy.

Some of the reactions to CTM are normal autonomic responses such as pleasant fatigue, bowel movements and diuresis. Oedema is markedly reduced and hormonal distribution is seen to achieve a degree of balance. Aspects of CTM are similar to NMT, and the 'skin rolling' methods used in some body areas are virtually identical in application. The effects are therefore interesting from a comparative point of view.

A Scottish hospital undertook a trial in which a small group of patients, attending a general psychiatric outpatient clinic, were treated with connective tissue massage. The group selected presented with symptoms of impaired peripheral circulation, muscular tension, and pain. A frequent complaint was of sleep impairment, which was not associated with any particular pathology, and which was resistant to even large doses of hypnotic drugs. Those selected for the trial responded poorly to drugs, and were unable to learn standard relaxation techniques. Connective tissue massage (CTM) was applied as follows:

Research Evidence into Clinical Effectiveness of Connective Tissue Massage in Cases of Anxiety

An initial diagnostic assessment was made, using a specific massage stroke, applied systematically to the back. This was a form of subdermal traction, or deep stroking, which stimulates the autonomic branch of the nervous system. Patients reported a slight sensation of scratching or cutting. Where tissues which were particularly tense when treated in this way, the sensation was stronger, being described as deep-dull pressure, or a sharp cutting sensation, both unrelated to the actual pressure being applied. A flare reaction of the tissues followed, and in some cases a weal developed. This sometimes persisted for some hours. The treatment proper consisted of a series of strokes which moved systematically through the back, each treatment lasting some 30 to 45 minutes, followed by a period of rest. Patients reported a feeling of warmth, and of being 'peaceful', and frequently fell asleep immediately. The nights' sleep following treatment were reported generally to be deep and refreshing. The usual length of a course was ten treatments, and these ceased when patients reported either disappearance of symptoms, or when no further improvement was seen to be forthcoming. A positive response often involved profuse sweating during treatment, and this was sometimes unilateral. A number of measurements and tests were conducted during the rest phase, after treatment. Arousal was tested by the playing, over a period, of twenty loud noises.

The physiological responses of the patients were recorded. Among the findings were that four out of five patients had a reduction in response to stress (randomly occurring loud noises) after CTM. This was of significant proportions. EMG activity, recorded on the frontalis muscle, showed that there was a significant decrease in response in three cases. Skin resistance was measured every minute during the rest period, and during the periods of stimulation with noise. EMG measurements were also recorded on the forearm extensor muscles. The findings were that in two subjects there was a significant increase in skin resistance, indicating lowered arousal, and two other subjects showed reduction in forearm extensor EMG activity. The other patient showed inconclusive effects. All subjects showed a significant response in one or more of the psychophysiological parameters. After cessation of treatment, 3 out of 5 patients ceased use of drugs completely, and the other two required diazepam in only small doses. All reported diminution of symptoms. The researchers report that the differences noted in response, between EMG findings in the frontalis muscle and forearm extensor, is of interest, since the former is more reactive in depressive illness, and the latter in more so in cases of agitation.

It is of importance to note that patients responded in their own way. There were no consistant findings, apart from overall reduction in evidence of symptoms. This supports the hypothesis that each individual has a unique pattern of response to stress, and that this pattern is consistent, regardless of the type of stress, endured. The response to non-specific therapy, such as CTM, allows the reponse of the individual to continue to be individual. They therefore utilize the beneficial aspects of the therapy in their own way, to meet the needs of their unique physiology.

The evidence resulting from this trial is that CTM is a useful tool in dealing with the consequences of psychiatric disturbances, anxiety and agitation. Experience indicates that similar results may be assumed for NMT. These findings were reported in *The Journal of Psychosomatic Research*, in an article entitled 'Anxiety States: preliminary report on the value of connective tissue massage'. The research was carried out at Bangor Village Hospital, Broxburn, West Lothian, Scotland (*The Journal of Psychosomatic Research*, Vol. 127, No. 2, pp125-129, 1983).

Chapman's Reflexes
A further reflex pattern has been described by Chapman and Owens. In an earlier work[12] I described these as follows:

> The reflexes of Chapman that I intend to discuss now are not the whole picture—they are only a part of the visible portion of the iceberg—but of immense value nonetheless.
>
> Drs Chapman and Owens first reported on Chapman's original findings in the late 1930s. A revised edition of their work has recently been published by the Academy of Applied Osteopathy.
>
> The surface changes of a Chapman's Reflex are palpable. They may best be described as contractions located in specific anatomical areas and always associated with the same viscera. In describing each organ reflex Chapman normally indicated tissue reflex areas, occurring anteriorly and posteriorly. These reflexes found in the deep fascia are described as 'gangliform' contractions. These contractions vary in size from a pellet to a large bean and are located anteriorly in the intercostal spaces near the sternum. Similar changes are found in those reflexes occurring on the pelvis. The tissue changes found in reflexes located on the lower extremeties are described as 'stringy masses' or 'amorphous shotty plaques'. Those reflexes occurring posteriorly along the spine, midway between the spinal processes and the tips of the transverse processes are of a more oedematous nature.
>
> *The Value of the Reflexes*
> Since the location of these palpable tissue change is constant in relation to specific viscera it is possible to establish the location of pathology without knowing its nature. The value of these reflexes is threefold:
> 1. As diagnostic aids.
> 2. They can be utilized to influence the motion of fluids, mostly lymph.
> 3. Visceral function can be influenced through the nervous system.
>
> *The Mechanism of the Reflexes*
> As to the mechanism whereby these reflexes act, it would appear that, in so far as the intercostal reflexes are concerned, stimulation of the receptor organs which lie between the anterior and posterior layers of anterior intercostal fascia acts through the intercostal nerve which enervates the external and internal intercostal muscles and thus, through the sympathetic fibres, affects the intercostal arteries, veins, lymph nodes, etc. Stimulation thus causes afferent and efferent vessels draining these tissues to increase or decrease, permitting lymph flow to be increased or decreased thus affecting the drainage of the

entire lymph system in the area. Through the sympathetic fibres associated with these tissues the lymph nodes of the vital organs are also affected.

Explaining Results of Neuro-muscular Technique
In my own mind I have no doubt that a knowledge of these reflexes goes a good way to explaining the sometimes startling results obtained through Neuro-muscular Technique. Stanley Lief placed great emphasis on the intercostal spaces and the paravertebral areas; he also stressed the importance of not over-treating, a consideration which cannot be repeated too often.

Research Evidence Supports Chapman's Reflex Usefulness
In a trial conducted in order to assess the effects of forms of manipulation on blood pressure, one of the methods used was stimulation of a Chapman's reflex (Mannino, R., 'The Application of Neurological Reflexes to the Treatment of Hypertension', *Journal of the American Osteopathic Association*, December 1979, pp225-230). A specific effect, attributable to this treatment was noted. The point chosen for treatment was the one related to adrenal function. The trial involved treatment of this point, or a sham point, in which pressure was applied to either the real or a false point, for a total of two minutes, in a make or break circular motion. The point is located in the intertransverse space, on both sides of the 11th and 12th thoracic vertebrae, midway between the spinous processes and the tips of the transverse processes. The sham treatment involved the area between the 8th and 9th thoracic vertebrae (this point relates to small intestine problems, and would have no effect on the sort of condition being assessed in these trials).

The results showed no effect on blood pressure, but did indicate fascinating alteration in aldosterone levels. Many hypertensives are shown to have low renin/high aldosterone levels. This has an effect on the renal tubules, which causes retention of sodium. Abnormalities in aldosternone levels have been shown in populations with essential hypertension. There was a demonstrable and consistent fall in aldosterone levels, within 36 hours of stimulation of the Chapman reflex for the adrenals, but no change at all in the levels when the sham points were stimulated. The delay in response, suggested that the treatment had a tendency to interrupt, or damp down, a feedback to the adrenal medulla by the sympathetic nervous system. This could decrease the circulating amount of catecholamines, thereby diminishing their effect on the cardiovascular reflex which in turn exerts an influence on the renin-angiotensin-aldosterone axis. The question is raised as to why, if this effect is the result of the manipulation of a Chapman's reflex, there was no observed lowering of blood pressure? The researchers considered that this may have been the result of an inadequate time allowance for the development of a lowering effect. In the use of drugs which effect aldosterone levels, blood pressure is not lowered for between five and seven days. Whether or not this suggestion is valid, the effect on aldosterone levels, via stimulation of the adrenal point, shows that these reflexes have a potent and predictable effect.

An element of disinformation has been forthcoming regarding the so-called neurolymphatic reflexes of Chapman, and it is important that this be corrected. Raymond Nimmo and James Vannerson, writing in *The Receptor*, the journal of the organization which teaches Nimmo technique (Receptor-Tonus Technique) a valuable method of soft-tissue manipulation, with more than a passing similarity to aspects of NMT, stated in 1971 (Vol. 12, No. 1, p 47): 'Research has not borne out the presumption (by Chapman) of a neurolymphatic reflex. Muscle fibres, which alone have the specific function of constricting vessels, do not exist in the walls of lymph vessels, except for a few fibres in the thoracic duct, and a few large trunks. These are sparsley located, and have little effect in lymph fluid propulsion.'

These two authors then castigate Chapman's assertion that the reflexes could exist at specific sites, which they term 'fantastic'. The first part of their statement is in contradiction to *Gray's Anatomy* (35th Edition, Longman, 1973, pp715). This tells us that lymph moves in a number of ways. Filtration occurs, generated by filtration of fluid from the capillaries. There is also a degree of movement engendered by contraction of surrounding muscles, which compress lymph vessels, the movement of which is determined by the presence of valves. This muscular contraction is dependent upon normal activity, and muscular contraction-relaxation sequences. Lymph is further capable of being moved, in such regions, according to Gray, by massage movements. Pulsating arterial vessels, in close proximity, also assists lymph movement, as does respiratory movement. Finally, and in contradiction of Nimmo and Vannerson, Gray states: 'The smooth muscle in the walls of the lymphatic trunks is most marked just proximal to the valves; stimulation of sympathetic nerves accompanying the trunks, results in contraction of the vessels; the intrinsic muscle of the vessels thus probably aids the flow of the lymph.' Since we may note that stimulation of cutaneous structures (see page 39) is capable of producing marked sympathetic responses, the possibility certainly exists that the term 'neurolymphatic reflex', as described by Chapman, may indeed be an accurate description of the phenomenon.

Beryl Arbuckle D.O. writes of Chapman's reflexes (*The Selected Writings of Beryl Arbuckle*, National Osteopathic Institute and Cerbral Palsy Foundation, 1977): 'The diagnostic value of these reflexes is amazing. For instance, a female having severe pain in the right lower quadrant of the abdomen, presents several possibilities, but the offending organ may well be located by means of the reflexes, the positive one showing whether the disturbance is due to appendix, cecum, tube or ovary.' She continues: 'With a degree of understanding of the interrelation of the endocrine glands, and of the important of the lymphatics and the autonomic distribution, the therapeutic value of these considerations can be shown clinically. There is a definite sequence which must be followed, in the management of these reflexes, to produce desired results, and, if not so applied, just as surely as the misapplication of any other therapy, further confusion of the body mechanism will result.'

The second point made by Nimmo and Vannerson is valid, inasmuch as we must be fully aware of the factor of anatomical individuality. Points of the body surface are never likely to be precisely identifiable by description of anatomical position. However, a general identification as to site is possible. McBurney's point for example, if present in appendicitis, is usually located within a few degrees of its commonly described location. There are exceptions of course, and in the inscrutable manner of the Orient, the Chinese have taken this well into account, in describing the locations of acupuncture points. The invention of the 'human inch', which uses the individual anatomical proportions of each person, allows for such individualization. In terms of the charts and maps, to be found in this text, the same factor should be borne in mind. The positions are approximate, and there will be great variations found.

Dysfunction in soft tissues is, however, palpable, and not dependent upon maps. Thus the general guidelines, provided by charts, are useful, but cannot take the place of palpatory skills.

Reference to these reflexes will be found in the chapter on treatment techniques.

The soft tissues are of major importance to the body's economy, structural integrity and well being. They are also a major source of pain and dysfunction and, as must now be obvious, of reflex disturbances.

A wide degree of clinical experience resulted in an American Chiropractor, Dr Terrence Bennett, reaching the conclusion that there were a group of previously unknown reflexes, available for diagnostic and therapeutic use, which he termed neurovascular reflexes. He described his work in a series of lecture notes, which were compiled into the book *Dynamics of Correction of Abnormal Function* (edited and published by Ralph Martin D.C., Sierre Madre, California, 1977) after Bennett's death. The major points are listed below.

Bennett's Neurovascular Reflex Points

Bennett describes the tissues which are palpated as altered in texture, being contracted or indurated, in much the same way as Chapman's reflexes. His method of treatment calls for a slight degree of pressure, which he describes as 'only minimal, enough to render the tissues semi-anaemic, which is adequate stimulus.'

Experience indicates that the light pressure should be accompanied by slight stretching of the skin. In accordance with the views of Dr Karel Lewit, this induces reflex activity (discussed in more detail under the heading of 'Hyperalgesic Skin Zones' on page 89).

The skin is stretched with the minimum of force, so as to take up the slack, by the fingertips being drawn lightly apart. In most cases, if the area involves any degree of soft-tissue dysfunction, a lack of anticipated elasticity will be noted in the skin as this distraction takes place. By maintaining the light stretch on the tissues, a yielding occurs, and it is after this that pulsation should normally be felt.

John Thie D.C. describes this in the following words: 'A few seconds after contact is made, a slight pulse can be felt, at a steady rate of 70 to 74 beats per minute. This pulse is not related to the heartbeat, but is believed to be the primitive pulsation of the microscopic capillary bed, in the skin' (*Touch for Health*, DeVorss, California, 1973).

Bennett insists that the contact be maintained until a response is noted in the form of the tissue altering, relaxing and, most importantly, the operator becomes aware of the presence of pulsation. This could arrive within a few seconds or take some minutes to emerge. The variable will be the patient and his/her condition. He terms the pulsation felt as the 'arteriole pulse' because, he states, 'it is the beginning of the system, at the junction of the artery and the arteriole, that controls the metabolism.' Tiny plexuses at the junction, connect either reflexey or directly with the aorta. The changes may occur within the area of a group of arterioles, or in a limb or an organ, through impulses reaching the aortic sinus. That in turn causing a correction of the circulation either way in the structure, as it receives these messages. 'The sensation of pulsation is essential,' he states. 'It has to be there, or else we are not accomplishing anything.' Together with this the change in tissue feel is important. 'The tissues under your fingers begin to relax as you

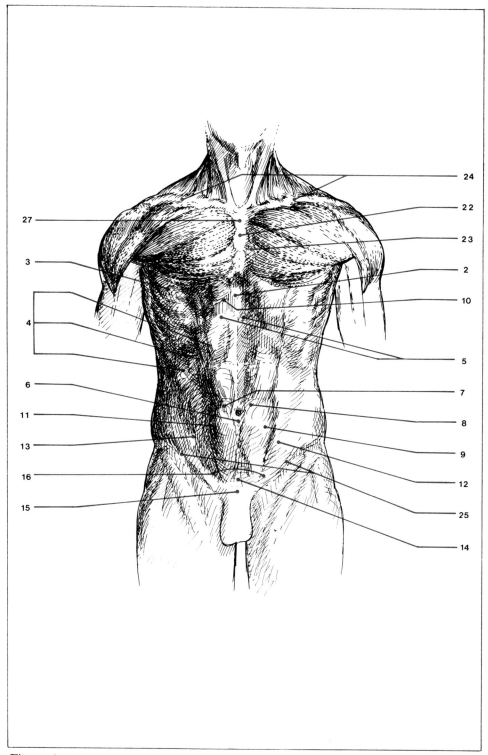

Figure 2a Bennett's Neurovascular Reflex Points. (See pages 60 and 61 for legend.)

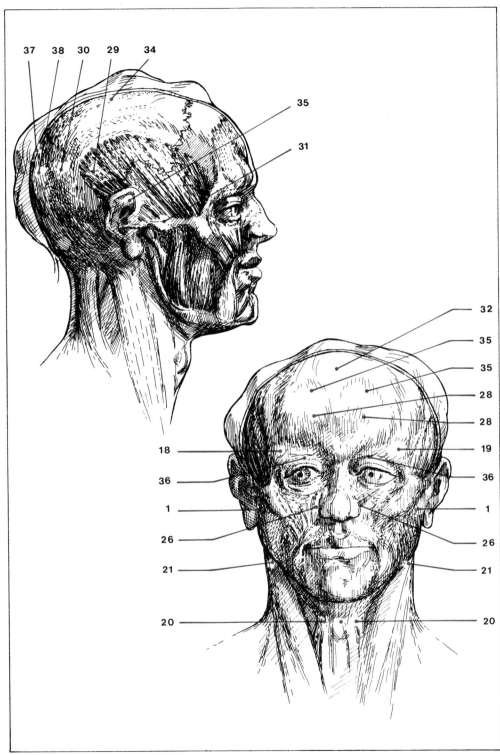

Figure 2b   Bennett's Neurovascular Reflex Points. (See pages 60 and 61 for legend.)

Bennett's Neurovascular Reflexes (Note these will be sensitive to light pressure if active). (*See Figures 2a and 2b.*)

Reflex name	Site	Notes on Use
1. Parotid gland	Raised area on masseter when jaw clenched.	Diagnostic and treatment point (prostate problems, mumps, premenstrual mastitis, lymphatic stasis.
2. Cardiac sphincter	Tip of xyphoid process.	Diagnostic and treatment point. If sensitive may relate to incompetent sphincter, heartburn etc.
3. Liver	Midclavicular line; right 5th costal interspace.	Diagnostic and treatment point.
4. Gall bladder	Just below costal cartilages of 9, 10, 11th ribs on right side.	All points mentioned are treatment points; only 11th rib point is diagnostic. Pain may be noted as far lateral as midaxillary line.
5. Pancreas	Medial to 6th and 7th rib heads. Aprox. 1in. below xyphoid process.	Diagnostic point is 5th and 6th costal cartilages right and left. Treatment points as described (site).
6. Pyloris	Lower border of umbilicus.	Diagnostic and treatment point.
7. Second segment of duodenum	One inch and 45° above umbilicus on right.	Diagnostic and treatment point.

Note: Order of treatment in this region should follow sequence of pyloris-duodenum-pancreas-liver-gallbladder.

Reflex name	Site	Notes on Use
8. 3rd portion of duodenum	One inch and 45° above umbilicus on left.	Diagnostic and treatment point.
9. 4th portion of duodenum	One inch and 45° lateral to, and below, umbilicus (left).	Diagnostic and treatment point.
10. Kidneys	Tip of 8th rib. Bilateral.	Diagnostic and treatment point.
11. Iliocecal valve	On right side midway between anterior-superior iliac spine and umbilicus.	Diagnostic and treatment point.
12. Internal rectal sphincter	On left side midway between anterior superior iliac spine and umbilicus.	Diagnostic and treatment point.
13. Appendix	Directly over the organ.	Diagnostic and treatment point.
14. Bladder	Just above pubic arch on midline.	Diagnostic and treatment point.
15. Prostate/uterus	Symphasis pubis.	Diagnostic and treatment point.

Reflex name	Site	Notes on Use
16. Spermatic cord/ovary	Approx. 1-1½ inches either side of bladder reflex.	Diagnostic and treatment point (note thyroid to be treated when ovaries receiving attention).
17. Suprarenal	One finger width below tip of 12th rib.	Diagnostic point is tip of 12th rib.
18. Anterior Pituitary	Right, lateral aspect of eyebrow.	Diagnostic and treatment point.
19. Posterior pituitary	Left, lateral aspect of eyebrow.	Diagnostic and treatment point.
20. Thyroid	Over the organ.	Diagnostic and treatment point.
21. Carotid sinus	On carotid artery, just below angle of jaw.	Diagnostic and treatment point.
22. Aortic sinus	Manubriosternal junction on ridge, or just inferior.	Diagnostic and treatment point.
23. Heart tone	Sternal end of 3rd rib. Contact on cartilage (left).	Diagnostic and treatment point.
24. Subclavian lymphatics	Just inferior to and slightly medial to midpoint of clavical.	Diagnostic and treatment point.
25. Femoral Lymphatics	On Poupart's ligament. Midway between symphasis pubis and anterior superior iliac spine.	Diagnostic and treatment point.
26. Maxillary sinus	Lateral to nares; bilaterally.	Diagnostic and treatment point.
27. Bronchial region	Midway between manubrium sternum and episternal notch.	Diagnostic and treatment point.
28. Frontal-emotional	Frontal eminences of forehead.	Diagnostic and treatment point.
29. Vagal	2 inches superior and 2 inches posterior to external auditory meatus.	Diagnostic and treatment point.
30. Parietal	2 inches superior and 3 inches posterior to external auditory meatus.	Diagnostic and treatment point.
31. Temporal-emotional	Midway between outer aspect of eye and external auditory meatus. Just superior to zygomatic bone.	Diagnostic and treatment point.
32. Anterior fontanel	Over anatomical area.	Diagnostic and treatment point.
33. Midsylvian	One inch superior to anterior aspect of external auditory meatus.	Diagnostic and treatment point.
34. Fissure of Rolando	Aprox 1½ inches posterior to anterior fontanel.	Diagnostic and treatment point.
35. Frontal eye fields	1½ inches superior to frontal eminences.	Diagnostic and treatment point.
36. Extrinsic Eye muscles	Superior to eyelids with closed eyes.	Diagnostic and treatment point.
37. Posterior fontanel	Over anatomical area.	Diagnostic and treatment point.
38. Menopause-glandular	½ inch inferior and lateral to posterior fontanel.	Diagnostic and treatment point.

All the points on the cranium are useful for treating emotional and stress conditions. Those marked 'emotional' are the strongest. Light pressure only is suggested.

work for a few moments; you sense the degree of tension releasing. When it releases that is all you can do.'

Some points are purely diagnostic, others are used for treatment, and some are both. For example, the coronary reflex in the 2nd thoracic interspace on the left, which is a palpable area of tissue change and which is sensitive to the patient, is diagnostic only (not illustrated). Awareness of Bennett's reflex areas may be found to be a useful addition to the range of available therapeutic and diagnostic knowledge. In using Neuro-muscular Technique, in its diagnostic mode, the tissues being evaluated will yield a multitude of sensitive points. Some of these may correlate with Bennett's findings, and they may then be used as part of an overall assessment, as to the nature of the dysfunction affecting the patient. They may, of course, also be used, as Bennett intended, as a system in their own right, for assessing and treating visceral and functional physiological changes, and pathology. A number of Bennett's points have been incorporated into the methods of Applied Kinesiology, notably the points on the cranium, which are used for treating emotional disturbances.

Among the cautions issued by Bennett are: do not overtreat the points on the cranium (two to three minutes is a maximum); in hyperthyroid cases, do not treat the thyroid and pituitary reflexes at the same visit (one should be treated, and alternated with the other at a subsequent visit); if the heart is enlarged then the third rib, at the midclavicular line, should not be treated; aortic sinus reflex should be treated before any of the brain reflexes are contacted; if the ovary is being treated then the thyroid should receive prior attention.

Acupuncture Points

Soft tissue changes often produce organized discrete areas which act as generators of secondary problems, it would be advantageous to examine briefly another aspect of 'trigger' points, that is, the existence of a network of points which is supposedly constantly capable of reflex activity. This network is, of course, the pattern of acupuncture points. What is of interest is that the location of these fixed anatomical points is capable of corroboration by electrical detection, each point being evidenced by a small area of lowered electrical resistance.

When 'active', due presumably to reflex stimulation of some kind, these points become even more detectable, as the electrical resistance lowers further. They also become sensitive to pressure and this is of value to the therapist since the finding of sensitive areas during palpation or treatment is of diagnostic interest. Sensitive and painful areas that do not have detectable tissue changes as part of their make-up may well be 'active' acupuncture points (or *Tsubo*, which means 'points on the human body' in Japanese). Not only are these points detectable and sensitive but they are also amenable to treatment by direct pressure techniques. They are, therefore, well worth some study.

One of the leading oriental experts on pressure techniques is Katsusuke Serizawe M.D. who, in his book on the subject (*Tsubo: Vital Points for Oriental Therapy*,

Japan Publishing Co.), discusses his nerve-reflex theory for the existence of these points.

The nerve reflex theory holds that, when an abnormal condition occurs in an internal organ, alterations take place in the skin and muscles related to that organ by means of the nervous system. These alterations occur as reflex actions. The nervous system, extending throughout the internal organs, like the skin, the subcutaneous tissues, and the muscles, constantly transmit information about the physical condition to the spinal cord and the brain. These information impulses, which are centripetal in nature, set up a reflex action that causes symptoms of the internal organic disorder to manifest themselves in the surface areas of the body. The reflex symptoms may be classified into the following three major groups: (a) sensation reflexes; (b) interlocking reflexes; (c) autonomic system reflexes.

(a) Sensation reflexes. When an abnormal centripetal impulse travels to the spinal cord, reflex action causes the skin at the spinal column affected by the impulse to become hypersensitive. This sensitivity to pain is especially notable in the skin, subcutaneous tissues, and muscles located close to the surface, since these organs are richly supplied with sensory nerves.

(b) Interlocked reflexes. An abnormality in an internal organ causes a limited contraction, stiffening, or lumping of the muscles in the area near the part of the body that is connected by means of nerves to the affected organ. Stiffness in the shoulders, back, arms, and legs are symptoms of this kind. In effect, the interlocked reflex actions amount to a hardening and stiffening of the muscles to protect the ailing internal organ from excess stimulus. When the abnormality in the organ is grave, however, the stiffening of the muscles is not limited to a small area, but extends over large parts of the body.

(c) Autonomic system reflexes. Abnormalities in the internal organs sometimes set up reflex action in the sweat glands, the sebaceous glands, the pilomotor muscles, and the blood vessels in the skin. The reflex action may cause excess sweat or drying of the skin as the consequence of cessation of sweat secretion. Its effect on the pilomotor muscles may be to cause the condition known as goose flesh. The sebaceous glands may be stimulated to secrete excess sebum, thus causing abnormal oiliness in the skin; or they may stop secreting sebum, thus making the skin abnormally dry. The reflex action may cause chills or flushing because of its effects on the blood vessels in the skin.

I have discussed the ways in which abnormalities in internal organs cause changes in the conditions of the surface organs of the body. But the intimate relation between internal organs and external ones has a reverse effect as well; that is, stimulation to the skin and muscles affects the condition of the internal organs and tissues, since impulses from the outside are transmitted to the inside by means of the spinal cord and the nervous system. For instance, stimulation transmitted to the spinal cord sets up a reflex action in the internal organ that is controlled by the nerves at the level of the spinal column corresponding to the height of the place at which the external stimulus was applied. Stimuli of this kind instigate peristaltic motion or contraction in the organ. The effect of such external stimulation on blood vessels and on the secretion of hormones has been scientifically verified.

Quite obviously there may be more effective ways of dealing with these points than by pressure techniques. However, since the study is concerned basically with manual treatment it is worth incorporating into our scheme of treatment the knowledge accumulated by the Chinese and Japanese over many centuries.

An attempt to correlate the various reflex systems and methods has been made by the American Chiropractor Dr George Goodheart. His system of Applied Kinesiology involves testing muscle groups for weaknesses and then, depending upon the results of such tests, using various massage and pressure techniques to normalize function. These points correspond to Chapman's reflexes, acupuncture points and other less well known reflex systems. It is not my intention to delve into Goodheart's techniques and theories, some of which seem far-fetched to a practical observer—he claims that muscles can be strengthened by passing a hand along the line of the 'energy' flow of an acupuncture meridian, without even touching the patient. However, where his methods support and utilize methods that are in line with Neuro-muscular Technique these will be mentioned in the treatment section.

It has been shown that the pain threshold can be dramatically elevated by pressure techniques on specific points. In complex experiments the research group of acupuncture anaesthesia, Peking Medical College, showed that finger pressure acupuncture caused a rise of 133 per cent in pain threshold of rabbits (using radiant heat as the painful stimulus). When cerebrospinal fluid was perfused from one rabbit to another after such experiments the recipient rabbit was found to have achieved a rise in pain threshold of up to 80 per cent. This suggests the presence of hormone-like substances produced by the brain in response to the original acupressure stimulus. These substances, now thought to be enkephalin and endorphin, may well play a role in NMT pain control. The point used in these tests was equivalent to the acupuncture point known as Bladder 60, posterior to the ankle (externally) and just anterior to the Achilles tendon.

Acupuncture Points and Trigger Points: Are They the Same Phenomenon?

We have previously noted that many of the different reflex systems have points which are interchangeable, and that many of these are traditional acupuncture points. In terms of local pain the view of Chifuyu Takeshige, Professor of Physiology, School of Medicine, Showa University (*Acupuncture and Electro-Therapeutics Research*, Vo. 10, pp195-203, 1985), is that: 'The acupuncture point of treatment of muscle pain is the pain producing muscle itself.' Respected acupuncture clinicians, such as George Ulett suggest: 'Acupuncture points are nothing more than time honoured muscle motor points.' C. Chan Gunn, however, finds this too simple an explanation, and states: 'Calling acupuncture points, motor points, or myofascial trigger points, is too simple. They are Golgi tendon organs.' These, and other researchers, are quoted by Stephen Botek M.D., Assistant Professor of Clinical Psychiatry, New York Medical College (*Acupuncture and Electro-Therapeutics Research*, Vo. 10, No. 3, pp241). He believes that 'myofascial needling', is the term of choice to define that type of acupuncture which dispenses with traditional explanations as to acupuncture's effects. Monique Ernst M.D., Research Fellow for the French government, studied the effects of stimulating two important acupuncture points electrically and manually. (*Acupuncture and Electro-Therapeutics Research*, Vol. 8, No. 3/4, 1983, pp343).

The points were Large Intestine 4 (Hoku) in the web between thumb and the first finger; and Stomach 36 (Tsu san li) below the knee. The study recorded skin temperature of the face, hands and feet. It was found that, as compared to a resting period, both manual and electrical stimulation of both points induced a general warming effect. This was immediate in the face, and after 10 to 15 minutes in hands and feet. The temperature increase was notably more marked after manual acupressure, than electrical stimulation. A number of hypothetical correlations between the sympathetic effects noted in this study, and the effects of acupuncture analgesia, were made as a result of this research. Pressure on these points is again shown to be more effective than other forms of stimulation.

George Lewith M.D. and Julian Kenyon M.D. (*Soc. Sci. Med.*, Vol. 19, No. 12, pp1367-1376, 1984) point to a variety of suggestions having been made as to the mechanisms via which acupuncture, or acupressure, achieve their pain relieving results. These include neurological explanations such as the 'gate control theory'. This, and variations of this theme, look at the various structures of the central nervous system, and the brain, in order to define the precise mechanisms involved in acupuncture's pain relieving action. This in itself is seen to be an incomplete explanation, and humoral and psychological factors are shown also to be involved in modifying the patient's perception of pain.

A combination of reflex and direct neurological elements, as well as the involvement of a variety of secretions, such as enkephalins and endorphins, are thought to be the modus operandi of acupressure, and probably of all of the various systems of reflex activity discussed in this section (Neurolymphatics etc.).

Felix Mann, one of the pioneers of acupuncture in the west, has entered the controversy as to the existence, or otherwise, of acupuncture meridians (and indeed acupuncture points). In an effort to alter the emphasis which traditional acupuncture places on the charted position of specific points, related in channels of activity, he stated the following, at the International Conference of Acupuncture and Chronic Pain, held in New York in September, 1983:

> McBurney's point, in appendicitis, has a defined position. In reality it may be 10cms higher, lower, to the left or right. It may be one centimeter in diameter, or occupy the whole of the abdomen, or not occur at all. Acupuncture points are often the same, and hence it is pointless to speak of acupuncture points in the classical traditional way. Carefully performed electrical resistance measurements do not show alterations in the skin resistance to electricity, corresponding with classical acupuncture points. There are so many acupuncture points mentioned in some modern books, that there is no skin left which is not an acupuncture point. In cardiac disease, pain and tenderness may occur in the arm. This does not occur more frequently along the course of the heart meridian, than anywhere else in the arm.

Hence, he concludes, meridians do not exist. If all the multitude of points described in acupuncture, traditional and modern, together with those points described by Travell and co-workers, Chapman, Jones, Bennett, etc., etc., are placed together on one map of the body surface, then truly we have to come to the conclusion that the entire body surface is a potential acupuncture point.

It is interesting to note that many of the points of referred pain and tenderness, used in Western medical diagnosis, are acupuncture points. Head's zones, for example, could be shown to include any acupuncture points, especially the Alarm and Associated points (given below). The points noted as being 'tender' in appendicitis, such as McBurney's, Clado's, Cope's, Kummel's, Lavitas', are on the stomach, Spleen and Kidney meridians of traditional acupuncture, and these are used in treating appendicitis by acupuncturists. Gastric ulcer patients produce tenderness at a site known as Boas' point, and this is precisely on Bladder point 21, which is the Associated point of the Stomach meridian. Brewer's point, in Western medicine, is noted in kidney infection, and this is Bladder point 20, the

Associated point for the Spleen (in traditional acupuncture this has a controlling role over water, the element of the kidneys). The degree of overlap between these well known points is also noted in comparing other systems, and charts of points.

Ah Shi Points

Acupuncture methodology also includes the treatment of points which are not listed, but which are known as Ah Shi points. These include all painful points which arise spontaneously, usually in relation to particular joint problems or disease. For the duration of their sensitivity they are regarded as being suitable for needle or pressure treatment. These points may therefore be thought of as identical, in all ways, with the 'tender' points described by Lawrence Jones in his Strain-Counterstrain methods (See Chapter 10).

Speransky and Selye: Common Findings

Speransky in his classic book, *A Basis for the Theory of Medicine*, points out that, after many years of work, he concluded the following: 'From any nerve point it is easy to bring into action nerve mechanisms, the functioning of which terminates at the periphery, in changes of a bio-physico-chemical character.' He then states: 'Justification exists for the thesis that any nerve point, not excluding peripheral nerve structures, can become the originator of neurodystrophic processes, serving as the temporary nerve centre of these processes.' These thoughts lead on to evidence which shows, says Speransky, that: 'It is obvious from this that the irritation of any point of the complex network of the nervous system, can evoke changes, not only in the adjacent parts, but also in remote regions of the organism.' The final conclusion, which Speransky offers us, and which is pertinent to acupuncture and *all methods of physical treatment*, is the following: *'Hence we obtain the rule that only weak degrees of irritation can have a useful significance; strong ones inevitably do damage.'*

These words should be burned into the consciousness of all therapists, of whatever school. The term 'irritation', is used by Speransky, and this is of interest, since a little thought will indicate that whatever is being done to a patient, in terms of therapy, involves to a greater or lesser extent an element of stress (or irritation). Stress, in this sense, being defined as any stimulus, pleasant or unpleasant, which calls upon the body to respond, or adapt, in some manner.

Manipulation, acupuncture, pressure techniques, use of heat and cold, hydrotherapy, electrical and mechanical therapies, surgery, and indeed the whole gamut of medications, whether they be drugs or homoeopathic dilutions of herbal substances, all call for a response on the part of the body. All are, therefore, to a degree, 'stress' factors. Speransky insists that only mild irritants can have a useful role to play in evoking a positive (i.e. healing) response. Hans Selye has come to precisely the same conclusion in his important research into stress. In experiments carried out in his extensive studies, Selye produced subcutaneous sacs in experimental animals by injecting a given volume of air under the skin. This was followed by the insertion of an irritant of some sort. He first demonstrated that the amount of exudate, and the thickness of the sac wall varied, as one might anticipate, with the strength and concentration of the irritant substance. He followed this by introducing a form of stress, such as intense cold, heat or forced immobilization.

The response of the animals varied greatly. In those that had been initially injected with a weak irritant, the stress which was then added seemed to aid the recovery, as evidenced by resolution of the irritated area, and inhibition of tissue fibrosis. Those animals, however, which had had strong irritants injected into the subcutaneous sacs, responded to the subsequent stress factor by showing an increase in inflammation, widespread necrosis, and often death. Selye concluded with these words: 'This was the crucial experiment, showing that *stress can either cure or aggravate a disease, depending upon whether the inflammatory response to a local irritant is necessary or superfluous.*' We now have Speransky's and Selye's combined evidence, that what we do to a patient, in terms of therapy, can be beneficial or harmful, and that this to a great extent will depend upon the degree of the irritation involved in the treatment, whatever form it takes.

Speransky's work further teaches us that Mann's words are true, and that *any part of the surface of the body* can be an initiator of a process involving neurological changes, which can be pathological or therapeutic. The classifying of certain points as being trigger points, others as being acupuncture alarm points, and yet others as being neurolymphatic or neurovascular, or any other, points, is merely a matter of convenience. It helps us to make a degree of sense out of the enormous amount of information available to us. That, to an extent, these points may be interchangeable, is obvious. For many are patently found in the self-same position, on different 'maps' of points. There are subtle variations in the behaviour of some points, such as has already been described with trigger points having a reference area (target area) and other points being found in pairs etc. This is a matter of practical classification, and interpretation of the characteristics of different points. They are all to some extent interchangeable, however, and a latent trigger point, which may be identified as sensitive but with no referral capabilities, might become an active trigger by the simple introduction of a chill, or a strain, to that area. Bearing in mind therefore that the distinction between the points discussed is man-made, we will continue to classify them in these ways for the convenience which this provides. It should also be borne in mind that whenever acupuncture points are mentioned, the availability of these for manual treatment (pressure, chilling, heating, etc.) remains. There is some evidence that needling can achieve particular effects, not available to pressure techniques, but this is equivocal, and for the purposes of soft-tissue manipulation, pressure can usually be shown to be as effective as needling, with the one major drawback, that only a limited number of points can be contacted by hand at any one time, as compared with the multiple needling which is possible in acupuncture.

Alarm Points, Associated Points, Akabane Points

There are, in traditional acupuncture, a number of key points which are more likely to become painful, in relation to particular visceral dysfunction. These have been classified as Alarm Points. These are presented below, and the following general information may make their employment and significance easier.

The Alarm Points are found only on the ventral surface of the body, each point being associated with one of the 12 meridians and its functions. Six of the points are on the mid-line, the others are bilateral. Tenderness elicited by palpation of an Alarm point may indicate dysfunction of the organ related to the point. In traditional acupuncture, if sensitivity is noted on light pressure, there is an associated

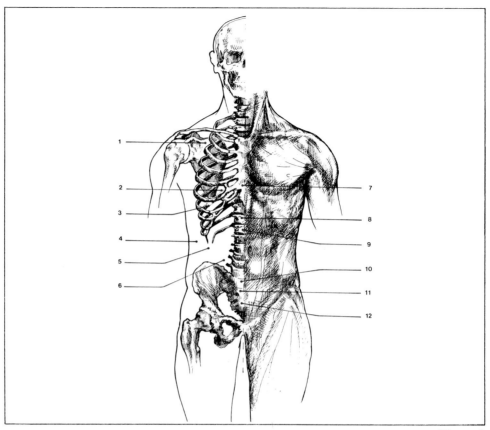

Figure 3

Location of Alarm points

These points are on the anterior surface of the body. Spontaneous pain at any point indicates disorder of the affiliated meridian. If tenderness is elicited on light pressure then this indicates a deficiency of energy in the meridian. Tenderness elicited on heavy pressure indicates an excess of energy in the meridian.

		Acupuncture point
Point 1 Lung		LU 1
Point 2 Liver		LV 14
Point 3 Gall Bladder		GB 24
Point 4 Kidney	bilateral	GB 25
Point 5 Spleen		LV 13
Point 6 Large Intestine		ST 25
Point 7 Heart Constrictor		VC 17
Point 8 Heart		VC 14
Point 9 Stomach		VC 12
Point 10 Triple Heater		VC 5
Point 11 Small Intestine		VC 4
Point 12 Bladder		VC 3

These are reflex points for meridian function and awareness of the roles played by the various meridians in body energy economics is necessary to evaluate the significance of reactions which produce tenderness in Alarm points.

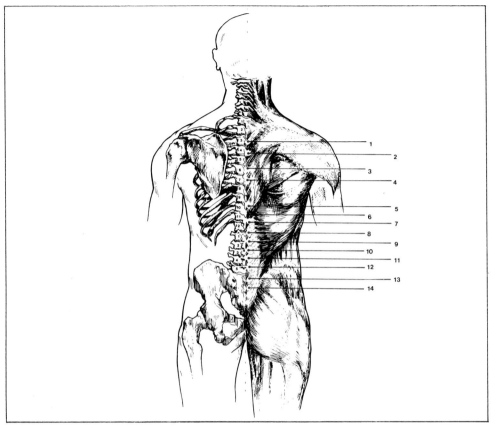

Figure 4

Location of Associated points
These points are on the dorsum of the body. Spontaneous pain indicates a disorder in the meridian associated with it. Tenderness elicited on light pressure indicates a deficiency in energy in that meridian. Tenderness elicited on heavy pressure indicates an excess of energy in the associated meridian. These points are all on the Bladder meridian and their associations are as follows:

	Meridian	*Bladder meridian point*
Point 1	Lung	13
Point 2	Heart Constrictor	14
Point 3	Heart	15
Point 4	Governor Vessel	16
Point 5	Liver	18
Point 6	Gall Bladder	19
Point 7	Spleen	20
Point 8	Stomach	21
Point 9	Triple Heater	22
Point 10	Kidney	23
Point 11	'Sea of Energy'	24 (Extra associated point)
Point 12	Large Intestine	25
Point 13	Small Intestine	27
Point 14	Bladder	28

These points are slightly lateral to the median line bilaterally and are also reflex points for the meridians with which they are associated.

energy (chi) deficiency. If heavy pressure is required, then the condition relates to an energy excess. On the back of the body are found the *Associated Points*, and these are all on the Bladder meridian, which runs parallel to the spine, bilaterally. Each Associated Point is related to one of the meridians and its function. The same assumed relationship with energy deficit or excess exists, as in Alarm Points (sensitivity on light pressure = deficiency, and vice versa). There are also a few Extra Associated Points, as illustrated. Spontaneous pain at any of these listed points indicates a disorder in that meridian, and its associated organ or function.

A number of important areas related to traditional acupuncture meridians are described as *Akabane Points*, and these are found on the fingers and toes, being the terminal points of the meridians. Sensitivity of any of these is said to relate to dysfunction and imbalance of energy in that meridian. The comparative degree of sensitivity, of these points, shows the relative imbalance between organ systems. Electronic measurement of these points is performed in a number of modern electro-acupuncture systems such as EAV. Manual testing is common, and was obviously the method used before electrical methods arrived on the scene. These points are all bilateral.

Melzack, Stillwell and Fox ('Trigger Points and Acupuncture Points of Pain', *Pain*, Vol. 3, pp3-23, 1977) have assumed that acupuncture points represent areas of abnormal physiological activity, producing a continuous, low-level input into the CNS. They suggested that this might eventually lead to a combining with noxious stimuli from other structures, innervated by the same segments, to produce an increased awareness of pain and distress. They found it reasonable to assume that trigger points and acupuncture points, although discovered independently and labelled differently, represented the same phenomenon. They found that the location of trigger points on Western maps, and acupuncture points used commonly in painful conditions, showed a remarkable 70 per cent correlation as to position.

It is interesting that the link between the source of pain or tender points- and the referred area of pain, noted in trigger points, in many instances seems to travel along the routes of traditional acupuncture meridians. The diagnostic value of palpation of acupuncture points is of great potential. Spontaneous pain in such a point, according to acupuncture tradition, indicates the need for urgent attention. It is not the intention of this book to provide instruction in acupuncture methodology, nor to necessarily endorse the views expressed by traditional acupuncture in relation to meridians and their purported connection with organs and systems. However, it would be shortsighted in the extreme to ignore the accumulated wisdom which has led many thousands of skilled practitioners to ascribe particular roles to these points (Alarm, Associated and Akabane). As far as a manual therapy is concerned, awareness of these roles, and the incorporation of their possible involvement into diagnostic and therapeutic considerations, is seen to be desirable. As we palpate and search through the soft tissues, in basic neuro-muscular technique, we are bound to come across areas of sensitivity which relate to these points. They are also often found to overlap with Neurolymphatic and Neurovascular points, as described elsewhere in this text. For example, reflex number 19 in Chapman's reflexes (neurolymphatic point, see page 165) which relates to the urethra, is identical to the neurovascular point of the Bladder, and the acupuncture alarm point of the Bladder meridian. Careful comparison will show many such overlaps. General guidance as to how to treat acupuncture points, which

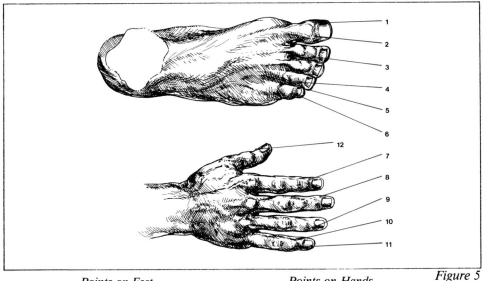

Figure 5

Points on Feet
1. Spleen
2. Liver
3. Stomach
4. Gall Bladder
5. Kidney
6. Bladder

Points on Hands
7. Large Intestine
8. Heart Constrictor
9. Triple Heater
10. Heart
11. Small Intestine
12. Lung

Location of Akabane points
These represent the terminal points of the meridians. Sensitivity of these relates to imbalance in the energy of the meridian. Comparative sensitivity shows relative imbalance in organ (energy) systems. Manual or electronic testing is possible.

are sensitive, must relate to whether a stimulating or sedating effect is desired. The body will utilize therapeutic stimulation to its best advantage. Homoeostatic mechanisms are at work, in which there is a constant effort to restore normality, and provided any stimulus is appropriate, and not excessive, the response will be beneficial. In accord with the methods used in treating neurolymphatic and neurovascular points (described elsewhere) it is suggested that, to some extent, the 'feel' of the tissues be allowed to guide the operator. A change, in the sense of a release of tension, or a softening, or a sensing of a gentle pulsation in the tissues, is often an indication of an adequate degree of therapy. In order to sedate what is an overactive point, up to five minutes of sustained or intermittent pressure, or rotary contact, may be required. For stimulation the timing could involve between twenty seconds and two minutes. By this time some degree of change should be palpable. As must be clear, if pressure is sustained beyond a certain point quite the opposite effect will be achieved. This is a natural phenomenon which occurs in response to all factors in life, which are initially stimulating. If prolonged, they become enervating or exhausting, and in terms of therapy this is undesirable unless anaesthesia is required. A short cold application for example will stimulate, a long one will sedate and too much can kill. Speransky's and Selye's words should be recalled, and the minimum effort used, consistent with achieving a response.

**The
Morphology of
Points**

Melzack, and other researchers, maintain that there is a little, if any, difference between acupuncture points and trigger points. Since all sensitive points are capable of becoming trigger points, this suggests that there is only one major type of point amenable to therapeutic usage, although depending upon its location, and the morphology of the tissues over which it lies, it could have a variety of effects. The morphology of acupuncture points has been studied, notably by Jean Bosey M.D., Professor of Anatomy at Montpellier University, France. He has described some of his findings (*Acupuncture and Electrotherapeutic Research*, Vo. 9, No. 2, 1984, pp79-106). In summary these are some of the major conclusions:

Points are situated in palpable depressions ('Cupules'). The skin (epiderm) over the point is a little thinner at the cupule level, under which lies a fibrous cone in which there is frequently found either a neurovascular formation, or simply a cutaneous neurovascular bundle. Free nerve endings are noted, and the presence, beneath the point, of Golgi endings and Pacini corpuscles is common. Connective tissues lie below at varying depths. Fascia and aponeurosis are noted and, it is stated: 'A passage of vessels and nerves, through the fascia, is very often found under the acupuncture point.' An anatomical study of 100 acupuncture points showed that they overlay large nerve trunks in 42 per cent of cases, large veins in 40 per cent and cutaneous neurovascular pedicals in 18 per cent. The effect, in deeper structures, of stimulation of muscle and tendon receptors, is noted, but this is thought to be indirect, rather than direct, because of the extremely small size of, for example, muscle spindles and Golgi tendon organs. The practice of manipulating the needle, thus imposing a degree of traction on the underlying (muscular) tissue, is noted, and this would, it is observed, impose stimulation on such receptor organs. Fat is also a common factor in the morphology of points, and this, and the connective tissue, are thought to be key factors in the achievement of the 'acupuncture sensation' which accompanies successful treatment. The conclusion reached is that a number of tissues are simultaneously affected by any particular acupuncture needle, *and, the author stresses, by strong finger pressure.*

Some points dissected show that neurovascular structures lie immediately below the point, and this may result in the particular effects noted by such points being treated. This is of interest to those using Bennett's Neurovascular points. The implications for those practitioners not employing needles, and who rely on pressure techniques in order to provide stimulus or sedation to such areas, is that, if accurately applied, the effects should be identical (to needle acupuncture), especially in relation to pain control.

**Electro-
acupuncture and
Trigger Points**

Kleyhans and Aarons ('Myodysneuria and Acupuncture', *Digest of Chiropractic Economics*, September 1974) discuss the factors which initiate, and which disperse, trigger points. They believe that electro-acupuncture owes much of its efficacy to the fact that galvanic dispersement of trigger points occurs with its use. They maintain that most, of not all, trigger points can be dispersed by 'pressure techniques, ultra-sound or galvanism, without recourse to the use of procaine injections or the use of chilling techniques.' Having palpated and located the trigger point, and proved its ability to reproduce pain or other symptoms in a target area, stimulation of the point (i.e. pressure, MET, etc.) is carried out to disperse it. Among the symptoms they list as possibly deriving from trigger points are the following:

deep aching pain; headache; parasthesia; menstrual pain; giddiness; weakness; shortness of breath; spasm; swallowing difficulty; blurred vision; sensitivity to light; tinnitus; anorexia; nausea; palpitation; oedema; excessively dry, oily or moist skin; depression; tension and poor concentration.

The various theories, methods and descriptive terminologies relating to the foregoing systems are of some general interest in as much as Neuro-muscular Technique overlaps and incorporates many aspects that are similar. This should not be confusing as there are many ways of looking at the same phenomena.

Neuro-muscular Technique, Muscle Energy Techniques and Strain-Counter strain methods can (with other modalities such as chilling agents) be used as an effective measure to detect and eliminate noxious trigger points and areas which generate dysfunction. Such dysfunction can take the form of muscular weakness, muscular contraction, pain, vaso-dilatation, vaso-constriction, tissue degeneration, gastro-intestinal, respiratory and a myriad other disorders including emotional and 'psychological' disorders.

These noxious points may reside in hypertonic or hypotonic muscle or in ligamentous or fascial tissues, or in apparently normal tissues. When active, they will always be sensitive to correctly applied pressure and can often be neutralized by manual pressure or a combination of chilling and manual pressure and stretching.

We now know what these triggers are, and the types of problems they can cause. In the treatment section we will discuss how to locate and treat them.

[1] Travell, Dr J., 'Symposium on Mechanism and Management of Pain Syndromes', *Proc. Rudolph Virchow Medical Soc.* (1957).

[2] Webber, T. D., 'Diagnosis and Modification of Headache and Shoulder, Arm, Hand Syndromes', *Journal of the American Osteopathic Association*, Vol. 72 (March, 1973).

[3] Mennell, Dr J., 'The Therapeutic Use of Cold', *Journal of the American Osteopathic Association*, Vol. 74 (August, 1975).

[4] Gutstein, R., 'The Role of Craniocervical Myodysneuria in Functional Ocular Disorders', *American Practitioner's Digest of Treatments* (November, 1956).

[5] Cornelius, A., *Die Neurenpunkt Lehre Vol. 2* (George Thins, Liepzig).

[6] Travell, J. and Bigelow, N., 'Role of Somatic Trigger Areas in the Patterns of Hysteria', *Psychosomatic Medicine*, Vol. 9, No. 6.

[7] Evans, J., 'Reflex Sympathetic Dystrophy', *Annals of Internal Medicine*.

[8] Dittrich, R. J., 'Somatic Pain and Autonomic Concomitants', *American Journal of Surgery* (1954).

[9] Blashy, M., 'Manipulation of the Neuromuscular Unit via the Periphery of the CNS', *Southern Medical Journal* (August, 1961).

[10] Hagbarth, K., 'Excitatory Inhibitory Skin Areas for Flexor and Extensor Motoneurons', *Acta Physiologica Scandinavia* (1952).

[11] Bishof, I. and Elmiger, G., 'Connective Tissue Massage', *Massage, Manipulation and Traction* (Licht, 1960).

[12] Chaitow, Leon, 'An Introduction to Chapman's Reflexes', *British Naturopathic Journal* (Spring, 1965).

Chapter 3

Diagnostic Methods

In the previous chapters we have dipped into the vast amount of information that exists relating to the neuro-muscular component of the human framework. An equally great number of diagnostic aids exist for the researcher into the ills of the body. The great beauty of Neuro-muscular Technique, as devised by Lief, is its combining of diagnostic and therapeutic movements. The thumb as it glides close to the spinal attachments of the paraspinal musculature is assessing the tissue tone, density, temperature etc., and at the same moment is treating those tissues that indicate dysfunction, by means of variable pressure. The response of the searching digit to whatever information the tissues impart, is immediate. Greater or lesser pressure, varying in its direction and duration, allows the practitioner to judge and treat at the same time and with great accuracy.

In a general sense, on a level involving the whole of an area or the total body picture, a diagnostic or assessment plan is required. Whilst the individual muscular indurations and dysfunctions will become apparent as treatment progresses, an overall diagnostic picture is required to enable prognosis and progress to be judged.

There is no valid substitute for skilful palpatory diagnosis in ascertaining the relatively minute structural changes—primary or reflex—that often have far-reaching effects on the body's economy.

It is generally agreed that the pads of the figures are the most sensitive portion of the hand available for use in diagnosis. Indeed the combination of the thumb and first two fingers is the finest mechanism, and can be adapted to vary with the area under palpatory consideration as to the practitioner's own preference.

Palpatory Diagnosis

The most successful method of palpatory diagnosis is to run lightly over the area being checked, seeking changes in the skin and the tissues below it. After localizing any changes in this way, deeper periaxial structures can be assessed by greater pressure. There are a number of specific changes to be sought in light palpatory examination. This applies to both acute and chronic dysfunction. Among these are:

1. *Skin changes.* Over an area of acute dysfunction, skin will feel tense and will be relatively difficult to move or glide over the underlying structures.

2. *Induration.* A slight increase in diagnostic pressure will ascertain whether or not the superficial musculature has an increased indurated feeling. When

chronic dysfunction exists the skin and superficial musculature will demonstrate a tension and immobility indicating fibrotic changes within and below these structures.

3. *Temperature changes*. In acute dysfunction a localized increase in temperature may be evident. In chronic lesion conditions there may, because of relative ischaemia, be a reduced temperature of the skin. This usually indicates fibrotic alterations in the underlying structures.

4. *Tenderness*. Tenderness can be misleading as it may indicate local or reflex problems in acute or chronic dysfunction. Its presence should be noted but not necessarily considered to be important. In acute joint dysfunction the superficial musculature and skin usually palpates as tender.

5. *Oedema*. An impression of fullness and congestion can be obtained in the overlying tissues in acute dysfunction. In chronic dysfunction this is usually absent having been replaced by fibrotic changes.

In deep palpation the pressure of the palpating fingers or thumb increases sufficiently to make contact with deeper structures such as the periaxial (paravertebral) musculature. Amongst the changes noted may be immobility, tenderness, oedema, deep muscle tension, fibrotic and interosseous changes. Apart from the fibrotic changes, which are indicative of chronic dysfunctions, all these changes can be found in either acute or chronic problems.

As Peter Lief D.O., son of the innovator of Neuro-muscular Technique, explains:

Palpation is the main method of detection. Gross lesions are easily palpable but sometimes they are so minute that their detection presents considerable difficulty, especially to the beginner. It sometimes takes many months of practice to develop the necessary sense of touch, which must be firm, yet at the same time sufficiently light, in order to discern the minute tissue changes which constitute the palpable neuro-muscular lesion.

The presence of a lesion is always revealed by an area of hyper-sensitivity to pressure, an area which may be better described as being a painful spot. After these have been detected and noted, specific attention is given to them in the subsequent treatments.

Brian Youngs D.O. has described what it is that the palpating fingers are seeking and finding and, since in NMT diagnosis and treatment often take place together, what they are achieving.

The changes which are palpable in muscles and soft tissues associated with such reflex effects have been listed by Stanley Lief. They are essentially 'congestion'. This ambiguous word can be interpreted as a past hypertrophic fibrosis. Reflex cordant contraction of the muscle reduces the blood flow through the muscular tissue and in such relatively anoxic regions of low pH and low hormonal concentration, fibroblasts proliferate and increased fibrous tissue is formed. This results in an increase in the thickness of the existing connective tissue partitions—the epimysia and perimysia—and also this condition probably infiltrates deeper between the muscle fibres to affect the normal endomysia. Thickening of the fascia and subdermal connective tissue will also occur if these structures are similarly affected by a reduced blood flow. Fat may be deposited, particularly in endomorphic types, but fibrosis is most pronounced in those with a strong mesomorphic component—a useful pointer for both prognosis and prophylaxis.

Fibrosis seems to occur automatically in areas of reduced blood flow, e.g., in a sprained ankle—where swelling is marked and prolonged, in the lower extremities where oedema of any origin has been constant over a period, in the gluteals where prolonged sitting is a postural factor, and in the neck and upper dorsal region where psychosomatic tension is frequent to a marked degree—depending upon the constitutional background. Where tension is the etiological factor, fibrosis seems teleological. Many devices have been developed to ease the strain on muscles which tend to be permanently contracted, e.g., locking of the knee joint, or the exact balance of the head on the shoulders, where only gentle contraction is needed to maintain postural integrity. If postural integrity is lost through some cause or another then the strain on the muscle may be eased by structural alteration and the increase of fibrous tissue in the muscles acts to maintain normal position of the head. Fibrous tissue can then take the strain instead of the muscle fibres. It is this long-term homoeostatic reflex which apparently operates in all cases of undue muscle contraction, whether due to strain or tension.

From this one can amplify Mr Lief's beneficial effects of neuro-muscular treatment as follows:

1. To restore muscular balance and tone.

2. To restore normal trophicity in muscular and connective tissues by altering the histological picture from a patho-histological to a physiologic-histological pattern with normal vascular and hormonal response.

3. To affect reflexly the related organs and viscera and to tonify them naturally.

4. To improve drainage of blood and lymph through the areas subject to gravitational or postural stasis, e.g., abdominal vessels not necessarily connected with viscera.

5. To reduce fatty deposits.

Thus the hyperaemia resulting from treatment automatically operates to reverse the original patho-histological picture and consequently normality will be approached.

The position of the practitioner and the patient and the various body structures, areas and tissues will be discussed in a later chapter. Apart from the tissue changes as mentioned above there should be an awareness of the reflex pathways and activities affecting and affected by each area being worked on. In this way the hands of the operator will yield a great fund of knowledge of the body which they are working on, as well as directly and reflexly aiding the achievement of homoeostatic equilibrium.

In seeking the cause of pain and other symptoms knowledge of the patterns of reflex activity and 'target areas' is obviously a useful diagnostic aid. There is clinical evidence that trigger points have a consistent localization and their localization can be predicted by studying the patterns of referred dysfunction and pain to which they give rise. These patterns of referred pain are, of course, predictable if the trigger point is found. Thus the point at which the patient feels pain and the point at which the pain originates are often not the same. This emphasizes the importance of accurate palpation in physical examination. Whether treatment is going to consist of anaesthetic injections, acupuncture, cryotherapy or pressure and stretch techniques (NMT) the diagnostic aspect remains the same. Deep palpation and pressure must reproduce the symptoms in the target area by irritating the trigger point.

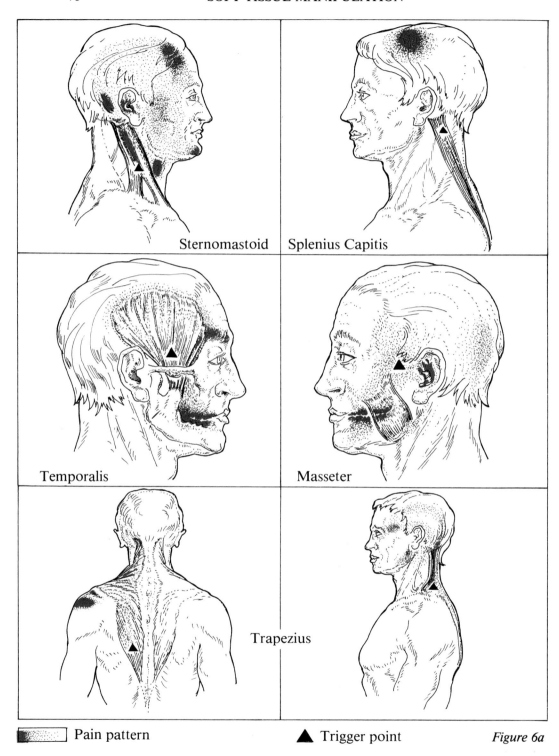

Sternomastoid   Splenius Capitis

Temporalis   Masseter

Trapezius

Pain pattern   ▲ Trigger point   *Figure 6a*

Myofascial trigger points and usual areas of referred pain.

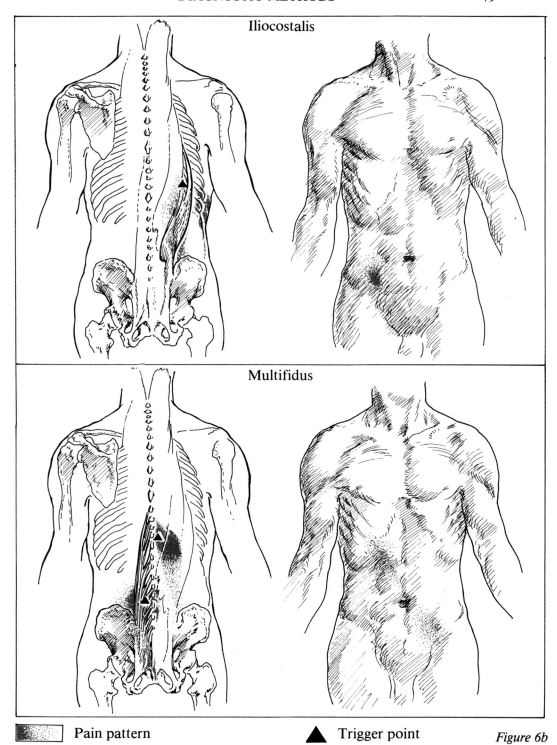

Iliocostalis

Multifidus

■░░ Pain pattern   ▲ Trigger point

Figure 6b

Myofascial trigger points and usual areas of referred pain.

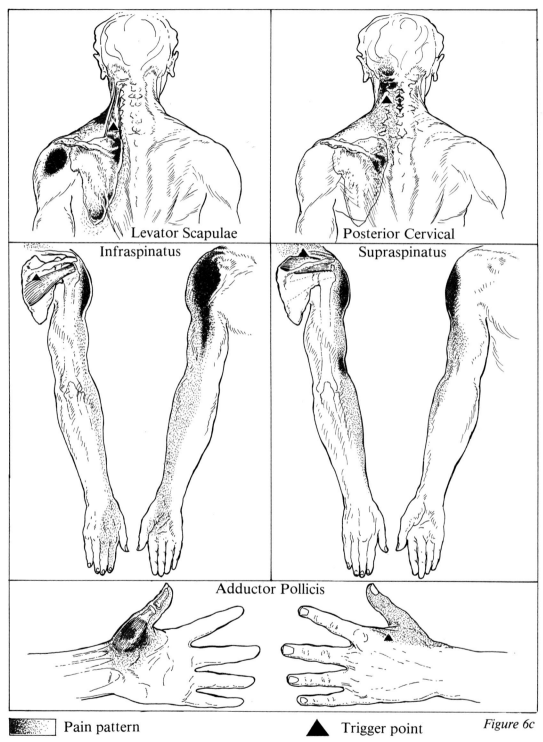

Levator Scapulae

Posterior Cervical

Infraspinatus

Supraspinatus

Adductor Pollicis

▨▨▨ Pain pattern

▲ Trigger point

Figure 6c

Myofascial trigger points and usual areas of referred pain.

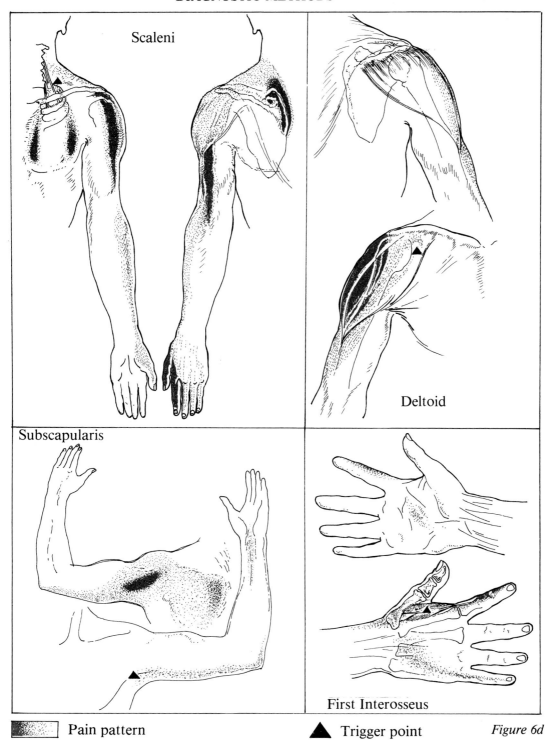

Scaleni

Deltoid

Subscapularis

First Interosseus

▨▨▨ Pain pattern   ▲ Trigger point   *Figure 6d*

Myofascial trigger points and usual areas of referred pain.

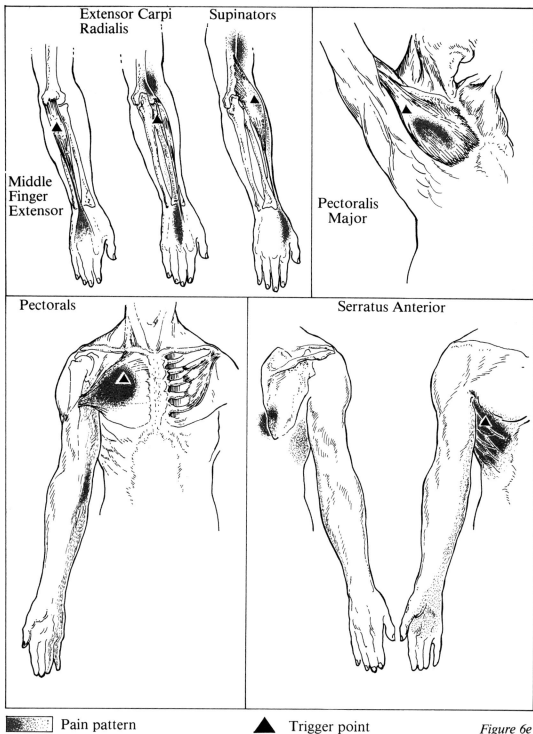

Extensor Carpi Radialis

Supinators

Middle Finger Extensor

Pectoralis Major

Pectorals

Serratus Anterior

Pain pattern   ▲ Trigger point

Figure 6e

Myofascial trigger points and usual areas of referred pain.

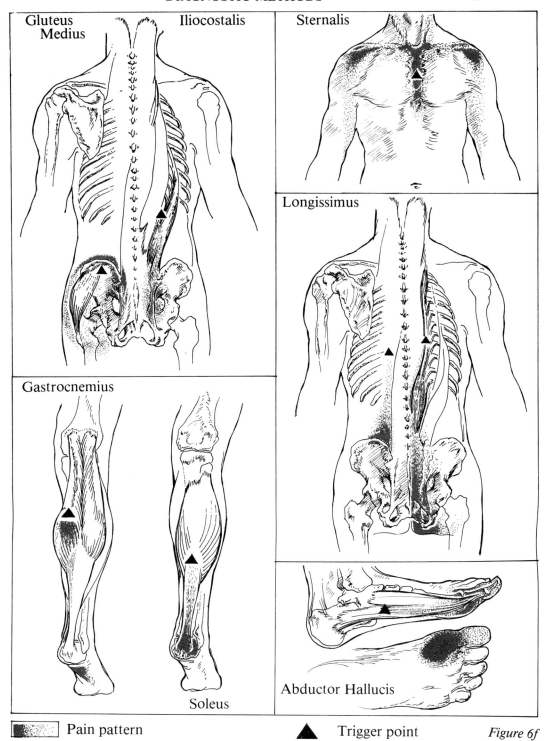

Gluteus Medius

Iliocostalis

Sternalis

Longissimus

Gastrocnemius

Soleus

Abductor Hallucis

Pain pattern   ▲ Trigger point   *Figure 6f*

Myofascial trigger points and usual areas of referred pain.

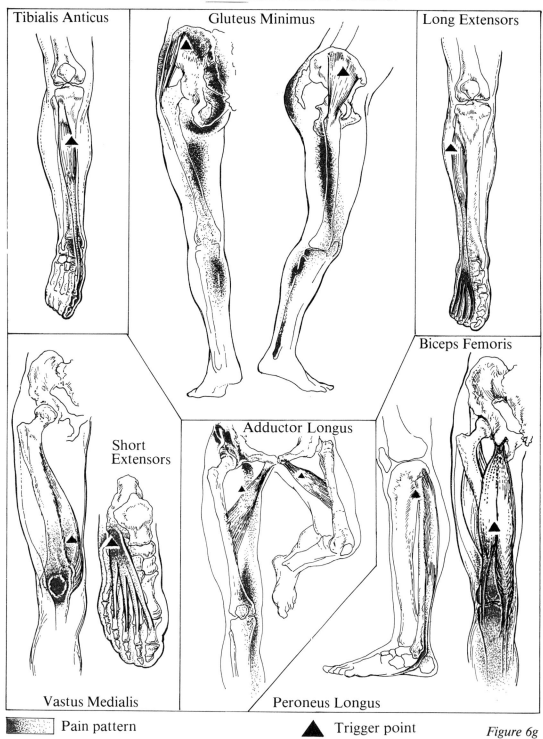

Tibialis Anticus

Gluteus Minimus

Long Extensors

Biceps Femoris

Short Extensors

Adductor Longus

Vastus Medialis

Peroneus Longus

■ Pain pattern   ▲ Trigger point

Figure 6g

Myofascial trigger points and usual areas of referred pain.

Dr Janet Travell was the main charter of these points and their target areas. As well as the trigger points discussed above there exist a number of palpable and often visible zones of altered soft tissue resulting from disturbed organs and functions. These areas lend themselves to neuro-muscular treatment, especially Lief's basic spinal treatment (to be discussed later). Some of these zones overlap and incorporate 'trigger' points. A general awareness and knowledge of their existence is certainly vital to an adequate understanding of what is being achieved in treatment. Since organs mainly receive their autonomic supply homolaterally, changes of a reflex nature will normally be found on the same side of the body surface. On the right side will be found the reflex zones from the liver, gall bladder, duodenum, appendix, ascending colon and ilium etc.

On the left side will be found the reflex zones from the heart, stomach, pancreas, spleen, jejunum, transverse colon, descending colon and rectum etc. Central zones occur as a result of dysfunction in the bladder, uterus and the head. Changes on the corresponding side of the body occur due to dysfunction of the lungs, suprarenal glands, ovaries, kidneys, blood vessels and nerves. According to Ebner[1] these changes in the connective tissue and muscles can take any of the following forms, drawn in bands of tissues, flattened areas of tissue, elevated areas, giving the impression of localized swelling; muscle atrophy or hypertrophy; osseous deformity of the spinal column.

Teiriche-Leube[2] and Ebner describe some of these zones in the following terms:

Table 2. Altered Soft Tissue Zones Resulting from Disturbed Organs and Functions, Giving Location and Symptoms

Illustration	Zone	Location	Symptoms
1	Bladder	Small, 'drawn in' area above anal cleft. Iliotibial tract may be drawn in. Swelling lateral aspect of ankles.	Bladder dysfunction. Cold feet and legs (below the knee). Rheumatic diagnosis.
2	Consti-pation	'Drawn in' band 2 to 3 inches (5-8cm) wide running from middle third of the sacrum downwards and laterally.	Tendency to or actual constipation.
3	Liver and gall bladder	Large 'drawn in' zone over right thoracic region and a band along lateral costal border on the right side. Small 'drawn in' area between lower vertebral border of scapula to spine at the fifth and sixth dorsal level. Seventh cervical area appears swollen or congested.	Liver and gall bladder dysfunction and anyone who has suffered from hepatitis.

Illustration	Zone	Location	Symptoms
4	Heart	Tension over left thoracic region including lower costal margin. If hepatic circulation is involved right costal margin will also be affected. The area between the left scapula and second and third dorsal vertebrae will be indurated. Posterior aspect of axilla appears thickened.	Coronary and valvular diseases of the heart.
5	Stomach	Overlapping the heart zones (above). Localized tension area below lateral aspect of the left scapular spine.	Stomach dysfunction. Gastric ulcer and gastritis.
6	Arterial disease of legs	A V-shaped configuration of the buttocks when sitting is noticed rather than the normal rounded shape.	Circulatory disturbance accompanied by angiospasm.
7	Arms	'Drawn in' areas over scapula extending over posterior deltoid.	Circulatory arm and hand problems. Neuritis paraesthesia etc.
8	Head	Thoracic area between scapulae. Lower third of sacrum just above bladder zone. Just below origin of trapezius.	Insomnia and all types of headache. Headaches related to digestive dysfunction. Headaches due to tension.
9	Venous lymphatic disturbance of the legs.	A tight band from middle third of sacrum, parallel to iliac crest laterally and anteriorly over gluteus medius.	Cramp. Swollen legs in summer etc., varicose veins and paraesthesia.

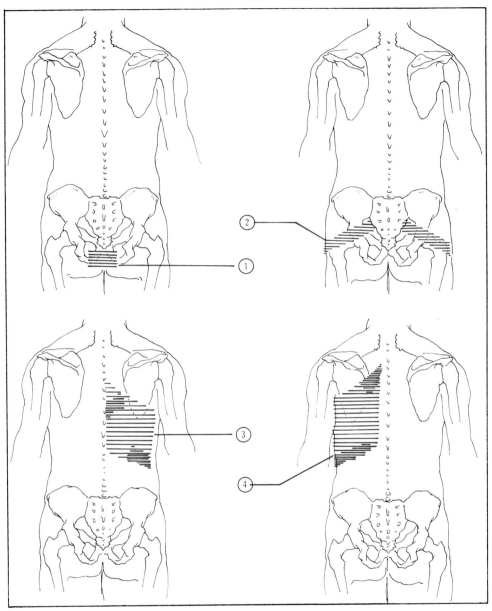

Connective tissue zones (after Ebner). 1. Bladder. 2. Constipation. 3. Liver and Gall Bladder. 4. Heart.

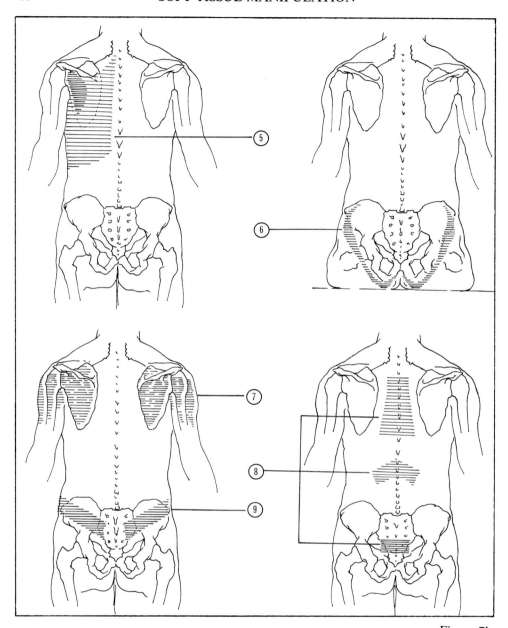

Figure 7b

Connective tissue zones (after Ebner). 5. Stomach. 6. Arterial disturbance of the legs. 7. Circulation of arms. 8. Head. 9. Venous lymphatic disturbances of the legs.

With Neuro-muscular Technique these and other areas of s ·ft tissue dysfunction may be found and treated with no obvious symptoms being present. It is clear that tissue changes often precede the appearance of symptoms of underlying pathology and in this alone the diagnostic value of these zones are evident. It is often possible to improve markedly symptoms of organ dysfunction and to improve the function of these organs (liver, stomach etc.) by releasing the congested fibrotic reflex zone. This is not, however, to be considered an end itself since it is clear that underlying causative factors (nutrition, infection etc.) must be dealt with. However, the value of the neuro-muscular tool should not be minimized.

Mackenzie's Abdominal Reflex Areas

Youngs[3] points out that Sir James Mackenzie established a clear relationship between the abdominal wall and the internal abdominal organs. Mackenzie[4] showed that organs which cannot react directly to painful stimuli (i.e. the majority) react by producing spasm and paraesthesia in the reflexly related muscle wall (the moytome) often augmented by hyperaesthesia of the overlying skin (dermatome).

The reflexes involved occur via the autonomic nervous system and can be viscerosomatic *or*, as has been evidenced by many researchers, including Lief, the origin can be somatic and the reflex therefore somatico-visceral.

Mackenzie's abdominal reflex areas are as indicated (*see Figure 8*). There is sometimes a degree of individualization. However, it is reasonable to state that the presence in abdominal muscles and connective tissues of contracted or sensitive areas indicates (in the absence of recent trauma or strain) some underlying dysfunction which is causing or resulting from the soft tissue lesion.

Skin: Reflex Effects and Hyperalgesic Skin Zones (HSZ)

Kiyomi Koizumi, of the State University of New York Department of Physiology, has studied the relationship between the skin surface and the internal structures of the body ('Autonomic system reactions, caused by excitation of somatic afferents: study of cutaneo-intestinal reflex', pp219-227, *The Neurobiological Mechanisms in Manipulative Therapy*, Plenum Press, 1978).

He studied a variety of animals, and it was found that stimulation of the skin of the abdomen produced profound inhibition of intestinal movement. He notes that this is a strong effect, and the intestine often became completely quiescent. Stimulation of the skin produces an increase in sympathetic fibre activity innervating the intestine, thereby inhibiting the mobility of the region. Stimulation of other skin areas, notably the neck, chest, fore and hindlimbs, inhibited the sympathetic activity, and therefore augmented intestinal motility. Vagal involvement in these changes was thought to be minimal, for when the vagi were sectioned the same responses were still noted. Reflexes disappeared, however, when the sympathetic nerve supply to the intestine, the splanchnic nerves, were sectioned. The somatic sympathetic reflex from the abdominal skin is a spinal reflex, whereas the reflexes originating from the other skin areas were thought to be a supraspinal reflex. The researcher points out that, whereas the parasympathetic system plays little part in these reflexes, its involvement increases aspects of emotional reactions. If we consider the involvement of these mechanisms in affecting internal function, via stimulus applied to the skin, we may better appreciate the findings of Chapman, Bennett and others, in their work on the multitude of reflex areas, which they

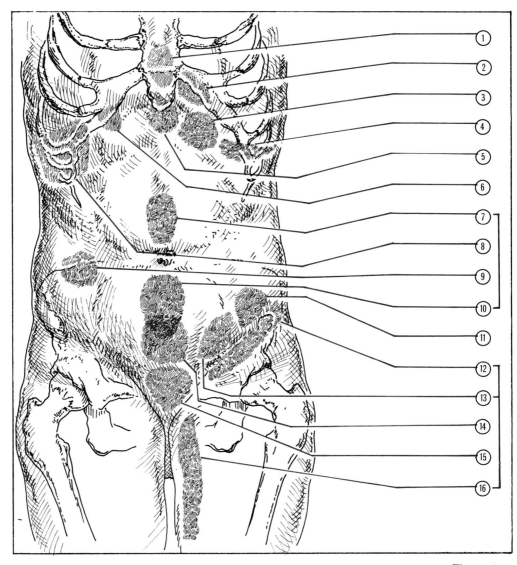

Figure 8

Reflex abdominal areas (after Mackenzie). 1. Oesophagus. 2. Stomach. 3. Solar plexus. 4. Spleen. 5. Duodenum. 6. Gall bladder. 7. Ilium. 8. Liver. 9. Caecum and Appendix. 10. Ilium. 11. Ovary and Descending colon. 12. Ureter. 13. Ureter. 14. Colon. 15. Bladder. 16. Ureter.

have so painstakingly charted, and which are available to us.

The sometimes dramatic effects obtained by the use of connective tissue massage methods can be seen to also relate to the pattern of therapeutic and diagnostic opportunities, which this knowledge opens. A number of techniques are available to us in diagnosing from, and treating, the cutaneous structures for reflex effect. These include skin rolling as well as the delicate 'skin distraction' or stretching method, advocated by Lewit (see also page 125). He discusses hyperalgesic skin zones which, if we reflect, are likely to be present in the skin overlying most, if not all, areas of reflex activity. Lewit points out a major advantage which awareness of Hyperalgesic skin zones (HSZ) offers. This is that, unlike the elliciting and mapping of areas, points or zones, which relies upon the subjective reporting of the patient, these areas are palpable to the operator. A popular method of noting relative tension in skin is to 'roll' it. A fold of skin is formed, and this is rolled between the fingers (*see Figure 15*, page 125). This method may produce some discomfort, or even transient pain, but is useful in that the increased tension and visibly thicker skin fold thus produced (as compared with surrounding tissues) is diagnostic of a HSZ.

The methods used in connective tissue massage are designed to obtain a picture of the mobility of the various layers of the connective tissue, as well as an idea of their consistency. One such method involves the lifting of skin folds, with the patient sitting. The skin is gripped between thumb and fingers, with care being taken not to pinch the fold. The fold comprises sufficient tissue to allow it to be lifted away from the fascial layer. This is usually performed, starting at the lower costal margin, and going up as far as the region of the shoulders. In some areas,

Lifting Skin Folds (Diagnostic)

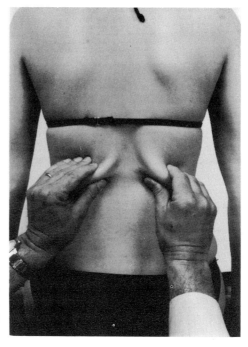

Figure 9

Skinfolds are lifted away from the fascial layer. Restriction in elasticity will be noted, if dysfunction exists locally or is affecting these structures reflexly.

especially overlying the mid-dorsal region, if there is any dysfunction involving the liver, gall bladder, stomach or heart, restriction of tissue elasticity will be noted. By lifting two folds simultaneously, right and left, it is possible to compare the relative freedom of these tissues.

Stretching Superficial Tissue (Diagnostic)

A second method may be used, in which relatively smaller areas are assessed. With fingers lightly flexed, and using only enough pressure to produce adherence between the fingertips and the skin, a series of short pushing motions are made, simultaneously with both hands, which stretches the tissues. Usually the pattern of testing goes from inferior to superior, sometimes in an obliquely diagonal direction. The patient is seated, and the operator works from behind, testing tissues from the buttocks to the shoulders.

Areas investigated, direction of stretch of tissues, and implications of reduced elasticity are:

1. The buttocks; stretching tissue from the ischial region, towards the lateral borders of the sacrum (arterial and constipation zone, see *Figures 7a and 7b*).
2. From the posterior aspect of the trochanters, towards the iliac crests. (Venous lymphatic and arterial disturbances of legs).
3. From the trochanters, towards sacro-iliac joints (venous lymphatic zone).
4. Over the sacrum, working from the apex towards the upper sacral segments (bladder and headache zones).
5. Over the lumbar region, on either side of the spine, working upwards (kidney zone).
6. Bilaterally up the spine, from lower costal region to the mid-thoracic level (liver and gall bladder zone (right side), and heart, stomach (left) and pulmonary dysfunction (on either side)).
7. Between the scapulae (headache zone).
8. Over the scapulae, from inferior angle, towards spine of scapula (arm zone).

Normal variations will exist independent of reflex activity. In individuals carrying increased adipose tissue, there will be a generally greater degree of tension or adherence noted, as compared to a thinner individual. An older person's skin will feel looser, in comparison to a young persons. The skin over the lumbar region is naturally less mobile than other regions. Adherence is being assessed, and this may or may not be accompanied by sensitivity. In connective tissue massage an assessment of this sort is made regularly, as it is diagnostic and prognostic, showing the rate of progress, and providing a unique insight into visceral and functional status.

Skin Distraction (Diagnostic and Therapeutic)

Lewit describes a 'new' method, which he finds reliable, painless and therapeutically very useful. Any area of skin may be thus assessed, large or small, with fingertip or hand contact.

In a small area, the fingertips (both index fingers) or index and middle finger tips of both hands, are placed close together, resting on the tissues to be tested. By separating the fingers the skin is stretched. A minimum of force is used, in order to simply take out the slack in the skin. The end-position is noted, as is the degree of 'springing' in the tissues. This is compared in several directions, over the area, and comparison is also made with the presumably healthy tissue, on the contralateral side. If a HSZ is present, then a stiffer degree of resistance will be noted, after the slack has been taken up. Where there is such resistance, if the end position of stretch is held for approximately ten seconds, the resistance will be felt to ease, and the normal physiological degree of springing will then be noted. This is measurable, and by marking the first stretch position with a skin pencil, and that available after 'release of the tissue', a measureable improvement will usually be noted.

The techniques may be used even for small areas (e.g. between the toes). These may be stretched by fingertip (light) pressure and separation. Larger areas are contacted by the ulnar border of the hands. The hands are crossed and placed on the tissue to be tested. Separation of the hands introduces stretch to take up the slack.

Having introduced this initial degree of stretch, resistance (end-feel) is then noted. If the tissues are resistant to stretch, and springiness is absent, the maintenance of the stretch (painless) achieves a release of the tissues.

All trigger points, tender points, connective tissue zones, Mackenzie's abdominal areas etc., are characterized by the presence of HSZ in the overlying tissues. This can provide identification of reflex activity and is itself an ideal form of treatment of these reflexes, and further provides accurate evidence of the subsequent situation. This is a very useful tool indeed, and should not be underestimated. Techniques for treating skin and superficial tissue are further discussed in Chapter 5.

Scar tissue often results in the presence of HSZ's around the scar. These are noted to be focal points of reflex activity. Acupuncture is a useful method of treating any very sensitive aspect of the scars themselves.

The reflexes described by Chapman are now commonly termed as neurolymphatic reflexes. These can be used in diagnosis and treatment and as a guide to the effectiveness of treatment. In 1965 I described[5] the technique for using these as follows:

Treatment applied through these reflexes, as advocated by Chapman and Owens, consists of a firm but gentle rotary pressure imparted by the index or middle finger. The finger should not be allowed to slip. As these areas are acutely sensitive great care should be taken not to overtreat as the reflex will become fatigued and no benefit will be derived.

My own view coincides with the above method except that I use a variable thumb pressure which fits in with the general neuro-muscular technique. Knowledge of the exact location of the reflexes is of primary importance.

By gentle palpation the operator should first ascertain the presence of involved reflexes. The anterior reflexes should be tested first. If found to be present the anterior reflex should be treated first, then the posterior counterpart of the involved anterior reflexes should be treated. The anterior reflex has, therefore, a dual role, namely, for diagnosis and then to initiate the reflex treatment. The anterior reflex is later of value to ascertain the effectiveness of treatment (after both anterior and posterior reflexes have been treated).

If, on repalpating the reflexes, there is no change in the feel or tenderness, the treatment should be repeated. If there is again no change it indicates either that the pathology is too great for rapid change, or that pathology is irreversible. It may also indicate that some musculoskeletal factor is maintaining the reflex. Primary treatment should then be directed at this factor rather than the reflex. The degree of treatment should be ascertained by palpation. Chapman and Owens described dosage of treatment in terms of seconds, but in practice I feel that anyone experienced in neuro-muscular treatment would have the degree of sensory awareness required to 'feel' when sufficient treatment has been given.

I would stress that I have found the reflexes of Chapman useful in differential diagnosis and in the treatment of various conditions from spastic constipation to migraine—but always as a part of a broad approach to the patient as a whole. That they can influence lymphatic drainage dramatically, I have no doubt—I am less sure of the effect on visceral conditions but have found that the reflexes themselves provide an excellent guide to progress. If they are no longer present then invariable the condition is progressing well.

The illustrations will aid the practitioner in locating these useful diagnostic and therapeutic areas.

Knowledge of Chapman's neuro-lymphatic areas, Bennett's neurovascular reflexes, Mackenzie's reflex areas, connective tissue zones and trigger points might appear a massive task for the memory, and so it is. However, the application of the general knowledge of their existence enables treatment to be effective even without precise knowledge of all the individual reflexes involved. In other words they can be used in diagnosis, if that is the aim. On the other hand they can be treated simply by locating them by palpation and treating whatever is found.

A general neuro-muscular treatment will elicit many such tender areas and the treatment or the use of Muscle Energy Technique will eliminate a number of them, thus aiding the general body economy. It is not essential, although it is desirable, for the practitioner to know what the various reflex points and areas are. The diagnostic and therapeutic aspects of this method overlap and as a result a number of diagnostic indications will be found in the chapters dealing with treatment. The aim of this chapter has been to try to classify some of the more obvious diagnostic indicators so that the practitioner's awareness can be broadened as to the range of diagnostic and therapeutic possibilities.

Etiology Speransky[6] has stated that the nervous system contains a record of the past history of the organism. The signs present in the muscuoskeletal system constitute the map which the practitioner has of past and present dysfunctions. It presents him with the opportunity to treat, alleviate and prevent further dysfunction.

Apart from palpation for tissue changes and reflex trigger areas, diagnosis should involve an evaluation of the gross stress patterns and postural factors. Each patient is an individual challenge and indeed this challenge is renewed at each visit. Thus, whilst the mechanics of treatment are similar the emphasis will probably be different at each visit. It is important that the patient understands this, and the nature of the problem as well as the goal desired. A co-operative patient will accept the time and effort required to achieve that goal.

Observation of the dynamic posture or body in motion gives an idea of balance, posture, gravitational stress, gross structural anomalies etc. Observation of certain body areas in individual movement will then help the visualization of their stress patterns, restrictions etc. Any trained physician, of whatever school, should then be able to decide the direction in which the myofascial tissues require guidance towards the achievement of normal functional integrity. Postural integrity will be considered in a later chapter. The body should also be observed in static positions such as sitting, standing, lying etc.

It is not the role of this work to instruct in postural assessment. The practitioner must learn to appreciate the arrangement of the various body structures and their inter-relationships. The myofascial tensions can then be visualized. When these gross and local postural patterns in active and passive modes have been observed an overall impression can be added to the palpatory impressions, both superficial and deep, which the hands can evaluate with the patient standing, supine or prone. By lightly passing the hands over the various structures alterations in tissue density and configuration can be felt. The deeper palpation to localize the dysfunction can then be performed or left to the neuro-muscular treatment where diagnosis coincides with treatment.

Obviously a history will have been taken prior to observation, palpation, and mobility tests. Such history should be comprehensive and should take note of traumatic incidents, habits, occupational positions and postures, emotional state and history, congenital deformity, surgery and of course general medical history and specific details of the presenting problems.

Mobility tests form, of course, part of the diagnostic procedures in soft tissue assessment. Since all physical therapists are concerned with joint mobility these tests will also be part of any overall assessment. Numerous works exist to instruct in this field. See Chapter 4 for appropriate tests.

Assessing Dominant Eye

In making a structural diagnosis it is important for the operator to be sure of the information he is acquiring. Dr Stiles makes a valuable contribution to this area by pointing out that it is often for reasons of position, in observing structure, that a student or practitioner fails to see what is obvious.[7] By being so positioned as to bring into play the non-dominant eye this becomes far more likely. The orientation of the subject in the field of view is determined by the position of the dominant eye, and thus it is essential to initially assertain which eye this is.

Hold your hands straight out in front of you. Palms facing each other. Bring them together to make an aperture (gap) about one to two inches across. Looking through this aperture focus on an object across the room from you. Close first one eye and then the other. When the non-dominant eye is closed the image you see through the aperture will not change. When you close the dominant eye the image shifts out of the field of vision. The dominant eye is not always on the same side as the dominant hand. If dominant hands and eyes are on different sides, this can lead to problems of accurately assessing palpatory findings, and the advice given is to palpate with eyes closed, where possible, in such cases.

When assessing visually, make sure that the dominant eye is lined up with the area or object being viewed. In an example where assessment of the chest is being made, Dr Stiles suggests that since most accurate visual information will be gained when the dominant eye is over the midline, the observation of the supine patient should be from the head of the table, and this should be approached from the side which brings the dominant eye closer to the patient.

Active motion, which is movement of one part of the body in relation to another, powered by conscious muscular effort; as well as passive motion in which an outside force acts on the body to induce movement, are both of diagnostic importance. Gradually it is possible to learn to distinguish between healthy tissue and tissue in which there exists dysfunction. This can only be learned by experience.

Observation, static and active; palpation, superficial and deep; a comprehensive and detailed history; mobility tests as required; localization of trigger areas; re-evaluation during the course of treatment; and an intelligent co-operative understanding of the patient and his problems are the diagnostic tools with which to understand the task in hand.

[1] Ebner, M., *op. cit.*

[2] Teiriche-Leube, H., *Grundriss der Bindesgewebs Massage* (Fisher, 1960).

[3] Youngs, B., 'NMT of Lower Thorax and Low Back', *British Naturopathic Journal*, Vol. 5, No. 11.

[4] Mackenzie, J., *Symptoms and Their Interpretation* (1909).

[5] Chaitow, Leon, *op. cit.*

[6] Speransky, A. D. *A Basis for the Theory of Medicine* (International Publishers, New York 1943).

[7] Edward G. Stiles D.O., lecture demonstration reported in *Patient Care*, 15 May, 1985.

Chapter 4

Postural and Emotional Considerations (Including Tests and Exercises)

Posture represents the sum of the mechanical efficiency of the body. It may be read as a book to assess the integrity, potential and, to some extent, the history of the individual.

The ideal posture is one in which the different segments of the body, the head, neck, chest, and abdomen are balanced vertically one upon the other so that the weight is borne mainly by the bony framework with a minimum of effort and strain on muscles and ligaments.

For such posture to be maintained special postural muscles must be in a state of constant activity. These have a special physiological property called 'postural activity'. These muscles include the sacrospinalis, psoas, quadriceps, sartorius and, to some extent, the calf muscles.

Correct posture is one in which the head is centred over the pelvis, the face directed forward, and the shoulder girdle approximately on the same plane as the pelvis.

The individual with poor posture may be described as one whose head is carried forward, whose scapulae are held in abduction, giving the shoulders a rounded appearance, whose dorsal curve is increased, and whose chest is flattened. Lordosis and prominence of the anterior abdominal wall below the level of the umbilicus is accompanied by an anterior tilt of the pelvis, the knees being slightly extended.

Even the slightest alteration in the normal balance of the various spinal segments is accompanied by some degree of soft tissue change. Poor posture may not produce immediate pathological symptoms but must be considered as a potential cause of trouble later.

Structure and Function Relationship

The inter-relationship between structure and function is total. The way the human machine is used and misused will greatly influence its structures. The structural changes engendered by postural and other, perhaps traumatic, insults will determine its ability to function mechanically. The soft tissues are the supporting structures which connect, bind, support and which provide stability and allow free motion to the articulations of the body.

The ability to contract and relax are the major attributes of most soft tissues. As a result of injury, disease or wrong use these soft tissues can undergo changes which include shortening, thickening, calcification and erosion. Changes in tension within fascial and connective tissue will occur depending upon the stresses imposed upon it by postural and other activities. This will result in reinforcement, shortening and thickening of these tissues. Excessive thickening can occur and this will accompany shortening, restriction of normal motion and probably alteration of positional integrity.

Postural defects can be shown to produce an accumulation of strain in the soft tissues (muscles, fascia, articular structures etc.) which predisposes towards dysfunction, pain and tenderness, especially in areas of bony attachment, areas of calcification and in areas where stress forces converge. When the deep fascia is subject to stress forces collagenous fibres will be deposited which may create stress bands along the lines of force. Excessive tensions exerted by fascia and muscles on an area of articular dysfunction may make manipulative correction difficult or impossible.

The position of the bony framework is determined by the soft tissues which invest, support, bind and move it. Faulty tensions in these soft tissues will lead to abnormalities in the skeletal structure and therefore of its function, and possibly of the organs and functions (blood vessels etc.) which are also supported by connective, fascial tissue and muscle. Not only is the soft tissue subject to gravitational stress but also to a battery of postural and occupational stresses overlaid with the normal contraction that comes with age. The spinal muscles deserve a degree of particular attention. As has been indicated, there is a general opinion that these may be divided into two groups. The first being the mainly phasic muscles, which have an inbuilt tendency to inhibition and hypotonia, and the predominantly postural muscles, which have the opposite tendency, to become shortened and hypertonic, in response to dysfunction, disuse and pathology. (These and other aspects of muscles in general, are discussed more fully in Chapter 1.) As far as postural considerations are concerned, Isaacson ('Living Anatomy; An anatomic basis for osteopathic theory', Journal of the American Osteopathic Association, Vol. 79, No. 12, pp752-9, 1980) also divides spinal muscles into two groups, using different considerations. He calls one type, the prime movers, (extrinsic) and the other type, the stabilizers (intrinsic). Among the stabilizers of the spinal column, are the erector spinae muscle mass.

He tells us, regarding these, that although often thought of as discrete entities (multifidus, intertransverse, interspinal, etc.) this is inaccurate. He states: 'various functions have been assigned to these intrinsic muscles, on the assumption that they actually move the vertebrae; however, the arrangement and position of the muscle bundles, making up this group, would seem to make it improbable that they have much to do in this regard.' They are, rather, stabilizers and proprioceptive sensory receptors which facilitate the co-ordinated activity of the vertebral complex. The force required to move the vertebral column comes from the large, extrinsic, muscles. Analysis of the multifidus group, which is particularly thick in the lumbar region, indicates that its component fascicles could not be prime movers, and that they serve effectively as maintainers of position, normal or abnormal, in which the prime movers place the vertebrae.

The same finding is made relating to the semispinal muscles, and the erector spinae groups. The first are frequently responsible for compensatory lesions, derived from vertebrae above or below, by virtue of the arrangement of groups of pairs of stabilizing muscle fascicles. These groups of muscles are, he maintains, responsible, in large part, for the co-ordinated, synchronous, function of the spinal column. This is a complex of the two functions of the different types of muscles in the region, those that stabilize, and those that move. Thus the vertebral column, and the body must be viewed as a functional unit, and not as a collection of parts and organs, functioning independently of each other. This is a concept which, while obvious, is often neglected in therapy.

Knowledge of the anatomical considerations discussed, and of the different ways in which the different muscle types react to dysfunction (hypertonia or hypotonia) helps us to appreciate that stress or strain applied to the body as a whole, or the spine in particular, will, regardless of cause, involve other areas of articulations, to some extent. This could involve muscular tone, body mechanics, and aspects of the circulatory and nervous system, as well as visceral function. In terms of soft-tissue manipulation, initial assessment of such function often relates to physiological alterations, as the body attempts to compensate for whatever changes have been imposed upon it. Later these become pathological, when the compensatory ability is exhausted. This is in line with Selye's general and local adaptation syndrome, (see page 16).

All such early changes, whether the result of trauma, repetitive postural or occupational strains or emotional stresses, will initially manifest themselves in the soft tissues. They are therefore accessible to skilled diagnostic assessment, as well as therapeutic intervention, which should take into account the totality of the body. Isaacson's injunction to consider the body, and the vertebral column, as a functional whole, is a timely reminder of what should be obvious, that the treatment of local dysfunction, without regard to the larger picture of causation, and interacting structural, mechanical and functional relationships, is bound to produce inferior results.

Postural Fascia

There are specializations of fascia, such as plantar, iliotibial, gluteal, lumbodorsal, cervical and cranial which stabilize and permit maintenance of the upright posture. Some of the fascial specializations of the body are referred to as 'postural fascia' because they have a special postural function and are among the first to show changes in the presence of postural defects. They assist in producing the necessary stabilization and, at the same time, permit motion initiated by muscular activity. Fascia is supplied with sensory nerves and many of its specializations previously mentioned are characterized by stress or tension bands of varying thickness.

Wherever the deep fascia is subjected to tension, it is reinforced in some way; for example, it may be further strengthened by deposition of paraneural bundles of collagenous fibres so that they form a definite aponeurosis. Dr Leon Page[1] points out:

The cervical visceral fascia extends from the base of the skull to the mediastinum and forms compartments enclosing the oesophagus, trachea, carotid vessels and provides support for the pharynx, larynx and thyroid gland. There is a direct continuity of fascia from the apex of the diaphragm to the base of the skull. Extending through the fibrous pericardium upward through the deep cervical fascia the continuity extends not only to the outer surface of the sphenoid, occipital, and temporal bones but proceeds further through the foramina in the base of the skull around the vessels and nerves to joint the dura.

Thus it can be seen that the respiratory movements or the positions of the head and neck could have an influence upon the intracranial structures purely through continuity of fascia as well as upon the thoracic visceral and vascular structures.

This provides part of the rationale behind cranial manipulative techniques. At birth much of the connective tissue is loose and poorly defined. Abnormal tensions during development may result from trauma, faulty nutrition, wrong use etc. and encourage posture bands to become fixed in states of unequal tension. This may result in shortening and thickening of fascia and of osseous structures into irregular patterns. Structural imbalance increases the load on postural muscles and fascia with consequent reinforcement of these abnormal states.

It should be recalled that in the human the degree of hip extension required for the upright posture is dependent on the hamstring and gluteus maximus muscles which also initiate knee joint extension together with the quadriceps femoris. The tensor fascia lata provides the opposing force for the hypertensors. These all deserve attention in diagnostic and therapeutic terms.

Low Back Pain In a major study of posture Lawrence Jones M.D., analyzed 500 cases of chronic low back pain. These cases included only those that had as their chief complaint chronic low back pain of at least ninety days continuous duration and which were intractable to previous treatment. Comparative study showed that this condition is a clinical rarity prior to the age of twenty. The main age for onset lies between thirty and sixty years of age indicating that 'the loss of elasticity of soft tissues and other changes that accompany age progression play a major role in bringing to the surface previously latent conditions'.[2]

It is significant that if individuals have not developed low back pain before the age of sixty, susceptability to this symptom almost disappears (apart from symptoms of organic origin).

Over 80 per cent of the cases in this study had had their symptoms for over five years. A generalized pattern of allied symptoms, indicated an essential unity of postural involvement. These allied symptoms include fatigue, general leg ache, sciatica and upper nerve root involvement. Jones considers generalized fatigue such a common accompaniment of chronic low back pain as to be considered as an outstanding diagnostic symptom of a postural etiology.

Jones' solution to the problem is by correction of the feet by means of a fixed postural shoe. He claims that 15 per cent of chronic cases are substantially relieved within ten days and over 40 per cent within a month.

In their classic *Essentials of Body Mechanics* Goldthwait et al show unequivocally the connection between the postural aspect and generalized ill health. To quote on just one aspect of this:

It has been shown that the main factors which determine the maintenance of the abdominal viscera in position are the diaphragm and abdominal muscles, both of which are relaxed and cease to support in faulty posture. The disturbances of circulation from a low diaphragm and ptosis may give rise to chronic passive congestion in one or all of the organs of the abdomen and pelvis, since the local as well as general venous drainage may be impeded by the failure of the diaphragmatic pump to do its full work in the drooped body. Furthermore, the drag of these congested organs on their nerve supply, as well as the pressure on the sympathetic ganglia and plexuses, probably causes many irregularities in their function, varying from partial paralysis to overstimulation. All these organs receive fibres from both the vagus and sympathetic systems, either one of which may be disturbed. It is probable that one or all of these factors are active at various times in both the stocky and the slender anatomic types, and are responsible for many functional digestive disturbances. These disturbances, if continued long enough may lead to diseases in later life. Faulty body mechanics in early life, then, becomes a vital factor in the production of the vicious cycle of chronic diseases and presents the chief point of attack in its prevention . . . In this upright position, as one becomes older, the tendency is for the abdomen to relax and sag more and more, allowing a ptosic condition of the abdominal and pelvic organs unless the supporting lower abdominal muscles are taught to contract properly. As the abdomen relaxes, there is a great tendency toward a drooped chest, with a narrowed rib angle, forward shoulders, prominent shoulder blades, a forward position of the head, and probably pronated feet. When the human machine is out of balance, physiologic function cannot be perfect; muscles and ligaments are in an abnormal state of tension and strain. A well-poised body means a machine working perfectly, with the least amount of muscular effort, and therefore better health and strength for daily life.

The Mind-Body Connection

The intimate relationship between the emotions and posture, and the mechanical use of the body, should be emphasized. Insofar as the soft tissues are concerned the relationship is a palpable one. Anyone who wishes to demonstrate this connection to themselves, need only sit for a moment or two and imagine an emotion, such as anger or disappointment, or any other strong feeling. Allow yourself to think and feel these emotions for some seconds, and become aware of the subtle, but noticeable, change which begins to occur in the muscles of the abdomen, the jaw, the shoulders, etc. Imagine then the effect of holding such emotions, not for a minute or two, but for months or years. The changes in the tissues would be dramatic, and would influence all function, and certainly posture.

Philip Latey, D.O., in his book *Muscular Manifesto* (Osteopathic Publications, London) describes three aspects of posture, which are observeable at examination of the patient. First we observe in the undressed patient, the 'image' posture. This being that self-conscious effort on the patient's part, which may be the image they wish to project to the practitioner (the patient is seldom aware of this). The request to 'let go', and relax completely, usually results in what Latey calls, the 'slump' posture. This presents us with the opportunity to see the effects of gravity on the less controlled muscle tone of the individual. There will be a generalized sagging as a rule. This also allows observation of particular areas which may be overactive such as hands, shoulders, jaw, etc. These may be clenched, hunched or moving, rather than part of the 'slump'. If the patient is then asked to lie down, we have 'residual' posture, and this is where we may begin to note those areas where the tension and contraction are almost permanently maintained. This will vary with the emotional state, and is accessible to palpatory skill and interpretation, as to its relevance to total body mechanics, as well as to psychological implications. Consideration of this aspect is not a part of this text, in any detail, but a few observations are of some importance.

Dr Wilfred Barlow tells us 'Anxiety and Muscle Tension Pain' (*British Journal of Clinical Practice*, Vol. 13, No. 5) that: 'There is an intimate relationship between states of anxiety and observeable states of muscular tension.' Electromyographic techniques have been used to demonstrate that muscular over-activity occurs in patients complaining of anxiety and tension. Wolff (*Headache and Other Head Pain,* Oxford University Press, 1948) noted that by far the largest group of patients seen by doctors is made up of those with 'marked contraction of the muscles of the neck. Such sustained contraction may be secondary to noxious impulses arising from disease of any structure of the head: more common, however, are the sustained contractions associated with emotional strain, dissatisfaction, apprehension and anxiety.'

We are aware of the term homoeostasis, which implies the return to a resting state of balanced equilibrium, after reacting to a disturbance. This may involve blood acidity, volume of blood, or the relaxed, resting state of muscles etc. Stress disorders may be thought of as the state of affairs which exists when the organism fails to return to a balanced resting state, after reacting to a given situation. Stress is therefore seen as a failure of homoeostasis to normalize tissues, or functions, after a responsive effort (which may be almost constant, in many cases). The involvement of the muscles in this sort of situation as a result of prolonged or repetitive physical or emotional stress, is a major cause of the changes noted in the musculoskeletal structures in general, and the soft tissues in particular. The muscles at first appear as though they have been activated, prior to any demand. As though they have been 'preset' for activity. This is an overalert situation which, in time, results in tissue changes of a chronic nature. It is imperative that such situations be normalized, not only by attention to the soft-tissue changes, which are palpable, but also by the patient's learning methods of relaxation and stress reduction. Examination of the patient should therefore include awareness of underlying tensions. The influence of such changes on posture are demonstrable.

Latey speaks of three primary areas of observeable dysfunction, relating to emotional involvement. These he terms the 'three fists'. Each being the equivalent of that area being maintained in a state of contraction, comparable to a clenched fist. There are the upper, middle and lower 'fists'. The *'lower fist'* is centred in the pelvic region and describes muscular changes, which are noticeable in the pelvis, low back, lower abdomen, and the lower extremities. The major structure which contracts in this region, Latey states, is the pelvic diaphragm, which forms the floor of the abdominal cavity. When this structure is contracted chronically it is often reinforced by contraction of the adductors of the thighs and the abdominal muscles. The effect on posture is to tilt the pelvis forward, with the legs rotated inwards. The pressure on the perineal area is then marked. The long-term postural response to these changes often involves a compensating shortening of the abductors of the legs, and the gluteals. A hyper-lordotic lumbar spine may then be observed. Any combination of variables in muscular contraction may be found, depending upon the manner in which compensation has been achieved. The emotional underpinnings of these changes should not be forgotten in any attempt to normalize the structural component. The physical signs, apart from palpable changes, might include 'knock-knees', 'pigeon-toes', 'flat feet', hip and low back pain, and restriction. Coccygeal inflammation, disturbed respiratory function, circulatory stasis, involving the lower limbs and the genital areas, gynaecological problems, urinary tract problems and difficulties in childbearing, are all possible eventualities. Spinal and pelvic joint problems are frequent.

One aspect of normalization, which Latey suggests in this region, involves teaching the patient to be aware of the subtle respiratory movement which should be present in the lower pelvic region, and which is lost when contractions, of the sort mentioned, are active. He says: 'I may try to teach the patient to relax his pelvic diaphragm. I find the easiest way to show a patient these pelvic movements is to ask him to lie on his front. If he now lifts one arm behind his back, and reaches down to cup his perineum with his hand, he can easily feel the movements of the pelvis with breathing. If he clenches his buttocks tight, he can feel how the movement is diminished. In this prone position, deep inspiration compresses the abdomen against the table, forcing the perineum to move.' By learning to relax these structures, the excursion of the movement increases, and the patient begins to relax the area in other positions. A symptom which indicates that desirable pelvic changes are occurring, is that the patient will begin to feel profound weakness in the legs.

Relaxing Pelvic Diaphragm

The *'middle fist'* is composed of two muscles. The first is the transversus thoracis, which lies inside the anterior part of the chest. It is attached to the sternum, and fans down and out to the inside of the ribcage. The lowest part of this inverted 'V', below the lower ribs, is often highly sensitive to pressure (where its name changes to transversus abdominus). Latey describes it as a remarkable muscle, capable of generating all manner of powerful sensations. These may range from nausea to weeping, sensations of choking, reflex contractions throughout the body, laughter, fear, etc. Physiologically relaxed breathing, he maintains, has as a central event, the rhythmical relaxation and contraction of this muscle. The other major muscle in this region is the serratus posterior-inferior, which runs from the lumbar spine upwards and outwards, to grasp the ribs from behind. Its contraction pulls them downwards, inwards and towards the spine. The emotional functions of the 'middle fist' are vomiting, laughing and weeping, all of which express an attempt to resolve internal imbalance. In all three functions the transversus alternates between full contraction and relaxation. Palpation of the movement of this component is achieved by having the patient sitting upright, or side-lying with knees drawn up so that the operator can palpate front and back simultaneously. By noting appropriate excursions of the lower ribs, below the sternum, movement may be assessed. A variety of emotional releases may occur in this position. Respiratory problems, notably asthma, are often a factor in which the 'middle fist' is involved. Relaxation of the spinal and neck areas, facilitates the restoration of function in these muscles. Gastro-intestinal symptoms are common.

The *'upper fist'* is characterized by the set of the neck and head, in relation to the body. Problems relating to the neck, shoulders and arms, and involving any of the organs of sense, and the head itself, are noted. Migraine is common. The emotional rigidity which accompanies the involvement of these areas relates to the patient's response to the outer world. The facial muscles may have a fixed character, and Latey points out that the expressions which are absent may be more important than the ones displayed. Those which are not expressed, in the facial muscles, may be expressed in the muscles of the scalp, and base of the skull.

TMJ problems may be found, as a set jaw with teeth clamped together is common. Anger and fear are the major emotions present in these characteristic tensions.

Treatment of all, or any, of these muscular manifestations of emotional stress, requires a comprehensive approach. Latey states the important instructions to all therapists: 'Techniques which blast their way through the patient's defences and resistances are nearly always worse than useless; they lead to withdrawal, shock and powerful rebound, in which the defences are re-established with additional restrictions, and preclude work at deeper, more complex and subtle, levels. Muscles must not be thought of as mechanical in function, they are at least as important when functioning as sensory organs.'

The research report in which connective tissue massage was shown to be of major value in treating anxiety problems (Chapter 2) is indicative of the value of reflex effects in such conditions. A direct attempt to normalize the entire soft-tissue component, such as might be used in Reichian or Rolfing methods, is one approach. A combining of attention to the musculoskeletal system, as well as aspects of psychotherapy and relaxation methods, which would help to deal with background causes and longterm management, would seem to be an ideal combination.

Alexander Technique A study of Alexander technique methods is suggested for the longterm postural reintegration of the individual (Barlow, Wilfred, *The Alexander Principle,* Arrow). Practitioners ought to be well aware of the implications of Alexander's revolutionary work. It is as useless to instruct a patient to 'stand up straight' as it is to instruct an anxious individual to 'relax'. They have no yardstick by which to measure what is straight or relaxed. Their subjective assessment of what is desireable, in these respects, is based on distorted information. What feels correct is patently not so, and all variations of posture, or degrees of relaxation, which they consciously impose on the phasic pattern of misuses, will be just as wrong in terms of what is desireable. The way we use ourselves is habitual, and acquired, and alteration of such patterns requires a relearning process. This is what Alexander Technique attempts, and it is a long and slow process. Without a good deal of preliminary soft-tissue work, and structural normalization, via the sort of methods outlined previously (MET, NMT etc.) this is a longer and more difficult process. Similarly, in attempting to learn relaxation methods, the tense, stressed individual, will be aided by complementary soft-tissue work. Once acquired, relaxation, like correct posture, and suitable 'use of the self', is not easily lost.

Hyperventilation Research has shown that the manner in which the individual uses his/her body, may have profound effects on health. Hyperventilation is an example of an incorrect use of respiratory function. Hyperventilation produces, in many individuals, phobic responses and panic reactions, of incapacitating dimensions. Trials reported in major medical journals indicate that the simple process of learning correct (diaphragmatic) breathing techniques, and simple timing of the inhalation-exhalation phases (exhalation should take marginally longer than inhalation) is all that is required to normalize many such, previously seriously handicapped people (agoraphobics in particular). (Research on this subject has been reported, in the *Journal of Psychosomatic Research,* Vol. 29, No. 1, p49-58. 'A controlled study of breathing therapy: treatment of hyperventilation syndrome'.)

Aerophagia Similarly, research indicates that aerophagia (swallowing air as a result of the nervous habit of frequent swallowing) is a major cause of exacerbation of hiatus hernia. Again the simple expedient of behavioural modification, by relaxation methods and improved breathing habits, is sufficient to normalize this, in most patients.

These two examples of the way in which functional misuse may be modified in response to the patient's needs, may help to make clear the intimate link between the physical structure, its function and what appear to be emotional (phobic behaviour) or mechanical (hiatus hernia) problems. Normalization of structure improves function; normalization of function aids in structural and symptomatic correction, both mental and physical. Both aspects, structure and function, require attention, if holistic ideals are to be achieved.

The pioneering osteopathic practitioner Carl McConnell (*1962 Year Book of the Osteopathic Institute of Applied Technique*, pp75-8) tells us: 'Remember that the functional status of the diaphragm is probably the most powerful mechanism of the whole body. It not only mechanically engages the tissues from the pharynx to the perinium, several times per minute, but it is physiologically indispensable to the activity of every cell of the body. A working knowledge of the crura, tendon, and the extensive ramification of the diaphragmatic tissues, graphically depicts the significance of structural continuity and functional unity. The wealth of soft tissue work centring in the powerful mechanism is beyond compute; and clinically it is very practical.'

Muscle Testing

In their study of posture Drs Kendall, Kendall and Boynton[3] have indicated that there exists a simple method of testing certain muscle groups in a postural context. Having repeatedly performed complete muscle tests on normal subjects they found certain groups that tended to show weakness in various particular postural or alignment problems. These muscles therefore represent the essential ones to be tested to assess the initial postural condition and to monitor progress.

It is not clear whether the postural faults precede or result from the muscle group weakness. Whenever muscle weakness exists some particular movement or degree of stability will be impaired. Tests as described are specific to the particular muscle. Where muscles that move the extremities are concerned the patient is required to hold the part in a specific position against the pull of gravity and against the maximum pressure exerted by the examiner.

In the case of small joints such as toes, gravity will play no part. A muscle that maintains its anti-gravity position against the operator's pressure is graded as 100 per cent. If the muscle holds its antigravity test position against medium pressure then an 80-90 per cent grade is given. A 50 per cent mark indicates that only the antigravity position is held but that no added pressure is exerted on the part of the operator. Less than 50 per cent indicates a very weak muscle and probably a degree of pathology outside the scope of normal manual therapy. In the case of the anterior trunk muscles gravity alone is used.

Pressure should always be applied gradually by the operator as even a strong muscle will give way to suddenly applied pressure.

If there exists a joint immobility which restricts the range of the part so that the test cannot be fully performed then the test should be carried out through the range that does exist.

Test for 'Lower' Abdominal Muscles

A person with 100 per cent 'lower' abdominal muscles is able to maintain the pelvis in a position of posterior tilt with the back flat while raising both legs from the table. The hands are placed behind the head. A narrowing of the costal angle indicates that the obliquus externus is contracting.

If the subject is unable to initiate leg-raising without allowing the back to arch, the legs are brought (with assistance) to a nearly vertical position and the subject is asked to hold the back flat while slowly lowering the legs. The angle between the legs and the table when the back just begins to arch off the table is used to determine the muscle strength grade. If the angle is about 80° the grade is 50 per cent; if it is about 60° the grade is 60 per cent; if about 40° the grade is 80 per cent.

When the 'lower' abdominal muscle test is given to patients with back pain an effort is made to avoid strain on the back. The attempt to do double leg-raising is omitted and the test is done by checking for pelvic tilt during leg-lowering, as described above. Also in such cases, the arms are usually crossed on the chest instead of being placed under the head.

It will be noted that the rectus abdominis is one of the muscles primarily concerned in both the 'upper' and 'lower' abdominal tests. This does not mean that the action is confined to the upper and lower aspects of the rectus respectively. The terms 'upper' and 'lower' refer not to location of the muscles, but to the section of the trunk which is chiefly involved in the movement.

The 100 per cent standard for lower abdominal muscles is primarily a standard for adult males. For other individuals normal strength according to age may be considered as follows: infants, test not used; aged 4-12 years, 60 per cent to 70 per cent; aged 12 years to adults, 70 per cent to 80 per cent; adult women, 80 per cent.

The tests for strength of 'upper' and 'lower' abdominal muscles are important in all routine postural examinations.

Trunk-raising Test of 'Upper' Abdominal Muscles

The starting position is supine with the hands clasped behind the head and the pelvis tilted backward to flatten the low back against the table. The subject should flex the trunk without jerking, raising first his head and then his shoulders. Through this arc, his feet should not come up from the table, but neither should they be held down by the operator. The change in the costal angle during the performance of abdominal tests indicates which of the oblique muscles is acting.

The second movement is flexion of the trunk on the thighs by the hip flexors. At this stage of the movement the legs may be held down if the weight of the legs does not counterbalance the weight of the trunk. If the hands are behind the head during the successful performance of the test a grade of 100 per cent can be given. A grade of 80 per cent is given if the movement can only be completed with the arms folded across the chest. For a 60 per cent result the arms would be extended diagonally forward during the movement. For a 50 per cent result the same arm position is used as for the 60 per cent but only the neck is capable of being raised by the patient, and not the shoulders.

If the subject with normal back flexibility is unable to perform to a grade of 50 per cent then the muscles are graded 'weak'. If the back muscles are very tight it must be determined whether abdominal weakness or back tightness has prevented completion of the test movement.

Patient supine, hands clasped behind the head. The examiner places the trunk in the exact test position of flexion and rotation, to an angle of 45° from the surface, and asks the subject to hold that position. If the strength of the muscles is 100 per cent the trunk will not drop or shift out of position. When the trunk is rotated forward on the right, the diagonal fibres of the right external and left internal oblique muscles are chiefly used. If the left side is rotated forward the left external and right internal oblique muscles are used.

Trunk-raising Test of Oblique Abdominal Muscles

The legs must be stabilized by an assistant during the performance of this test, and hip flexor strength must be adequate to stabilize the pelvis in this test position. For an 80 per cent test result the arms are folded on the chest and the shoulders are held only a few inches above the table. For a 60 per cent test result the arms are extended forward and the lower shoulder is barely lifted from the table. A 50 per cent result does not involve raising the trunk. With the examiner giving moderate resistance against a diagonally downward pull of the subject's arm, the cross-sectional pull of the oblique abdominal muscles should be very firm on palpation and should pull the costal margin toward the opposite iliac crest. The test may also be done by applying pressure against the thigh with the leg in about 60° hip flexion. The obliques should then pull the iliac crest toward the opposite costal margin. The test of the oblique abdominal muscles is most important in case of scoliosis.

The movement starts with the patient lying on his side. The upper arm is held along the side of his body. The lower arm is folded across the chest and the hand rests on the upper shoulder. Pillows are placed on top of and between the legs to prevent the discomfort of one leg pressing on the other as the operator stabilizes them by downward pressure. The subject raises the trunk by lifting first the head and then the shoulders sideways. There should be no rotation of the trunk. As the movement progresses, the upper side of the pelvis tilts downward a little to accommodate for the change in pelvic position. The examiner, in his effort to stabilize the legs, must not prevent the adjustment.

Test of Lateral Trunk Flexors

The ability to do this test movement correctly depends upon having a full range of motion in lateral trunk flexion as well as upon having adequate strength. The lateral trunk flexors are graded 100 per cent if the costal margin can be brought close to the iliac crest. If the lower shoulder is raised about four inches (10cm) from the table the muscle grade is 80 per cent. If the shoulder is raised only one to three inches (2.5-7.5cm) from the table the grade is 50 to 60 per cent. If the trunk fails to move through the full arc of motion the examiner must determine whether the primary reason is weakness of the muscles being tested or tightness of their opponents. The tests for strength of lateral trunk flexors are important in cases of lateral pelvic tilt and scoliosis.

Patient should be prone, with fists clenched and resting on the buttocks. Legs are stabilized by the operator whilst the patient lifts the head and thorax from the table. If the subject can hold this position against maximum pressure exerted downward on the upper dorsal spine by the examiner, the grade is 100 per cent. If the position is held against slight pressure the grade is 80 per cent. If the subject

Test of Back Extensor Muscles

almost completes the full movement the grade is 60 per cent. If he raises high enough to lift the lower end of the sternum from the table the grade is 50 per cent.

While exerting pressure on the upper back with one hand for the 100 per cent and 80 per cent tests, the examiner continues to stabilize the lower legs with the other hand.

The low back extensors are seldom weak in cases of typical faulty posture. However, since the erector spinae muscles are the most important of all trunk muscles, it is necessary to detect weakness when it exists. For this reason, and because the routine examination of back extensors will dispel the mistaken idea that most painful low backs are 'weak' this test is included in the group of postural cases.

Tests for Serratus Anterior

The serratus anterior holds the scapula close to the rib cage and rotates the inferior angle of the scapula forward. The sitting position is one of several which may be used for testing this muscle. The arm is placed in about 120° flexion and the examiner exerts downward pressure on the upper arm and backward pressure on the medial border of the scapula with the other hand. If the serratus anterior is weak the inferior angle of the scapula will rotate medially and the whole vertebral border of the scapula will stand out from the rib cage; the subject will be unable to hold the test position because of lack of adequate scapular stabilization.

Tests for strength of the serratus anterior should be done in cases of faulty scapular position, or in cases of pain in the area of the rhomboids since the latter may shorten and be painful in cases of serratus weakness.

Test of the Psoas Major

The subject is in a supine position. The examiner places the leg to be tested in a position of hip flexion, slight abduction and slight external rotation, and asks the subject to hold that position while he presses downward and slightly outward on the lower leg. The examiner stabilizes the opposite hip. The test for psoas major is of particular importance in cases of anterior deviation of the pelvis, lumbar kyphosis, or lumbar scoliosis. Weakness tends to be bilateral in cases of lumbar kyphosis, and unilateral in cases of lumbar scoliosis.

Test of Gluteus Medius (Posterior Part)

The subject lies on his side with the lower leg flexed at the hip and knee. The upper leg, which is the one to be tested, is placed in abduction, slight extension, and slight external rotation by the examiner, and the subject is asked to hold this position against pressure. Then the examiner uses one hand to help stabilize the pelvis while with the other he presses downward and slightly anteriorly on the lower part of the leg. Attempts by the subject to compensate by rotating the leg back into a neutral position, by rolling the upper hip backward or forward, or by bringing the thigh into flexion are common. The grade should be determined by the ability to hold against varying degrees of pressure in the designated test position. Tests for gluteus medius strength are of particular importance in cases of low back pain and in case of faulty alignment of the lower extremity.

Test of Gluteus Maximus

For this test the subject is in a prone position. With the knee bent to 90° or more the thigh is raised several inches above the table and the subject is asked to hold this position as downward pressure is exerted by the examiner on the lower part of the posterior thigh.

Testing for strength of the gluteus maximus is of particular importance in cases of anterior pelvic tilt and in cases of coccyalgia.

Test of Hamstring Muscles

With the subject prone, the knee is bent to about 45° angle. The subject is asked to maintain the position of knee flexion as the examiner exerts downward pressure on the back of the ankle.

Test for strength of hamstrings is of special importance in cases of anterior pelvic tilt and hyperextension of the knees.

Test of Soleus

The subject is prone with the knee flexed to at least a 90° angle. The foot is placed in plantar flexion and the subject is asked to hold that position. The examiner provides support for the leg with one hand while with the other he exerts pressure to pull the heel towards the planta.

This test is important for cases in which there is a deviation of the body forward from the plumb line. It is also advisable to test this muscle in cases in which there is an increase in the height of the longitudinal arch.

Tests for Toe Flexor Muscles

The test movement for the flexor hallucis longus is flexion of the distal joint of the big toe. The subject attempts to hold the position as the examiner applies pressure against the distal phalanx.

For the flexor digitorum longus test the subject bends the distal joints of the second, third, fourth and fifth toes and holds against pressure by the examiner.

In pronation of the foot, weakness is frequently found in these two muscles. They are more often weaker on the left than on the right because the left foot is generally more pronated than the right.

The flexor brevis is tested by having the subject flex the toes and hold against pressure applied to the middle phalanx.

The test for flexor brevis is important in cases of longitudinal arch strain. A point of acute tenderness is often observed at the place of origin of this muscle on the os calcis.

In the test for flexion by the lumbricales the subject flexes the metatarsal-phalangeal joints of the four outer toes and holds while pressure is applied against the proximal phalanges.

Tests for strength of lumbricales are particularly important in cases of metatarsal arch strain and in cases of hammer toes.

A number of patterns of postural deviation can result from, or in, particular muscle weakness. Where the pelvis is tilted anteriorly, producing a lordotic lumbar spine and an elevated thoracic cage, the rectus abdominis lying between the pubic bone and the sternum will be stretched and weak.

In the postural condition where the pelvis is tilted anteriorly and the hips are held in flexion with a hyperextended or lordotic lumbar spine, with a compensating dorsal kyphosis, there will be tension, tightness and great strength in the low back extensors and hip flexors while the muscles controlling the lower abdomen and the hamstrings will be stretched and weak.

In the half-stooped posture in which the legs are deviated posteriorly and the trunk has deviated anteriorly with a compensatory anterior tilt of the pelvis, the hip joint is in flexion and the lumbar spine slightly hyperextended. The hip flexors will have shortened and the back extensors will be contracted. Where there exists a flattened lumbar curve due to a pelvic tilt posteriorly, there is often a tightness in the hamstrings and weakness in the hip flexors or back extensors or both. The abdominal muscles may or may not be strong and tight.

Where the pelvis and upper legs have swayed forward in relation to the feet there will be hyperextension of the hip. The pelvis will be tilted slightly posteriorly and there is no increase in the lumbar curve. The anterior hip ligaments, the hip flexor and the external oblique abdominal muscles limit and maintain this position. All these will be stretched and weak. The low back and hamstring muscle will be short and strong. The upper back muscles will be weak and stretched and the upper abdominals will be strong and short.

Where the pelvis deviates right and tilts to the left, the right hip is in adduction.

The right gluteus medius will be weaker than the left. The left leg is in abduction and the left hip abductors, especially the tensor fascia lata, will be tight and strong.

If the individual has marked weakness of the right gluteus medius muscle the trunk will deviate towards the affected leg causing an abduction of the right leg and excessive weight bearing on it.

The relevance of these conditions and any muscular weaknesses that might be ascertained should be correlated with tests to determine the physiological state of tightness of these same and others postural muscles. The length or tightness of these should be assessed. (*See Figures 10a and 10b.*)

Tightness or shortness is of primary concern, and should be dealt with before any attempt is made to strengthen weak muscle groups. These will frequently normalize themselves once antagonists, which have shortened, are released and relaxed.

The following tests are used for assessing particular groups of shortened muscles. Some may also be used as MET positions for lengthening those found to be shortened, by the simple expedient of taking the muscles to their current physiological limit, and having the patient attempt to counter any restriction by pushing against the restraining counterpressure of the operator. Never use the full force of the patient's strength, but always a graduated degree of this, starting with a small effort. Full details will be found in Chapter 10.

1. The patient sits and bends forwards, in an attempt to touch the fingers to the toes, whilst maintaining straight knees. If he can do so, and also dorsi-flex the toes, the low back and hamstring muscles are probably not shortened.

2. If toe touching is possible, but the toes are plantar-flexed, then there is *probably tightness in the gastrocnemius-soleus* muscles.

3. If in the same position toe touching is difficult, or impossible, and the pelvis is relatively posteriorly tilted when the patient is at full stretch, then *the hamstrings are probably shortened.*

4. If in the same position the individual cannot lean forward, beyond an almost

vertical position of the spine, then *the low back muscles are tight.*

5. Unless: The individual can reach a far way down the leg, but observation indicates that most of this ability is the result of excessive flexibility in the upper back muscles, in which case *low back and/or hamstrings are probably shortened.*

6. But sometimes: The hamstrings may be stretched in compensation for tight low back muscles. This is unusual, and weakness of the hamstrings would indicate this.

7. If in the same position the individual is unable to sit, even with the spine vertical, but holds it in leaning backwards, when at full stretch towards the toes, then a combination of *tight low back muscles, tight hamstrings, and tight gastrocnemius-soleus, is likely.*

8. If in this same position, toe touching is almost possible, but the lumbar spine is not flexed, but remains lordotic, despite attempted flexion, then *the low back muscles are very tight.*

9. The patient lies down. If a leg can be raised whilst the opposite leg is kept flat on the table this is normal. This tests the hip flexors on the opposite side, as well as hamstring tightness, and pelvic tilting ability.

10. If the leg cannot be raised beyond about 45 degrees, but the spine remains flat against the table, and pelvic tilt is noted, then the *hamstring is tight on that side.*

11. If leg-raising again fails to reach beyond about 45 to 50 degrees and the low back arches, and the pelvis fails to roll posteriorly, this *indicates tightness of low back and opposite hip flexor muscles.* These are maintaining the pelvis in anterior tilt, when one leg is held to the table, and the other raised.

12. If the leg raises to about 45° but the pelvis tilts well posteriorly (while opposite leg fixed to table) this indicates *stretched low back muscles and tight hamstrings.*

13. If leg raising is beyond 90° and the low back stays flat, and pelvic tilt is normal *then the hamstring is stretched.*

14. If the leg raises to 90°, pelvis fails to roll posteriorly, and low back arches, this *indicates stretched hamstring, tight opposite hip flexor, and tight low back.*

15. Tensor fascia lata is tested by the patient side-lying, lower leg flexed comfortably. The upper leg extended so that the foot drops over the edge, behind the patient. The leg should be able to drop into adduction, towards the table. The trunk should remain in contact with the table and not arch upwards during this test.

16. If the leg fails to drop, when the pelvis is fixed, then there is *tension, in the iliotibial band and tensor fascia lata* (tensor fascia lata incorporates both tensor fascia femoris, and the lateral thigh fascia). See also page 156 for iliotibial band tests.

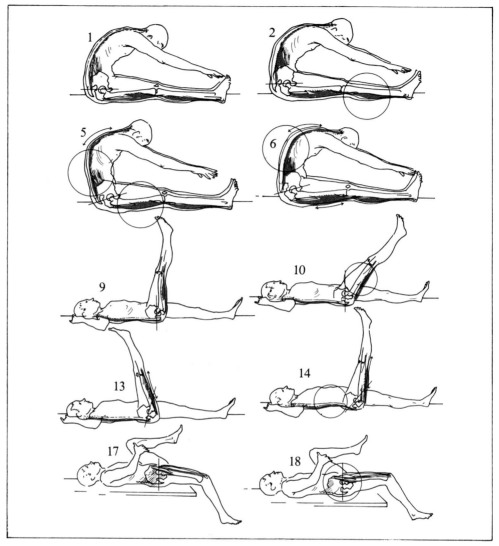

Figure 10a

Tests for Muscle tightness
1. Normal length of muscles of back and posterior thigh.
2. Tight gastrocnemius-soleus. The inability to dorsiflex the feet indicates tightness of plantar-flexor group.
3. Tight hamstring muscles. Pelvis is tilted more posteriorly due to this.
4. Tight low back muscles.
5. Tight hamstrings; slightly tight low back muscles and stretched upper back muscles.
6. Slightly tight low back, stretched upper back and slightly stretched hamstrings.
7. Tight low back, hamstrings and gastrocnemius-soleus.
8. Very tight low back muscles.
9. Normal hamstrings (right) low back and left hip flexor muscles.
10. Tight right hamstrings.

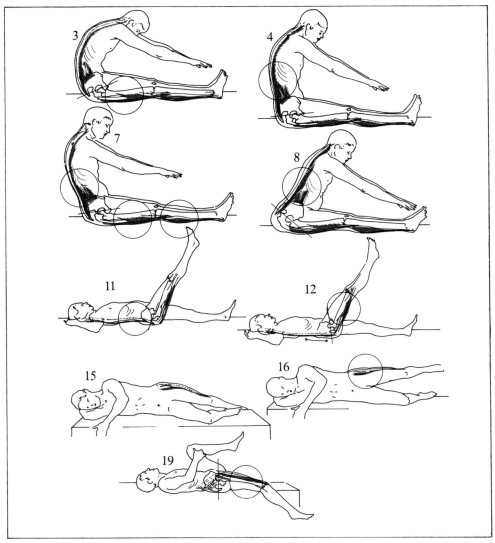

Figure 10b

11. Tight low back and left hip flexor muscles. Normal right hamstrings.
12. Tight right hamstrings; stretched low back and left hip flexor muscles.
13. Stretched right hamstrings, other muscles normal.
14. Stretched hamstrings, tight low back and left hip flexors.
15. Normal tensor fascia lata (includes lateral thigh fascia and tensor fascia femoris).
16. Tight tensor fascia lata.
17. Normal length of hip flexor muscles (includes ilio-psoas, rectus femoris, tensor fascia lata and sartorius). If back is flat against table, and thigh is able to touch along its length, then these are considered normal.
18. Tight hip flexor group.
19. Rectus femoris tightness. Right knee extends as left thigh brought down. Rectus femoris refers to the knee.

17. The patient is lying supine with the buttocks near the edge of the table. The flexed leg is held by the patient in maximum flexion (on the side not being tested), the other leg hangs over the edge. If the thigh can be held against the table in this position, the hip flexor group are probably normal.

18. If, however, the thigh cannot be brought down to the table *then the hip flexors are shortened.* (These include iliopsoas, Rectus femoris and TFL).

19. If the knee extends, as the thigh is brought to the table surface, then *rectus femoris tightness is probable.* The remaining hip flexors having allowed hip extension, but the thigh muscle having referred this to the knee.

Test for soleus. Patient squats and should be able to place whole sole of foot against floor, including heel. If heels leave floor, *soleus is shortened.*

Patient supine, leg straight. The foot is dorsiflexed, and may show limitation, which disappears when the knee is flexed. This is characteristic of *gastrocnemius shortening.*

Testing for tight erector spinae. The patient sits with legs over side of table and places hands on crest of ilium, fixing the pelvis. Patient attempts to flex spine to place forehead to knees. If the bend fails to reverse the lumbar curve, then the *erector spinae are shortened* in this region. (*See Figure 12.*)

Quadratus lumborum is assessed by comparing side-bending ability. Test first for any difference in leg length, which could confuse the assessment. Patient stands erect, feet slightly apart and attempts to bend sideways, running hand down lateral leg. *Quadratus is shortened* on left if limitation is noted on side-bending to the right, and vice versa.

The arms are stretched overhead with the patient supine. With the back flat, and the hips and knees flexed, the entire length of the arm should be able to contact the table. This assesses tightness in the adductors and internal rotators, which include pectoralis major and minor, lattisimus dorsi, teres major, subscapularis, and the rhomboids. (*See Figure 11.*)

   This is not a comprehensive list, but indicates the sort of testing which can isolate individual tight muscles and groups. Application of MET and NMT is indicated when these are found.

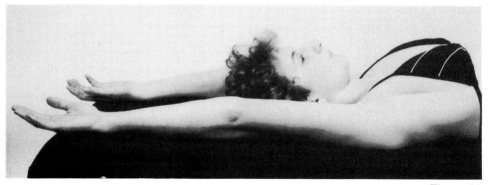

Figure 11

Right (*Figure 12*)   Test for erector spinae shortening: Patient sits on edge of table and places hands on crests of ilii, fixing pelvis. Patient attempts to flex spine to place head on knees. If the bend fails to reverse the lumbar curve the erector spinae are shortened in this region.

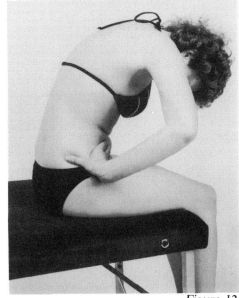

Below left (*Figure 11*)   Test for tightness of adductors and internal rotators of arms. The arms stretched overhead with the patient supine should be able to contact the table for their entire length, if no shortness in these muscles is present.

Figure 12

Objective assessment of the patient's posture combined with tests for muscle strength and muscle length (or tightness) provide the operator with the ability to concentrate on those areas of soft tissue dysfunction (too tight, too weak, too strong, too short etc.) which are present in any particular case. It should be borne in mind that posture represents not only the habitual manners of use, the occupational stresses and the inherited and acquired mechanical deviations but is also the mirror image of the total of psychic stress to which the individual has been and is being subjected. The degree of muscular guarding and built-in protective rigidity resulting from such stress presents a major area of dysfunction. The release of these tissues can often be of importance in normalizing emotional disturbances.

The operator has within the framework of the general and specific manoeuvres incorporated into NMT a method for dealing with the types of postural problems which result from or which cause soft tissue dysfunction. It goes without saying that other methods can and should be used as well in the ultimate correction of these conditions. These methods may include exercise, re-education, manipulation, corrective footwear etc. as indicated by the particular circumstances.

The use of NMT however gives an unequalled method for the normalizing and assessing of the soft tissue component.

A pattern of treatments over a series of ten to fifteen visits aimed at normalizing the spinal, abdominal and lower limb soft tissues, will effectively prepare the body for the correction of postural habits.

Rolfing techniques, which attempt to achieve similar results in eight treatment sessions, are notoriously painful, albeit successful. NMT need hurt no more than in a transient manner and it is at least as effective as Rolfing.

It is suggested that for postural correction, the first visit should deal with basic spinal and abdominal work, clearing up whatever is most obviously tense, contracted and painful. Following sessions should deal with the connective tissues and muscles of the feet and legs, the shoulders and the thorax, before returning to the spinal and abdominal tissues. Special emphasis should be applied to those soft tissues which postural patterns or muscle stretch or strength tests indicate to be most in need. After eight to ten sessions the patient should be demonstrably improved and retesting will give proof of this. At this stage postural re-education, exercises and breathing techniques all come into play. Until a moderate degree of soft tissue improvement has been achieved by this earlier treatment such additional measures would have less chance of success.

Stretching and Strengthening Exercises

Before any of these methods are employed, MET should be attempted in order to gain maximum length in shortened muscles. Muscle energy variations, in which the patient uses gravity as the counterforce, should then be introduced, as well as the stretching movements described below. Only after this should toning or strengthening exercises be introduced (see Chapter 10).

The following exercises will prove useful in stretching or strengthening particular muscles and groups as indicated in any given case.

Exercises should be done daily until normal length has been restored to tight muscles and until weak muscles have been strengthened. There will always be both weakness and tightness in opposing groups of muscles and both aspects must be dealt with. NMT provides the ability to normalize those aspects of the soft tissues that cannot easily be improved by exercise alone, no matter how specific these may be.

Low Back Stretching Exercise

Patient lies, face down, with a firm pillow under the abdomen and a small pillow or rolled towel under the ankles. The patient should relax in this position and then roll the pelvis inferiorly over the abdominal pillow by pulling down with the buttocks and hamstrings. The patient is trying to flatten the lumbar curve by tilting the pelvis posteriorly.

Lower Abdominal Exercise (1)

Patient lies supine with a rolled towel under the knees. The hands are placed behind the neck and the patient tilts the pelvis posteriorly to flatten the low back against the surface. This is achieved by pulling the lower abdominal muscles up and in holding this tension with the back flat whilst respiration continues deeply and slowly. The upper abdominal muscles should be relaxed and the chest should expand freely whilst the retracted muscles are held for at least a minute.

Lower Abdominal Exercise (2)

The position is as above but with the knees bent and feet close to buttocks. The back is held flat as the legs are slowly slid into a straight position. The back should remain flat during this manoeuvre and also as the knees resume the bent position, one at a time. Repeat eight to ten times.

Upper Abdominal Exercise

Patient lies on the back with a rolled towel under the knees and the pelvis tilted to flatten the lower spine. The arms are extended forward or placed behind the head and the patient lifts the head and shoulders approximately ten inches (25cm) from the surface and slowly returns to a lying position. Repeat eight to ten times.

Patient lies on the back, knees bent and the low back held flat to the surface, one or both arms are stretched above the head. The entire length of the arm should touch the surface with the elbow straight and as close to the side of the head as possible. This position is held for at least a minute while the patient breathes and relaxes.

Pectoral Stretch Exercise

Patient sits with legs extended and a rolled towel under the knees. The abdominal muscles are retracted and the patient reaches forward to grasp the toes (or the furthest point of the legs possible). This should cause a degree of stretch in the low back area and the back of the legs. This should be repeated ten to fifteen times and then maintained for at least a minute to complete the exercise.

Low Back and Hamstring Stretch

Same position as above but without towel under the knees.

Hamstring Stretch

The patient adopts a position similar to that of an athlete at the start of a sprint. The foot of the flexed leg should be placed on the floor and remain flat whilst the foot of the leg which extends posteriorly should be dorsiflexed and internally rotated so that weight is borne on the ball of the foot. The hands are placed on the floor immediately below the head. The major tension is applied to the anterolateral aspect of the thigh by flexing the forward knee so that the pelvis is moved down. A rocking motion is maintained to repetitively stretch these structures. It is important for the knee on the extended leg to remain fully extended during the exercise which should be repeated slowly and strongly fifteen to twenty times.

Anterolateral Thigh Stretch

The patient sits on a stool with the back against a wall. The hands should be placed palm forward beside the head. The low back should be flattened against the wall by retracting the abdominal muscles. An effort to push the body against the wall is made whilst of the head is stretched upwards with the chin pressed in and back. The elbows should be pressed back against the wall. This position should be maintained for not less than one minute.

Upper Back Trapezius Stretch (1)

The same position as above should be adopted but this time with the arms upwards and outwards so that they are stretched diagonally away from the midline at about 45° from the vertical. This position (abdomen retracted, chin in and crown of the head up) should be maintained for at least a minute. A few variations in arm position, to bring them directly above the head and then return to the diagonal position should be carried out during the exercise.

Upper Back and Trapezius Stretch (2)

The patient stands with feet twelve inches (30cm) apart and with the feet externally rotated to an angle of about 30° from the parallel. The heels remain flat on the floor throughout. In women accustomed to high heels this will not be possible and in this event shoes should be worn. At no point during this exercise should

Muscle Balance and Lumbosacral Flexion Exercise

the patient rise onto the toes. The spine should be flexed with head bowed, the arms should be pointed to the floor at a point between the toes.

A 'flat-footed' squat is then performed so that the buttocks approximate the heels and the fingers touch the floor, elbows between the knees. If there is a tendency to overbalance (as will be the case with long-femured individuals) a counter balance of about 8 lbs (3½kg) may be held. By attempting to reach the desired position repeatedly (ten to fifteen times) a degree of stretching will occur in the lumbosacral area and in the posterior calf. The quadriceps femoris and gluteus maximus will be strengthened.

Having reached the position of squatting, an up and down jigging movement is useful — this can be thought of as trying to 'tuck the tail between the legs'.

Foot and Knee Stretch

The patient stands with feet straight forward about two inches (5cm) apart. The knees should be relaxed, neither rigid nor bent. The foot and calf muscles that raise the arch should be contracted and the weight should be transferred slightly to the outer borders of the feet. The buttocks should be tightened to externally rotate the legs to the degree that allows the knees to point directly forward. This is to be repeated ten to fifteen times.

Depending upon the indications the appropriate exercises should be performed daily.

Conclusion

In the long run posture can only be corrected by the individual learning afresh how to use his body machines correctly. The breaking of old habits and the learning of new ones is not easy but the employment of NMT to normalize the soft tissues will increase the individuals awareness of his body's structures whilst at the same time removing restrictions which can often physically prevent correct use of a part of the body. If one part malfunctions then the whole will malfunction. In earlier chapters we have seen how posture, tension, dysfunction and emotional states are often intertwined. By breaking into this web of interconnecting factors and releasing soft tissue structures from the contractions and patterns of stress imposed upon them, many of the other aspects of the problem will become more easily soluble. Thus with soft tissue relaxation comes the chance for postural improvement as well as a re-education in muscular tension patterns and a reduction of fatigue and those psychological tension states that feed on these physical conditions.

In treating the individual for postural dysfunction, NMT, applied to spinal, abdominal and other regions (limbs for example), is of prime importance. Combined with this, MET methods are of value in removing areas of undue tightness. All other techniques, outlined in Chapter 5, may be employed as and when indicated. No attempt should be made to introduce exercise programmes for the strengthening of weak muscle groups until all efforts to release and stretch tight antagonists is completed. Using NMT and MET primarily, a series of ten to twelve treatments is usually adequate for the achievement of what one might term postural restructuring. A sequence of treatment to different areas might be carried out. The author has found the following pattern to be useful, at weekly intervals:

Treatment 1. NMT to superficial spinal and abdominal regions. Assessments of tight muscle groups.

Treatment 2. NMT to feet and entire legs, and assessment of tight muscle groups in this area.

Treatment 3. NMT to neck and shoulders. MET to areas found shortened on previous visits.

Treatment 4. NMT to thorax, anterior and posterior. Breathing function assessed. MET to areas found shortened on previous visit.

Treatment 5. NMT and MET to legs and pelvis, especially postural muscles (TFL, psoas, hamstring, etc.).

Treatment 6. ⎰ NMT and MET attention to spinal and abdominal musculature,
Treatment 7. ⎱ with attention to postural and trigger point factors.

Treatment 8. Concentration on balancing muscle groups which have tightened, mainly using MET. Breathing reassessed.

Treatment 9. Re-education regarding posture and habitual patterns of use. Basic exercise patterns to weakened structures, which have not strengthened after stretching of tight antagonists.

Treatment 10. General NMT to reassess soft tissues. Exercises and MET (and self-treatment with MET for any structures still shortened).

This would provide a basic normalizing influence on posture and function, but treatment at weekly intervals could be needed, for many months yet, depending upon individual problems.

[1] Page, Dr Leon, *Academy of Applied Osteopathy Yearbook* (1952).

[2] Jones, Lawrence, *The Postural Complex*, (Charles Thomas, Springfield, Illinois, 1955).

[3] Kendall, Kendall and Boynton, *Posture and Pain*, (The Williams and Wilkins Co., Baltimore, 1952).

Chapter 5

Techniques and Index of Neurolymphatic Reflexes

The thumb technique employed in NMT enables a wide variety of therapeutic effects **Thumb** to be produced by its different activities. The tip of the thumb imparts a varying **Technique** degree of pressure via any of four facets. The very tip may be employed or the medial or lateral aspect of the tip can be used to make contact with angled surfaces. For more general (less localized or less specific) contact, of a diagnostic or therapeutic type, the broad surface of the last phalange of the thumb is often used.

The hand is always spread so that the direction of the thumb stroke runs towards one of the fingertips. During the stroke, which covers between two and three inches (5-8cm), the fingertips act as a fulcrum point. The chief force is imparted to the thumb tip by the operator leaning onto the thumb in a controlled manner. The thumb thus never leads the hand but always trails behind the fingers, the tips of which rest just beyond the end of the stroke.

The extreme versatility of the thumb enables it to modify the direction of imparted force in accordance with the indications of the tissue being treated. As the thumb glides across and through those tissues it is an extension of the operator's brain. In fact, for the clearest assessment of what is being palpated the operator should close his eyes so that every minute change in the tissue can be felt and reacted to.

The thumb and hand seldom impart their own muscular force except in dealing with small localized contractures or fibrotic 'nodules'. In order that the force be transmitted directly to its target, the weight being imparted from the shoulder should travel in as straight a line as possible. To this end the arm should not be flexed at the elbow or the wrist by more than a few degrees. The positioning of the operator's body in relation to the area being treated is also of the utmost importance in order to facilitate economy of effort and comfort. In this regard both the optimum height *vis-à-vis* the couch and the most effective angle of approach to the various body areas must be considered. The descriptions and illustrations in the treatment sections will aid the operator in this respect.

The degree of pressure will depend upon the nature of the tissue being treated. The thumb will allow for a great variety of changes in pressure during its strokes across and through the tissues. The patient should not feel acute pain but a general degree of discomfort is usually acceptable as the thumb is seldom stationary. A stroke or glide of two to three inches (5-8cm) will usually take four to five seconds, seldom more unless a particularly obstructive indurated area is being dealt with.

Of course, if reflex pressure techniques are being employed, a much longer stay

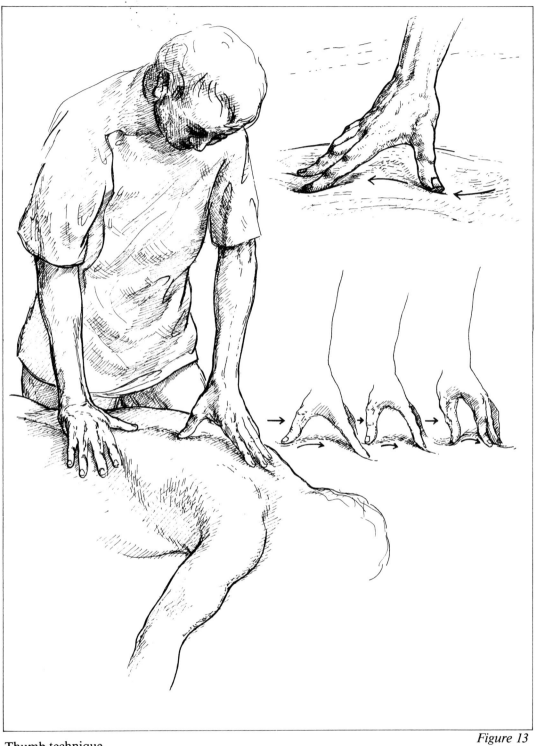

Thumb technique.

Figure 13

on a point will be needed, but in normal diagnostic and therapeutic use the thumb continues to move as it probes, decongests and generally treats the tissues. It is not, therefore, possible to state the exact pressures necessary. Obviously on areas with relatively thin muscular covering the pressure would be less than in thick, well covered areas such as the buttocks. Attention should also be paid to the relative sensitivity of different areas and different patients. The thumb is not just mechanically stroked across or through tissue but is an intelligent extension of the operator's diagnostic sensitivities and it should feel to the patient as though it is assessing every fibre of his soft tissues. Pain should be transient and no bruising should result if the above advice is followed.

In certain localities the thumb's width prevents the degree of tissue penetration suitable for successful treatment. The middle or index finger can be suitably employed in such areas. The most usual area for this is in the intercostal musculture and in attempting to penetrate beneath the scapula borders in tense fibrotic conditions.

Finger Technique

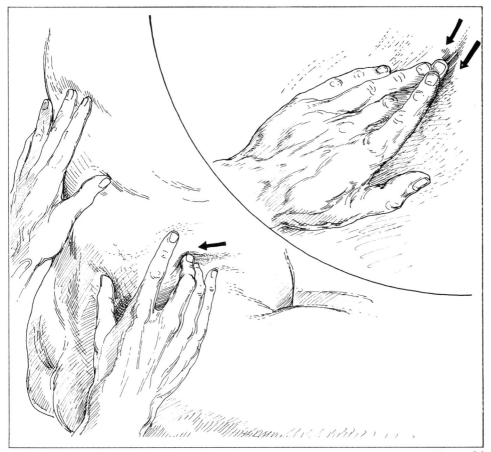

Finger technique.

Figure 14

The middle finger is slightly flexed and, depending upon the direction of the stroke, is supported by one of its adjacent members. As the treating finger strokes with a firm contact and usually a minimum of lubricant, a tensile strain is created between its tip and the tissue underlying it. This is stretched and lifted by the passage of the finger which, like the thumb, should continue moving unless or until dense, indurated tissue prevents its easy passage. These strokes can be repeated once or twice as tissue changes dictate.

The angle of pressure to the skin surface is between 40° and 50°. The fingertip should never lead the stroke but should always follow the wrist, the palmar surface of which should lead. It is possible to impart a great degree of pull on underlying tissues and the patient's reactions must be taken into account in deciding on the degree of force to be used. Transient pain or marked discomfort are to be expected but no more than that. All sensitive areas are indicative of some degree of dysfunction, local or reflex, and are thus important. This knowledge should be imparted to the patient so that a co-operative attitude is assumed.

Unlike the thumb treatment, in which force is largely directed away from the operator's body, in finger treatment the motive force is usually towards the operator. The arm position therefore alters and a degree of flexion is necessary to ensure that the pull or drag of the finger through the tissues is smooth and in order to protect the hand muscles from strain. Unlike the thumb, which makes a sweep towards the fingertips, whilst the rest of the hand remains relatively stationary, the whole hand will move as the finger pressure is applied. Certainly some variation in the degree of angle between fingertip and skin is allowable during a stroke and some slight variation in the degree of 'hooking' of the finger is sometimes also necessary. However, the main motive force is applied by pulling the slightly flexed middle finger towards the operator with the possibility of some lateral emphasis if needed. The treating finger should always be supported by one of its neighbours, usually the ring finger.

Skin Rolling Technique

This involves the use of either or both hands. The fingers draw tissue towards the operator whilst the ball(s) of the thumb(s) roll over the gathered mound of tissue. In this way the tissue is effectively lifted, stretched and squeezed. The most useful areas of application occur where the tissues lie tight to the underlying structures, such as directly over the shoulder joint and on the lateral aspect of the thigh. The squeezing pressure imparted by the roll of the thumb can be extremely uncomfortable and care should be exercised during its application. The angle of stretch, pull and roll may be varied and repeated several times to impart maximum stimulus to the reflex effects and to stimulate circulation and drainage. Stanley Lief and Boris Chaitow employed this simple, yet effective manoeuvre as part of their general treatment. The latter described its usefulness as follows:

> One of my favourite techniques to enhance nerve and blood circulation is 'skin rolling'. Between the skin and the muscular and bony structures it covers, is a veritable network of blood and nerve structures and functions which can, and often do, fail to achieve their full, effective circulation for high efficiency and health because the skin is often so adhered to its lower structures that circulation and function is appreciably reduced. This of course adversely affects the efficiency and health of the patient. There is probably no formula that will enhance this aspect of function more effectively than 'skin rolling'.

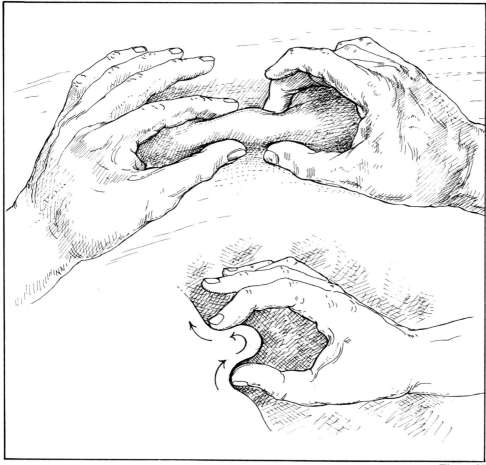

Skin rolling technique.   *Figure15*

A specific example of its effective benefit is to skin-roll a major joint such as a shoulder in conditions of articular rheumatism, arthritis, neuritis, frozen shoulder etc.

As noted in Chapter 2 the skin overlying regions, or points of reflex activity, will frequently be found to have markedly reduced elasticity, and to adhere to underlying structures. The assessment of these areas is described in Chapter 3. Treatment of HSZ involves the same procedure as is used for diagnosis. Fingertips, or the ulnar aspects of the crossed hands, are placed together on the skin surface. The tissues are stretched as the fingers, or hands, separate. In order to establish the presence or lack of physiological elasticity, the skin is stretched in various directions. If restriction is noted then the tissues are held in a painlessly stretched position, until a degree of release is noted. This should take no more than ten seconds. The same area may be stretched in this manner in various appropriate directions. The release of the tissues is itself the therapeutic effort, providing reflex stimulus. The subsequent maintenance of the free elastic state of the tissues is evidence of an improvement in the causative factors. Naturally,

Treating Hyperalgesic Skin Zones

if underlying factors maintain the reflex activity, whether this be musculo-skeletal or visceral dysfunction, the improvement will be shortlived. HSZ then become useful diagnostically and prognostically.

Lewit states: 'If pain is due to the HSZ, this method is quite as effective as needling, electrostimulation and other similar methods. Moreover, it is entirely painless, and can be applied by the patient himself.' Such zones are frequently noted with musculo-skeletal conditions, and in chronic pain syndromes. In cases of recurrent headache, HSZ are found medially below the mastoid process, at the temples and eyebrows, and on the forehead above the eyebrows, and on both sides of the nose. This correlates with many of Bennett's neurovascular reflexes.

Pinch-Roll Technique for HSZ

With the patient prone, the operator's hands are placed so that the fingers are more cephalid, and the thumb more caudad. The fingers draw skin towards the thumb, which lifts this fold. The tissue thus held, between the thumb and fingers, is then lifted away from the body, and rolled slightly upwards (towards the fingers cephalid). The degree of stretch, and/or pinch, employed, is a variable factor which the operator may decide upon depending upon the amount of stimulus called for. Either skin alone, or skin and underlying tissue, may be lifted, stretched and stimulated (pinched) in this way. Traditional Chinese medicine calls for this procedure to be undertaken from the base of the spine upwards, for a tonifying effect, and from the neck downwards, for a sedating effect.

Pressure Techniques

There are a number of different pressure techniques used for dealing with trigger points. Where underlying (i.e. bony) tissues allow direct pressure onto such points so that the trigger is squeezed between thumb and the underlying tissue, the variables will be the duration of such pressure and degree of continuous or variable pressure employed. Where no such suitable underlying tissues exist or where it would be dangerous to exert direct pressure through the muscle to the underlying structures (e.g. sternocleidomastoid) then squeezing or pinching techniques are employed. These will also vary with regard to the duration and nature (e.g. variable pressure) of the force imparted.

Chapman suggests a vibratory treatment, lasting ten to fifteen seconds, on the reflexes that he described (neuro-lymphatic). He used fingertip pressure to impart the required energy, although thumb pressure of varying intensity is just as effective. This can be applied as a gradually intensifying pressure building up over five to eight seconds, easing for two or three seconds and then repeated. Although this should not take more than half a minute. These points can be over-treated and the optimum time would seem to be from fifteen to thirty seconds with the pressure (or squeeze) of a variable nature. If the patient is able to report a referred pain resulting from the pressure then this can be continued for up to a minute, with fluctations in the degree of pressure, until the patient indicates a diminution in the referred pain or until the time has elapsed.

Use of skin stretching technique, and/or light digital pressure, is the suggested treatment of Bennett's neurovascular points. The successful application of therapy to these points is characterized by the sensation of pulsation, which should be felt on light palpation of the point after treating it.

As with other reflex areas, and trigger points, these will often have been identified during Neuro-Muscular Technique application. They have been noted as discrete areas of tissue alteration. They may palpate as being tender, or painful, to finger pressure, and will almost always be found to lie in muscle tissue, which is itself tense and shortened. If the points, thus located, refer sensations or symptoms, which may or may not include pain, to other areas, then they are trigger points. A point which refers symptoms to a target area of only weak intensity is termed a silent trigger, whereas one which refers strong sensations, and is itself very sensitive to pressure, is termed an active one. All other discrete areas of sensitivity, located in an assessment using NMT or palpation, but which do not refer symptoms elsewhere on sustained pressure, represent one of the other forms of reflex activity already outlined. Most such points will be found if in an active state of reflex activity, to have an area of cutaneous alteration overlying them, and this is the hyperalgesic skin zone, which may be treated as described. Most of the discrete areas which will be uncovered in this manner will be found to be lying in shortened musculature, and these tissues *must be restored to their full resting length* subsequent to, or as part of, any treatment method. Unless this is achieved the chances of obliterating the reflex activity is minimal. The methods of Muscle Energy Technique, as outlined in Chapter 7 should therefore form a part of any therapeutic intervention. The actual pressure techniques advocated in dealing with trigger points, active or silent, have been described by J. Vanneson D.C. (*Digest of Chiropractic Economics*, July/August 1977, pp55-64) as being, ideally, one of two forms of pressure. The first is a sustained static pressure, and the other a low firm gliding pressure which is applied to larger sensitized zones. Both methods are said to assist in the break up of circulatory stasis, caused by sustained vasoconstriction. The hydrodynamics of such pressure methods induce static fluids to be forced to move away from sensitized receptors. Such fluids also contain metabolic irritants. The amount of time involved should be determined by palpable easing of tension or the patient reporting a lessening of local and/or referred pains, sensations, or other symptoms.

This accompanies a lowered intensity of sensory stimuli, conveyed to the cord, and a complementary reduction in strong motor stimuli to the muscles in which the point lies. A combination of vascular and neurological changes, resulting from pressure techniques, is therefore responsible for reduction in pain, tension and reflex activity. At this point the muscle must be stretched to its full resting length whether this involves chilling and stretching, as described on page 160, or Muscle Energy Technique, or both, is a matter of personal choice by the operator. Both methods are successful. A far lesser degree of pressure is suggested in the treatment of neurolymphatic reflexes, as compared to trigger points.

It is important to realize that the objective 'feel' of these contractions is unlikely to change much during such treatment. Any changes resulting from the treatment will occur later, when homoeostatic forces have come into operation. The variation in pressure during the treatment is more desirable than a constantly held degree of pressure, which may irritate and exacerbate the condition. Mitchell, in the Foreword of *An Endocrine Interpretation of Chapman's Reflexes* (Academy of Applied Osteopathy, 1963) recommends that pressure be applied by the pad of the middle finger. This should be maintained as a light direct pressure in an effort to decongest the fluid content of the palpable reflex trigger. Mitchell believes that the determining factor for the amount of treatment to be whether a decrease in oedema takes place or there occurs a dissolution of the gangliform contraction, together with reduction in the sensitivity of the point over a period of between 20 and 120 seconds. The stimuli threshold is being raised in these points and inhibition of noxious impulses is being achieved. There is nothing to be gained from achieving local pressure anaesthesia (numbing) by exaggerated effort. Reflexes that are not painful should not be treated—only an active (and therefore sensitive) reflex point requires direction pressure as described. Any totally silent triggers may be dealt with by NMT, and subsequently with MET, which would normally correct the dysfunction locally as well as restoring normal length to the muscle.

Following treatment of reflex points (trigger points, myofascial triggers, myodysneuria, Chapman's reflexes, etc.) the muscles involved should be actively or passively stretched for up to half a minute each. Should this fail to result in the full resting length of the muscle being achieved, MET methods should then be employed.

Elbow Technique

In treating certain muscle groups, notably the gluteals and the sacrospinalis group, it is sometimes difficult, or impossible, to impart adequate force via the thumb due to the degree of resistance in the tissues involved. Elbow technique treatment should not be given at the same time as NMT but should be preparatory to it, on a number of occasions, so that NMT can subsequently be effectively applied. In treating sacrospinalis, for example, the entire spine should be well lubricated and the operator should stand on the patient's left side (patient supine, pillow under thorax).

The right elbow tip is placed just superior to the sacral base with the forearm at right angles to the patient's body. By flexing the knees slightly and allowing weight to be transferred via the elbow, the operator can apply controlled pressure to the muscles. The elbow is allowed to glide slowly cephalad. If pain is reported, lessen the pressure. Several glides or strokes along the full length of the spine will greatly relax even marked contractions. Similar techniques can be applied to the gluteal area.

Tissue Release Technique

In using NMT it is often helpful to apply a local 'tissue release' technique to areas of marked contraction or spasticity. In areas overlying bone the techniques suitable for use in the abdominal region are not applicable. The method recommended is as follows:

The contact on the tissues involved is made by extending the digits of either hand and making firm contact with the area between the first and second metacarpo-phalangeal joints. This contact is rotated clockwise or anti-clockwise in order to increase the tension in the underlying tissues. The other hand is then placed over the contact hand so that the downward pressure and rotation are reinforced. In addition, a further direction of stretch should be introduced by the second hand. The tissues are therefore receiving a direct downward pressure, a rotational stretch and a further degree of stretch, all maintained by the two treating hands.

The overlying hand should be placed in such a way that the radial border

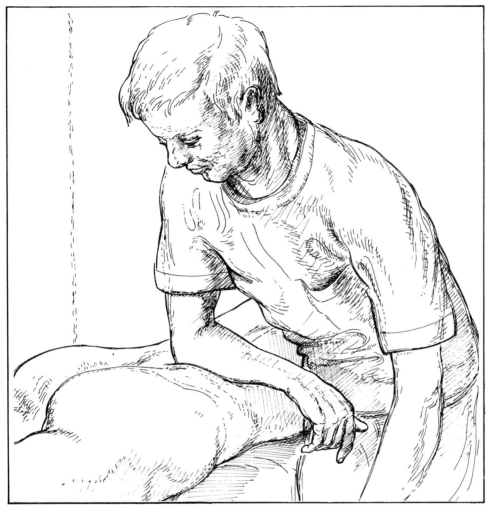

Elbow technique.

Figure 16

of the metacarpal base of the thumb is directly over the contact point of the first hand's contact (i.e. over the second metacarpal joint area). The fingers of the overlying hand should be tightly in contact with the lateral border of the contact hand. The final application of the release technique may be performed in one of two ways. The overlying hand executes a short sharp squeeze by flexing the middle finger against the metacarpals of the contact hand. The resulting pressure in the inter-metacarpal area provides the 'thrust' or release force. The line of force of this squeeze is towards the operator.

The second method of release, which is more suitable for deeper contractions of tissue, is applied via short sharp thrust by the overlying hand against the contact hand with a simultaneous medial rotation of the contact hand. The line of force in this technique is away from the operator.

Percussion Technique or Spondlyotherapy

In order to stimulate organs via the spinal pathways, direct percussion techniques have long been employed by Osteopathic and Chiropractic practitioners. A number of mechanical methods exist as does an effective manual system (Gregory's Spondylotherapy).

The middle finger is placed on the appropriate spinous process and the other hand concusses this with a series of rapidly rebounding blows for approximately five seconds. During this period about fifteen precussive blows should be applied. This technique is usually applied to a series of three or four (or more) adjacent vertebrae. An example of this is the treatment as above, of the fifth thoracic spinous process, proceeding downwards to the ninth, in the case of liver dysfunction. Treatment would only be applied if the area was painful to palpating pressure. Similarly concussion over tenth, eleventh and twelfth thoracic spinous processes would stimulate kidney function.

A mild 'flare up' of symptoms and increased sensitivity in the area treated would normally indicate that the desired degree of stimulation had been achieved. This form of manual spondylotherapy fits into NMT by virtue of its reflex effects and its easy application. Needless to say, a sound knowledge of spinal mechanics and neurological connections is a prerequisite of such a manoeuvre.

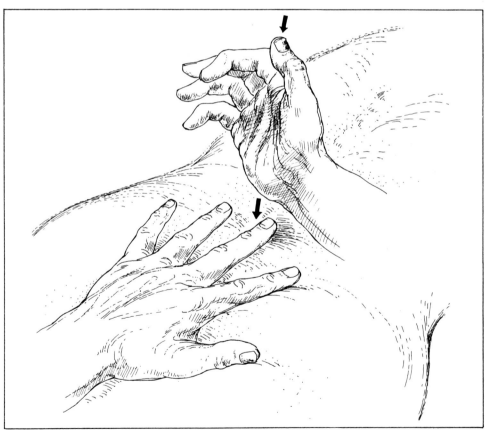

Figure 17

Percussion technique (Spondylotherapy).

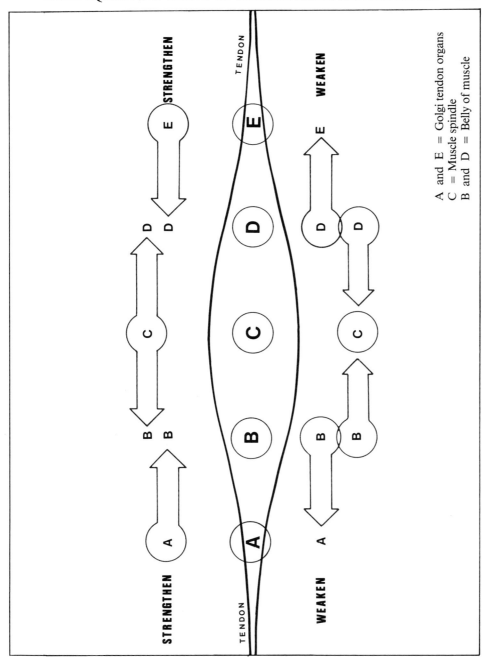

Figure 18

Proprioceptive Adjustment of Muscles and Tendons (Applied Kinesiology). Pressure directed away from the belly of a muscle in the region of the Golgi tendon organ produces relaxation of the muscle. Pressure towards the belly of a muscle, in the region of the Golgi tendon organ produces a toning effect. The opposite effect occurs if pressure is produced near the belly of the muscle. Pressure towards the centre, on the belly of the muscle, has a weakening effect, and pressure away from the spindle, in the belly of the muscle, produces a toning effect.

Proprioceptive adjustment (Applied Kinesiology)

Kinesiological correction utilizes two key receptors in muscles to achieve its effects. A muscle in spasm may be made to relax by the application of direct pressure (using approximately two pounds of pressure) away from the belly of the muscle, in the area of the Golgi tendon organs, and/or by the application of the same amount of pressure towards the belly of the muscle, in the area of the muscle spindle cells. Tendon organs, as the name implies, are found at the 'end' of the muscle, near the origin and insertion. Muscle spindles are found more predominantly near the central portion of the muscles.

The precise opposite effects (i.e. toning or strengthening the muscle) is said to be achieved by applying pressure away from the belly of the muscle, in the muscle spindle region, and towards the belly of the muscle in the tendon organ region.

The basic assumption of Applied Kinesiology is that attention to the weakened musculature should be primary. The strengthening of this results in a contribution towards normalization of contraction which will have taken place in the antagonists.

These principles should be borne in mind, and may be used by means of the simplified system described above, relating to Golgi tendon organs and muscle spindles, or by use of muscle energy methods which, via isometric and isotonic concentric contractions, can 'weaken' or 'strengthen' muscles as appropriate.

Many authorities, as we have noted, take the opposite view, and prefer to deal with the contracted, shortened musculature before paying attention to the weakened muscles, which should tone up in response to their antagonists being relaxed.

Specific Psoas Technique

In postural distortion such as scoliotis or marked lumbar lordotic conditions as well as in many acute low back and sciatic cases, the ilio-psoas muscle is found to be involved.

Lewit (*Manipulative Therapy in Rehabilitation of the Motor System* Butterworths, 1985) mentions that, in many ways the psoas behaves as if it were

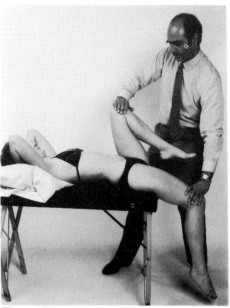

Figure 19

Treatment of psoas spasm: Patient lies with buttocks at edge of table, leg on unaffected side, flexed at knee and hip, leg on affected side hanging down. Operator fixes flexed knee and exerts downward pressure on the other limb as patient attempts to raise it. The isometric contraction is held for 5-10 seconds with minimal force being employed. After relaxation the leg should be able to hang further towards the floor if psoas relaxation has occurred. Repeat until maximum release achieved. Note that patient may hold the flexed knee.

an internal organ. Tension in the psoas may be secondary to kidney disease, and one of its frequent clinical manifestations, when in spasm, is that it reproduces the pain of gall-bladder disease (often after the organ has been removed). The characteristics of psoas problems are not difficult to diagnose, according to Harrison Fryette (*Principles of Osteopathic Technique*, Academy of Applied Osteopathy, 1954).

The distortions produced in inflammation and/or spasm in the psoas are characteristic and cannot be produced by other dysfunction, he maintains. The origin of the psoas is from 12th thoracic to (and including) the 4th lumbar, but not the 5th lumbar. The insertion is into the lesser trochanter of the femur, and thus, when psoas spasm exists unilaterally, the patient is drawn forwards and side-bent to the involved side. The ilium on the side will rotate backwards on the sacrum, and the thigh will be averted. When both muscles are involved the patient is drawn forward, with the lumbar curve locked in flexion. This is the characteristic reversed lumbar spine. The 5th lumbar is not involved, but great mechanical stress is placed upon it, when the other lumbar vertebrae are fixed in a kyphotic state. In unilateral psoas spasms a rotary stress is noted at the level of 5th lumbar. The main mechanical involvement is usually at the lumbodorsal junction. Attempts to treat the resulting pain, which is frequently located in the region of the 5th lumbar and sacro-iliac, by attention to these areas, will be of little use. Attention to the muscular component (see below) as well as the mechanical dysfunction at the lumbordorsal junction, is usually successful.

Apart from the direct pressure methods, described below, there are also a number of muscle energy methods, as described by Lewit and Grieve (*Mobilization of the Spine*, Churchill Livingstone, 1985). These will also be discussed below. Lewit maintains that psoas involvement is usually associated with spasm of the thoracolumbar erector spinae, and that relaxation of these will often release psoas spasm, and vice versa. A number of trigger points are likely to be found in the rectus abdominis muscles in such conditions.

The Test for Psoas Contraction

Measure for contracted psoas by standing at head of table, with patient lying supine and hands stretched overhead. Be sure to line the mid-line of the palms up with the nose, umbilicus and mid-point between the ankles. Grasp the wrists equally and, with equal tension, pull gently above head as far as possible. The short arm side indicates the side of psoas contraction. Be sure to repeat the test after relaxing psoas. If both arms are found to be of equal length but tension is felt to be equal in both shoulders, then both psoas muscles may be contracted. X-ray diagnosis is the only sure method of determining psoas contraction and its effects of spinal function. (See also Test 18 on page 114.)

Psoas Technique

(a) Patient lies on back with knees flexed, hands at side. Practitioner stands on side opposite contracted psoas. One hand presses down firmly through the linea alba, three to four inches (7-10cm) below the umbilicus until the probing fingers contact the body of the fourth to fifth lumbars. Then gently slide fingers laterally until the body of the psoas is felt and maintain firm but gentle pressure for about a minute. Check arms overhead and, if even, the psoas is relaxed.

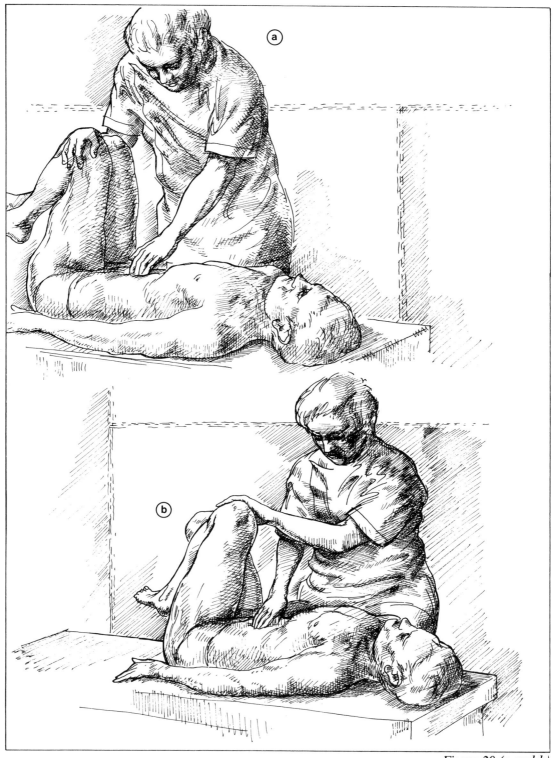

Figure 20 (a and b)

Psoas techniques.

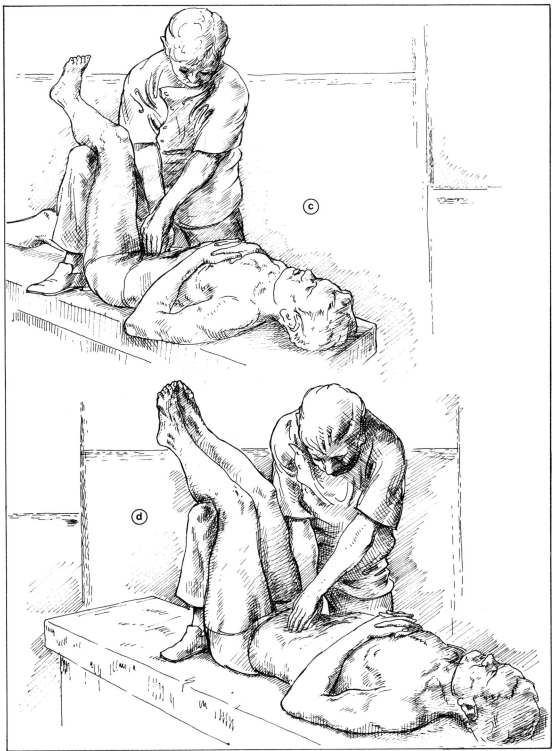

Figure 20 (c and d)

Psoas techniques.

(b) Same as (a) except practitioner is seated on opposite side of contraction. Same contact with fingers through linea alba but with the other hand bringing the flexed leg towards the opposite shoulder and rotating the pelvis against probing fingers.

(c) Same as (a) except the practitioner places his flexed leg on the table to support the patient's leg on contracted psoas side. In this manner, both hands are free to support each other as they penetrate heavier abdominals.

(d) Same as (a) except practitioner's flexed leg supports both patient's legs. This is especially useful when there exists a contraction of both psoas muscles.

Muscle Energy Techniques for Psoas Spasm: Lewit's Method

Lewit suggests the same position for treating the condition, as is used for examination. (*See Figure 19.*) The patient is supine with buttocks at the end of the table. The leg of the side to be examined (or treated) is over the edge. The patient grasps the flexed knee of the other leg, which is then pulled towards the chest so that the lumbar curve (if any) is flattened against the couch. If the iliopsoas is shortened, then the knee of the leg hanging over the edge will be raised, instead of being below, or on a level with, the patient's hip. *Note:* in this position, if the tensor fascia lata (see page 156) is shortened, the leg will be slightly abducted, and the patella will deviate slightly outwards.

The operator may now fix the flexed knee, and with the other hand exert pressure downwards on the knee of the side being assessed. This establishes the degree of shortening in the psoas. If at the same time the patient is able to exert upward pressure with the limb, and if an isometric contraction were maintained for some 5 to 10 seconds (not using full force, but a minimal contraction), then post-isometric relaxation will have been achieved, and some additional stretch should be forthcoming after the patient has suitable relaxed. This may be repeated several times. Alternatively the operator may attempt to resist the patient's effort to push the leg into a greater degree of extension, thus employing the antagonists. After some seconds of appropriate relaxation, there should be additional play in the muscle, achieved by reciprocal inhibition. This may be repeated several times, always commencing from the position of greatest stretch.

Self-Treatment of Psoas

Lewit suggests self-treatment in a position as above in which the patient, having taken the extended leg to the limit of its stretch, is told to lift it slightly (say 2cm) and to breathe in slowly, and then to slowly let the knee drop as he exhales. This is repeated 3-5 times. The counter-pressure, in this effort, is achieved by gravity. Those familiar with Yoga methods will recognize that it is in an identical manner that the slow progression is made, in which students are able to approximate some of the more difficult positions required.

Grieve's Psoas Method

Grieve suggests another manoeuvre involving post-isometric relaxation. In this the patient again lies at the edge of the table with the unaffected leg flexed, and the knee pulled towards the chest. The leg on the affected side is hanging over the edge, with the medio-plantar aspect resting on the operator's far knee or shin. The operator is standing sideways on to the patient, at the foot of the table, with both hands fixing the thigh of the extended leg (just above the knee) to the table. The operator's far leg is flexed slightly at the knee, so that the patient's foot can rest, as described. This is used as a contact with which resists the attempt of the patient to externally rotate the leg, which is made at the same time as he/she attempts to flex the hip. The operator resists both efforts and an isometric contraction of the psoas, and associated muscles, therefore takes place.

After some seconds of the isometric contraction, and with appropriate breathing (see Chapter 9) the patient's extended leg is taken into further extension, and the process is repeated three to five times. The degree of effort should not be great, and should begin with no more than 20 per cent of the strength of the patient.

Induration Technique

Since many patients are too frail or too ill to allow the full NMT treatment to be applied, a useful technique exists to aid in normalizing reflex and local areas of the para-spinal musculature. Stoddard has pointed out that protective spasm in muscle can often indicate underlying pathology (osteoporosis etc.). Deep pressure techniques would be contra-indicated in such conditions.

With the patient sitting or lying, the operator runs the finger tips longitudinally down the side of the spine over the transverse processes. Any spot or area of hardened or indurated tissue that also palpates as tender to the patient is marked for attention. This is applied by palpating the sensitive area with the tips of the fingers of one hand whilst applying light pressure towards the painful spot with the other hand which is resting on the spinous process of the vertebra alongside the indurated tissue. Direct pressure (light) towards the pain should lessen the degree of tissue contraction and the sensitivity.

If it does not do so then the angle of push on the spinous process towards the painful spot should be varied slightly so that, somewhere within an arc embracing a half circle, an angle of push towards the pain will be found to abolish the pain totally and will lessen the objective feeling of tension. A slightly increased push (not a thrust) is all that is required before moving on to the next indurated area. This technique can be used with NMT or instead of the deeper probing measures which for practical reasons may be contra-indicated (patient's condition or patient's inability to adopt prone position etc.).

Temperomandibular Joint Dysfunction Treatment

Dysfunction of the TMJ is a vast subject, and the implications of such problems have been related to a variety of other areas of dysfunction, ranging from cranial lesions to spinal and general somatic alterations and endocrine imbalance. The reader is referred, for a comprehensive analysis of the causes and clinical management of this condition, to a major book, edited by Harold Gelb D.M.D., entitled *Clinical Management of Head, Neck and TMJ Pain and Dysfunction*, (W. B. Saunders Company, 1977). Diagnosis of the particular pattern of dysfunction is, of course, essential before therapeutic intervention is possible. There are many possible causes of TMJ dysfunction, and a co-operative relationship with a skilled dentist is an advantage in such problems, since many aspects relate to the presence of faults in the bite of the patient.

A knowledge of cranial mechanics is desirable, and a history of trauma should be sought in those patients presenting with TMJ involvement. One common source of injury is the equipment used in applying spinal traction, in which a head halter with a chinstrap is used. This can cause the mandible to be forced into the fossae, impacting the temporal bones into internal rotation. A strap causing pressure on the occipital region could jam the occipitomastoid and lambdoid sutures, upwards and forwards, also resulting in internal rotation of the temporals. This can cause major dysfunction of cranial articulation and function. This would be further exaggerated were there imbalances present in these structures, prior to the trauma. Inept manipulative measures can also traumatize the area, especially thrusting forces, exerted onto the occiput, whilst the head and neck are in extreme rotation. Inadvertent pressure can also be applied to the mastoid portion of the temporal bone during manipulation. Any situation in which the patient is required to maintain the mouth opened for lengthy periods, such as during dental work, or when a laryngoscope is being used, may induce strain, especially if the neck is extended at the time. All, or any, such patterns of injury should be sought when T.M.J. pain, or limitation of mouth opening, is observed. Apart from correction of cranial dysfunction, via skilled cranial osteopathic work, the muscular component invites attention, using MET methods, and other appropriate measures. Gelb suggests a form of MET which he terms 'stretch against resistance' exercises.

MET Method 1
Reciprocal inhibition is the objective when the patient is asked to open the mouth against resistance applied by the operator's, or the patient's, own hand. (Patient places elbow on table, chin in hand and attempts to open mouth against resistance for ten seconds or so.) The jaw would have been opened to its comfortable limit before attempting this, and after the attempt it would be taken to its new barrier before repeating. This MET method would have a relaxing effect on the muscles which are shortened, or tight. (*See Figure 21*.)

MET Method 2
To relax these, using post-isometric relaxation, counter-pressure would be required in order to prevent the open jaw from closing (using minimal force). This would require the thumbs (suitably protected) to be placed along the superior surface of the lower teeth, whilst an isometric contraction was performed. In this exercise the operator is directing force through the barrier, (operator direct method) rather than the patient (patient direct, as in first example. (*See Figure 22* and Chapter 9.)

Exercise 1
Gelb suggests a retrusive exercise be used in conjunction with the above. Both methods being useful in eliminating 'clicks' on opening the mouth. The patient curls the tongue upwards, placing the tip as far back on the roof of the mouth as possible. Whilst this is maintained in position the patient is asked to slowly open and close the mouth (gently), to reactivate the suprahyoid, posterior temporalis and posterior digastric muscles (the retrusive group).

Exercise 2
The patient places an elbow on a table, jaw resting on the clenched fist. This offers some resistance to the slow opening of the mouth. This is done five times with hand pressure, and then five times without, ensuring that the lower jaw does not

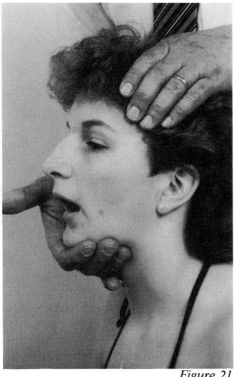

Figure 21

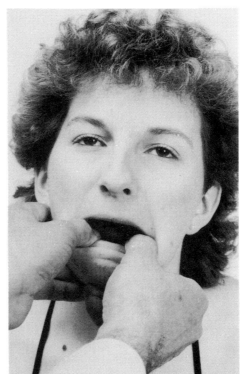

Figure 22

Above Tempero-mandibular dysfunction: Patient opens mouth against resistance applied by operator in order to induce reciprocal inhibition of tight musculature, preventing full opening of mouth. Self-treatment is possible by patient providing counterforce.

Above right Tempero-mandibular dysfunction: Patient resists operator's effort to force mouth open. Post-isometric relaxation results in improved ability to open mouth. Less than full force should be employed in all such methods.

Right Patient places elbow on table with chin resting on fist. This offers resistance to repetitive slow opening and closing of mouth. This is repeated five times against pressure, and then five times without. Lower teeth should remain behind upper teeth at all times, to avoid lower jaw coming forwards. Twenty-five such movements, morning and evening, help to restore normal function.

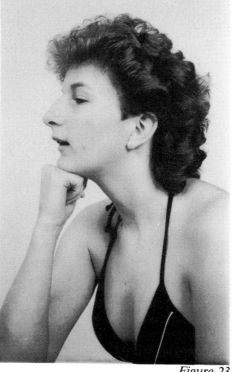

Figure 23

come forward. The lower teeth should always remain behind the upper teeth on closing. A total of 25 such movements are performed, morning and evening.

Exercise 3
Midline exercise: This calls for the placing of two halves of a round toothpick, between the upper midline teeth, and lower midline teeth. These act as markers, so that as the teeth are slowly separated and brought together (with opening and closing of the mouth) they can be seen to stay aligned. Use a mirror, and if deviation occurs the toothpicks should be realigned, and the exercise continued. This may at first mean that the patient cannot open the mouth very far, before deviation occurs. However, the corrective effect on the deviant muscles is such that this will progressively improve. The tight muscles will have to slacken, and the hypotonic ones will have to increase activity in response to the positional adjustments taking place during the exercise. This is repeated 25 to 50 times, twice daily. (*See Figure 24*.)

Below left Two halves of a rounded toothpick are placed between upper and lower midline teeth. As the teeth are slowly opened and closed the toothpicks are used as a guide to symmetry of motion, and can aid in realignment if deviation is noted in a mirror. Repetition helps to re-educate deviant muscles. Repeat 25-50 times daily.

Below right Tempero-mandibular dysfunction (jaw deviating to one side on opening). In treating a right side problem (jaw deviates to right on opening) the patient sits in front of operator, head turned to left. Operator stabilizes head against chest and cradles jaw. Patient's mouth is open and relaxed. Operator draws jaw towards his chest with his left hand imposing traction on right TMJ area. When slack has been taken out, patient offers resistance to further traction for 3 to 7 seconds. After relaxation PIR will ensure that greater excursion is possible laterally to the left. Repeat several times.

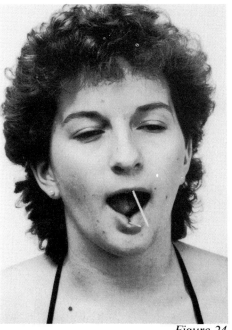

Figure 24

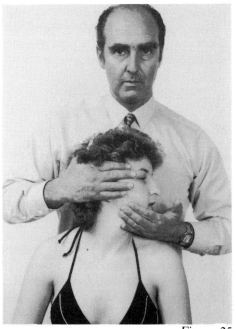

Figure 25

MET Method 3

Lewit suggests the following method of TMJ problems, maintaining that laterolateral movements are important, using post-isometric relaxation. The patient sits with the head turned to one side (say the left in this example). The operator stands behind her and stabilizes the patient's head against his chest. The patient opens the mouth, allowing the chin to drop, and the operator cradles the mandible with his left hand, so that the fingers are curled under the jaw, away from him. The operator draws the jaw gently towards his chest, and when the slack has been taken up the patient offers a degree of resistance to its being taken further, laterally. After a few seconds of gentle isometric contraction, the operator and patient relax simultaneously, and the jaw will usually have an increased lateral excursion. This is repeated three times. This should be performed so that the lateral pull is away from the side to which the jaw deviates, on opening. (*See Figure 25.*)

The principles of Muscle Energy Technique are simple, and the operator may use direct or indirect techniques involving isometric or isotonic, concentric or eccentric, contractions, to deal with the muscular components of any problem which can be identified as having soft-tissue involvement. See Chapter 9.

Applied Kinesiology

Applied Kinesiology founder, Dr George Goodheart states: 'Joint clicking on closing represents hypertonicity of the buccinator and masseter. This dysfunction could be facilitated by the origin and insertion of the masseter, internal pterygoid and buccinator being spread apart, stimulating Golgi tendon activity. This effectively restores lost vertical dimension.' In a similar manner, clicking on opening represents a unilateral or bilateral hypotonicity of the temporalis, which could be corrected by applying pressure into the posterior portion of the temporalis towards the condylar attachment, and reciprocating pressure on the condyle, resulting in tonus of the temporalis being increased, thereby reducing the relative protrusive position of the mandible.

This method is based on the principle of strengthening a muscle by pressure, applied to the area in which the Golgi tendon organ resides (near the origin and insertion) towards the belly of the muscle. To reduce the tone of a tense muscle, pressure (approximately two pounds) is applied towards to muscle belly in the region of the muscle spindles (nearer the midportion of the muscle). The reverse also applies (pressure away from belly of muscle in region of Golgi tendon organ, weakens it, and away from belly of muscle in region of spindles, strengthens it).

These are basic Applied Kinesiology Techniques, and can be seen to exploit the natural function of spindles and Golgi tendon organs, as does Muscle Energy Technique and much of NMT in its direct pressure methods.

Spontaneous Release Technique

In spinal and appendicular strains, injuries or lesions there is often an evidence distortion from the normal anatomical posture or position. This eccentric state is often relieved by placing the joint or patient in an exaggerated degree of the deformity found at examination. If this is held for 90 to 120 seconds a spontaneous release will often occur. Jones[1] states that this technique depends on the ability to produce relaxation of reflex muscle tension which limits and binds the joint(s).

The art is in finding the specific direction in which a painful joint can be moved which will release muscular tension and relieve pain. When passively placed in such a position for several minutes a lasting marked inhibition of painful stimuli will result with concomitant increase in motion. The evolvement of these ideas into a system, which Jones has entitled Strain-Counterstrain is detailed in the book of that title (Academy of Applied Osteopathy, 1981). This is described in Chapter 10. This method involves the identification of 'tender' points, which are associated with most joint dysfunction, and the positioning of the patient, or the part involved, in such a manner as to reduce the sensitivity noted in the palpated tender point. Jones declares that the points are purely diagnostic. However, since they may be equated with the spontaneous tender points, noted with joint problems in traditional acupuncture (Ah Shi points), it may be assumed that the maintenance of finger contact, and some degree of pressure on these points during the repositioning of the patient, or joint, involves some therapeutic input. A general guide to the position of the commonest points associated with joint dysfunction is given on pages 234 and 235. These should be seen as approximate, as the position of the soft-tissue response will, to a great extent, depend upon the precise position at the time of injury. Not only is relief usually achieved in an exaggeration of any distortion which may be present, but this is frequently a replication of the position in which the injury occurred.

Abdominal Techniques

Boris Chaitow, who worked closely with Lief wrote:

> Stanley Lief taught that manipulation (bony or soft tissue) should not only be confined to the spine itself but also locally to every possible area related to the particular symptom or stress. On the whole the Neuro-muscular Technique he devised is applied with the thumb, as this universally useful digit lends itself to the pattern of pressure and technique required, and is at the same time highly sensitive in diagnostic palpation.
>
> One of the areas of the body which Stanley Lief found uniquely amenable for his soft tissue technique, and can be used with dramatic results, is the abdomen. The enormous variations of functionally and structurally abnormal factors that can develop in the abdominal cavity are manifold. It can be safely asserted that there is no one in middle age and older who has not, unfortunately, developed some of the tensions, contractions, adhesions, nerve and muscle spasms in various parts of the gastro-intestinal tract and abdominal cavity so common today. All these would normally be outside the scope of the conventional manipulator. But, with the Neuro-muscular Technique, a practitioner can achieve almost dramatic benefits in local stresses and in health in general. He devised for the abdomen the special technique he called 'bloodless surgery' a method of breaking up deep-seated adhesions and contractions. It also enables the operator to improve function and circulation related to female problems such as dysmenorrhoea, menorrhagia and amenorrhoea, fibroids etc.

Specific Abdominal Release Techniques

In developing NMT Stanley Lief displayed an eagerness to learn methods from many sources. He was not content, however, to merely incorporate complementary techniques into his concept but developed and improved on the often crude ideas that others had originated. It was in this refining and adapting process that he showed his genius. During Lief's lifetime, and since his death in 1963, his cousin and former assistant Boris Chaitow has further enlarged on the basic technique and has brought NMT to the point where its application has reached a precise and refined use. As with all manual methods there is an indefinable element of art mixed with the mechanical and scientific aspects of its application. No one can acquire the art without practice and it cannot be taught. The basic mechanics, however, can be passed on by the written word and illustrations or, preferably, by demonstrations.

Lief used methods derived from an American system of manipulative or 'bloodless surgery' to amplify his abdominal techniques. His and Boris Chaitow's technique is presented here. These 'release' techniques can be applied to soft areas of the body (e.g. the throat) as well as to the abdomen. The original concept of 'bloodless surgery' was that adhesions were being 'peeled' away from their anchorage by the technique and in some cases this might have been so. However, its application is to any area of tight, fibrosed, spastic, contracted or adhering soft tissue in the abdominal region. The most dramatic improvements in function are noted after its use in such conditions as spastic or atonic constipation, visceroptosis, dysmenorrhoea, menorrhagia etc. as well as ill-defined abdominal congestion and pain.

Precisely what takes place after release technique is open to conjecture. An improvement in tone and circulation and usually of general function is the most obvious result. It is a matter of debate whether this is because of a release of a long-held contractive state in the soft tissues or because of an actual breaking of adhesions or because of some other mechanism. A general abdominal neuro-muscular treatment precedes the Specific Release Technique A. This serves to both relax and tone the area in a general manner whilst enabling the operator to localize areas which feel indurated or contracted objectively, as well as noting all areas of subjective sensitivity as reported by the patient.

It is these (a) tight, contracted and (b) sensitive areas that receive the release technique. The ability of the operator to localize accurately such areas is obviously critical and must be a matter for constant practice until the hands and fingers feel such abnormalities as a matter of course. To this end it is suggested that the middle finger of the right hand (in a right-handed operator) be trained to seek and mark those areas that will require specific release techniques. This requires practising the use of the hand in a position where the fingers are flexed so that the middle finger is slightly more prominent than its neighbours.

This aids its task of palpating specifically the tissues being probed. The non-searching fingers support the hand and are involved in assessing tissue tension as well as holding movable soft tissues as an aid to the palpating finger. The patient should be supine with knees flexed and feet as close to the buttocks as possible for maximum abdominal relaxation and with the head on a small pillow. The operator should stand facing the patient on the side opposite that being treated, i.e. to treat the left inguinal area the operator stands, knees flexed, leaning across from the patient's right side. This allows the tissues being manipulated to be drawn towards the operator in a controlled manner whereas such a procedure performed with the hands being pushed away from the operator, as would be the case if working from the side being treated, would cause a degree of pushing or gouging of the tissues resulting in pain and a lack of fine control.

Technique A

Having located an area of contracted (often sensitive) tissue the middle finger locates the point of maximum resistance and the tissues are drawn towards the operator, to the limit of pain-free movement. The middle finger and its neighbours should be flexed, fairly rigid and be imparting force in two directions at this stage, i.e. downwards (towards the floor) and towards the operator. (In 'bloodless surgery' techniques the right hand is always on the 'adhesion' and the other contact on the organ to which the lesion is attached.) With the fingers maintaining the above position the thumb of the left hand is placed almost immediately—no more than quarter of an inch (6mm) away—adjacent to the middle finger of the right hand in such a way that a downward pressure (towards the floor) will provide a fulcrum point against which force can be applied via the right hand in order to stretch or reduce the degree of contraction in the tissue (or indeed to break or 'peel' adhesions) The thumb should also be fixed and the contact can be via its tip or its lateral border or a combination of the two.

The idea of a fulcrum is important since the two points of contact are both on soft-tissue structures and the effect of the manipulation is achieved, not by

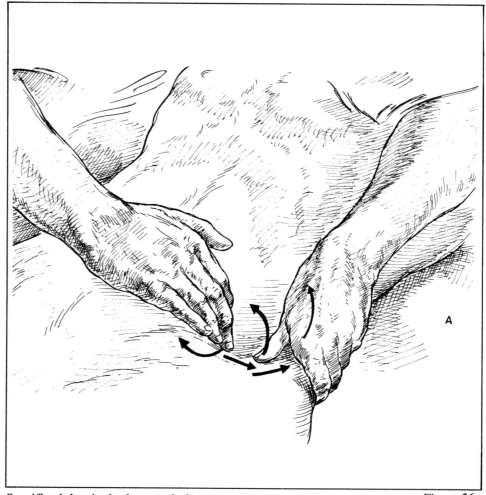

Specific abdominal release techniques.   *Figure 26a*

pulling or twisting these apart, but by a combination of movements which impart force in several directions at the same time. This is accomplished by a quick clockwise movement of the right hand (middle finger contact) against the stabilizing anchorage of the left thumb. Movement of the thumb during this release is not essential or necessary. However, Boris Chaitow does impart a degree of additional torsional force by releasing the thumb contact in an anti-clockwise direction at the moment of manipulation.

With both hands in contact, as described, and the contact digits flexed and rigid, the operator should be so positioned that he is leaning over the affected area, knees flexed with the legs separated for stability, elbows flexed and separated to a point of 180° separation. The force that will be present at the point of contact is a downward one, to which is added a slight separation of the hands, which increases the tension on the affected tissues. The manipulative force is imparted by a quick, flicking of the right contact in a clockwise direction whilst maintaining the left thumb contact (or taking it in an anti-clockwise direction).

The effect of the right hand movement would be to snap the right elbow towards the operator's side. If a double release is performed then both elbows will come rapidly to the sides. The amount of force imparted should be controlled so that no pain is felt by the patient. The essence of this technique is the speed with which it is applied and its success depends upon this as much as the correct positioning of the hands and the exact location of the area of tissue dysfunction. The same procedure can be repeated several times on the same area and the release of a number of such areas of contracted or indurated tissue, at any one treatment, is usual. The same thumb contact is often maintained whilst variations in the direction of tissue tension are dealt with by slightly altering the angle of the right hand contact and manipulative effort. If, after manipulation, no objective improvement is noted on palpation then the angle of the contacts should be varied. Nothing will be gained, however, by attempting to use excessive force in order to achieve results.

Since the degree of trauma to the patient is minimal, the after-effects should not include bruising or much discomfort. Any such after-effect would indicate undue pressure or force. Boris Chaitow describes the above method as follows:

> For the technique of NMT on the abdomen referred to already as 'bloodless surgery' palpate with the tips of the fingers of the right hand, and having located the area of abnormal feel, place those four fingers as a group at the distal border of the lesioned area and place the thumb of the left hand along the nails of the right fingers. Give a sharp flick with both hands simultaneously, the left hand thumb being twisted anticlockwise and the fingers of the right hand clockwise (difficult if not impossible to describe on paper). This achieves an appreciable breaking-up, without trauma or hurt to the patient, of tensions, adhesion, congestions etc., both on the wall of the abdomen and structures within the cavity. Obviously these flicks with the hands have to be repeated a number of times to feel a discernible difference in the lesioned tissue. Stanley Lief achieved dramatic changes in tissue structure and functional improvements in many types of abdominal stresses including digestive problems, gall bladder blockage, gall stones, constipation, spastic colon, colic, colitis, uterine fibroids, dysmenorrhoea, menorrhagia, small non-malignant abdominal tumours, post-operative adhesions etc.

Technique B
A second method for the release of tense, contracted, indurated connective and muscular tissue, is sometimes employed. This requires the same positioning of

the patient and the operator, as in method A. It is worth recalling that thickening will occur in fascia in accordance with the degree of stress imposed upon it. Since enormous gravitational stress occurs in the abdominal region, as a result of postural embarrassment, it is frequently the case that tight 'stress bands' will be felt inferior, superior or lateral to internal organs (e.g. intestinal structures) that have sagged and become displaced. Such contracted tissue is often the source of reflex trigger activity and is often, in itself, the cause of mechanical interference with normal venous and lymphatic drainage as well as being a possible source of pain. Any procedure that helps to normalize such tension should be accompanied by a programme of postural re-education and exercise if it is to have any lasting beneficial effects.

The operator's right hand, fingers flexed and middle finger slightly in the lead, probes through the surface abdominal musculature and attempts to 'lift' the structures beneath towards himself. In this way, areas of abnormal resistance will be quite easily traced by the tip of the middle finger of the right hand. The most inferior point of attachment of such a band is located and held firmly by this flexed

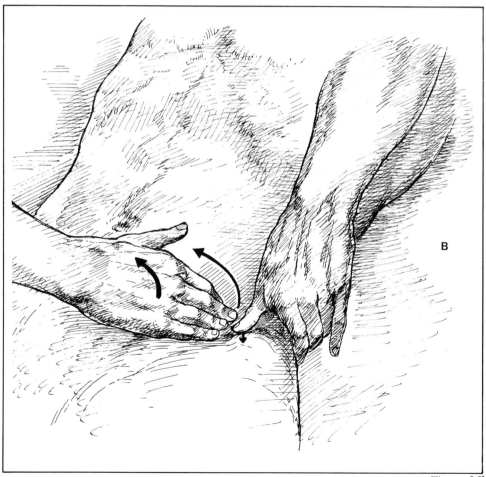

Specific abdominal release techniques.

Figure 26b

digit. The tip and lateral border of the thumb of the left hand is then placed adjacent to this contact so that the right hand contact is on the tension band and the left contact is on the structure to which it attaches. The manipulative force is achieved by a rapid, anticlockwise movement of the right contact whilst firm stabilizing pressure is maintained by the left thumb.

The closer the two contacts are to each other at the moment of release, the less force is required and the less danger of injury to the tissues there will be. It is suggested that by visualizing an attempt to tear an envelope held between thumbs and forefingers this concept will be better understood. The closer the holding digits are to each other the easier such an operation would be. Since the manipulative effort is attempting to, at least, stretch and, at most, separate the fibres involved it is necessary to impart a high velocity, low amplitude torsional force and not a vague stretching effort imparted over a large area of unyielding tissue.

The actual manipulative force is imparted by the tip of the middle finger of the right hand but is of course the result of the movement of the whole hand. The wrist snaps medially and the elbow outwards at the moment of release. This speedy 'flicking' action is one that should be practised over and over again so that its execution is a matter of routine. A release of contracted tissue will be followed by an immediate freedom of mobility of tissues and of organs formerly 'bound' and immobile. Such 'release' procedures (A or B) should be performed throughout the abdominal area and should be preceded by the general neuro-muscular treatment and be followed by a general procedure to 'lift' the abdominal contents back to a physiologically correct position. Abdominal and postural exercises on the part of the patient, combined with diaphragmatic breathing techniques, should also be carried out. A series of six to ten such treatments over a period of a month or so is suggested in chronic conditions involving visceroptosis and abdominal congestion. The application of these techniques to the hypogastric and inguinal regions will be found to be of immense benefit to patients suffering from menstrual irregularities. Local function will be greatly improved as a result of the structural and circulatory improvements following specific release techniques.

Splenic or Liver Pump Technique

This is a simple measure, via which function of either the liver or spleen may be enhanced. The operator stands on the side opposite the organ which is being stimulated (left side of patient, reaching across for the liver, and vice versa for the spleen). Patient is supine, knees and hips flexed. The operator's cauded hand is placed under the lower ribs, and the other is placed anteriorly, just medial to the costal cartilages of the lower five ribs (see Figure 27). Alternative bimanual compression should initially be carried out in a direct anterior-posterior direction. This is done approximately twenty times per minute, for one to two minutes. After this the direction of the pumping action should be more in an antero-lateral direction, for a further minute. The effect on the spleen is such as to increase the leucocyte count by an average of 2,200 cells per cubic millimeter. (Simon Fielding D.O., *Journal of Alternative Medicine*, December 1983, pp10-11).

Basic Soft Tissue Techniques Derived from Traditional Massage

Petrissage (kneading, wringing and stretching movements)
These techniques attempt to 'milk' the tissues of waste products, and assist in

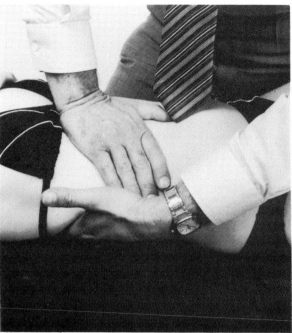

Figure 27

Liver pump technique: Patient is supine with knees and hips flexed. Operator stands at opposite side to organ to be 'pumped' (right side leaning across to stimulate spleen function, and left side to reach across to stimulate liver function). Operator's caudad hand is placed below lower ribs, and the other is placed just medial to costal cartilage of lower 5 ribs. Bimanual compression is carried out initially in a direct antero-posterior direction, at a rate of 20 per minute, for 1-2 minutes. Pressure is then directed antero-laterally for a further minute. When spleen pumping is carried out leucocyte count rises rapidly.

circulatory interchange. The manipulations press and roll the muscles under the hands. Petrissage may be performed with one hand, where the area requiring treatment is small, or more usually with two hands. In extremely small areas (base of the thumb for example) it can be performed by two fingers, or finger and thumb. It is applicable to skin, fascia, muscle, etc. In a relaxing mode, the rhythm should be around 10 to 15 cycles per minute, and to induce stimulation this can rise to around 35 cycles per minute. It is usually a cross fibre activity.

Unhurried, deep pressure is the usual mode of application in large muscle masses, which require stretching and relaxing. The thenar eminence or the hypothenar eminence, are the main strong contacts, but fingers, or the whole of the hand, may be involved. An example of this movement, as applied to the low back, would be as follows:

Both hands are placed on one side of the prone patient, one at the level of the upper gluteals, the other several inches higher, each hand will describe circles, counterclockwise, but they will do so in such a manner that as one hand moves laterally from the spine the other hand will begin to move towards the spine from a point a little higher on the back. The contact can be the flat hand, or the thenar or hypothenar eminences. The hands shape themselves to the contours of the back. The tissue between the hands, as they approximate each other, is lifted and pressed downwards and together. This squeezes and kneads the tissues. Each position receives three or four cycles of this sort before the lower hand takes the place of the upper hand, and it glides upwards to its next position. Little lubricant is required, as the hands should cling to the part being manipulated, lifting it, and pressing and sliding only when changing position. Even then a degree of deep stroking is used to move fluid contents.

One handed petrissage may involve treatment of an arm for example. In this the hand lifts and squeezes the tissues, making a small circular motion. Many other variations exist in this technique, which is mainly aimed at achieving general relaxation of the muscles, and improved circulation and drainage.

Effleurage (Stroking)

This is a relaxing drainage technique, which should be used, as appropriate, to initiate or terminate other manipulative methods. Pressure is usually even throughout the strokes, which are applied with the whole hand in contact. Any combination of areas may be thus treated. Superficial tissues are usually rhythmically treated by this method. Since drainage is one of its main aims, peripheral areas are often treated, in order to drain venous or lymphatic fluid towards the centre. Lubricants are usually used.

A useful low back variation is the use of stroking horizontally across the tissues. The operator stands facing the side of the patient, at waist level. The caudad hand rests on the upper gluteals, and the cephalid hand on the area just above the iliac crest. One hand strokes from the side closest to the operator away to the other side, as the other hand applies a pulling stroke, from the far side towards the operator. The two hands pass, and then without changing position, reverse direction and pass each other again. The degree of pressure used is optional, and the technique can be continued in one position for several strokes, before moving the hands upwards on the back.

This is but one of many variations on the theme of stroking; a technique which is relaxing to the patient and useful in achieving fluid alteration.

Vibration

This is used to reach below superficial tissues. It is performed by small circular or vibratory movements, with the tips of fingers or thumb. The heel of the hand may also be used. The aim is to move the tissues under the skin, and not the skin itself. It is applied, for example, to joint spaces, around bony prominences and near well-healed scar tissue to reduce adhesions. Pressure is applied gradually, until the tolerance of the patient is reached. The minute circular, or vibratory, movement, is introduced, and this is maintained for some seconds, before gradual release, and movement to another position. Stroking techniques are used subsequently, to drain tissues and to relax the patient.

Cross fibre friction involves pressure across the muscle fibres, and in this form the stroke moves across the skin, in a series of short deep strokes. One thumb following the other, in a series of such strokes, laterally from the spinous processes, aids in reduction of local contraction and fibrous changes. Short strokes along the fibres of muscle may also be used, in which the skin contact is maintained, and the tissues under the skin are moved. This requires deep short strokes, and is useful in areas of fibrous change. Thumbs are the main contact in this variation.

Another variation on the treatment of fibrocytic change, is the use of deep friction, which may be applied to muscle, ligament or joint capsule, across the long axis of the fibres, using the thumb or any variation of the finger contacts. The index finger, supported by the middle finger, or the middle finger with its two adjacent fingers supporting it, makes for a strong treatment unit (see *Figure 14*). Precise localization of target tissues is possible with this sort of contact.

The above is not a comprehensive description of massage-based, soft tissue techniques, but is meant to indicate the basic movements available, from this source. Some or all of these are bound to be of use, in any attempt to deal with the soft-tissue problems of patients.

Note

The enormous privilege which the patient allows, in permitting the practitioner to make physical contact in this way, also grants a degree of 'power' to the operator. Defences are lowered, and the patient is likely to be amenable to discussing areas of their emotions and thoughts, which they might resist in other situations. This presents opportunities for therapeutic intervention on other levels than the physical. The operator should be aware of the potent 'placebo' effect of which they are capable. Suggestions, and positive guidance, can have powerful influences on the patient, and thus care should be exercised, and diligent application of healing techniques undertaken, knowing that the recipient is, as a rule, receptive and highly suggestible.

'S' Contact Technique

The hands should be positioned in such a way as to allow basic thumb technique to be applied across the fibres of a contracted or indurated muscle or soft tissue area so that the thumbs are travelling in opposite directions to each other, about one inch part. In this way, as the short stroke is applied simultaneously with each thumb at a slow speed, the tissues between the two thumbs will be progressively stretched. This technique should be applied along the course of particularly spastic and hard unyielding tissues, as well as the basic thumb technique. It is called 'S' contact because the tissues being treated form that shape as the strokes are performed. The same procedure exactly may be used, but with a flicking action of the thumb to complete the stroke, once effective tension has been created in the tissues by the opposing thumbs. This 'springing' has the effect of stimulating local circulation most effectively and if the tissues are not too sensitive, may be effective in breaking down infiltrated or indurated tissues.

Piriformis Muscle Technique

The piriformis muscle syndrome results from contracture of the muscle which is usually traumatic in origin. The effects can be circulatory, neurological and functional, inducing pain and paraesthesia of the affected limb as well as alterations to pelvic and lumbar function. Diagnosis usually hinges on the absence of spinal causative factors and the distributions of symptoms from the sacrum to the hip joint, over the gluteal region and down to the popliteal space. Palpation of the affected piriformis tendon, near the head of the trochanter will elicit pain. The affected leg will be externally rotated.

The piriformis muscle syndrome is frequently characterized by such bizarre symptoms that they may seem unrelated. One characteristic complaint is a persistent, severe, radiating low-back pain extending from the sacrum to the hip joint, over the gluteal region and the posterior portion of the upper leg, to the popliteal space. In the most severe cases the patient will be unable to lie or stand comfortably, and changes in position will not relieve the pain. Intense pain will occur when the patient sits or squats since this type of movement requires external rotation of the upper leg and flexion at the knee.

A common sign of the piriformis syndrome is a persistent external rotation of the upper leg. This indication, which is known as the positive piriformis sign, is easily detected when the patient is examined in the supine position.

The buttock on the same side as the piriformis lesion is usually sensitive to touch or palpation. Severe pain may occur when pressure is applied to the area over the piriformis muscle and its tendinous insertion on the head of the greater trochanter.

Another diagnostic sign may be the shortening of the leg on the affected side due to contracture of the piriformis muscle. In cases where the leg on the opposite side appears shortened, it is probable that some other dysfunction exists and that the condition is not directly related to the piriformis syndrome.

In order to determine the effects of a piriformis muscle contracture on the sacrum, the patient should be examined in the prone position. In the case of a right piriformis muscle contracture, there will be a left oblique axis rotation of the sacrum. The sacral base on the right side will be seen to be anterior in relation to the posterior, superior iliac spine. The sulcus overlying this spine will be deepened because of the anterior rotation of the sacrum. The apex of the sacrum will be found to have moved to the left of the midline and more posteriorly at the level of the posterior inferior spine of the ilium. The sulcus on the left side will appear to be shallow because of the posterior movement of the sacrum at this point.

Additional findings that result from this oblique axis rotation of the sacrum include rotoscoliosis of the lumbar vertebrae and increased lordosis. There may be secondary or multiple lesion patterns that affect the entire vertebral column, including the atlanto-occipital region.

The patient also may mention pain that follows the distribution pattern of the sciatic nerve to the level of the popliteal space and sometimes to the more distal branches of this nerve. When the common perineal nerve is involved, there may be a paraesthesia of the posterior surface of the upper leg and some portions of the lower leg.

One of the most perplexing problems arising from the piriformis syndrome is the involvement of the pudendal nerve and blood vessels. This nerve with its branches, provides the major sensory innervation of the perineal skin and the somatic motor innervation of much of the external genitalia and related perineal musculature in both women and men. The pudendal blood vessels supply essentially the same areas. The pudendal nerve, after passing through the greater sciatic foramen, re-enters the pelvis by way of the lesser sciatic foramen. As it proceeds, it divides into three main branches. These are the inferior heamorrhoidal nerve, the perineal nerve, and the dorsal nerve to the clitoris (or penis) The perineal nerve divides into the posterior labia majora (or the scrotum) and the perineal body. The deep branch of the perineal nerve supplies the levator ani (in part), the transversus perinei superficialis and profundus, the bulbocavernosus, and the ischiocavernosus muscles. The branch to the bulbocavernosus further divides to supply the bulb. The dorsal nerve to the clitoris also supplies the crura, the prepuce, and the glans of the clitoris (or penis).

Compression of the pudendal nerve and blood vessels can result in serious problems involving the functioning of the genitalia on both sexes. Since external rotation of the upper legs is required for women during coitus, if there were interference with the blood supply and innervation of the genitalia, it is understandable that a female patient might complain of pain during sexual

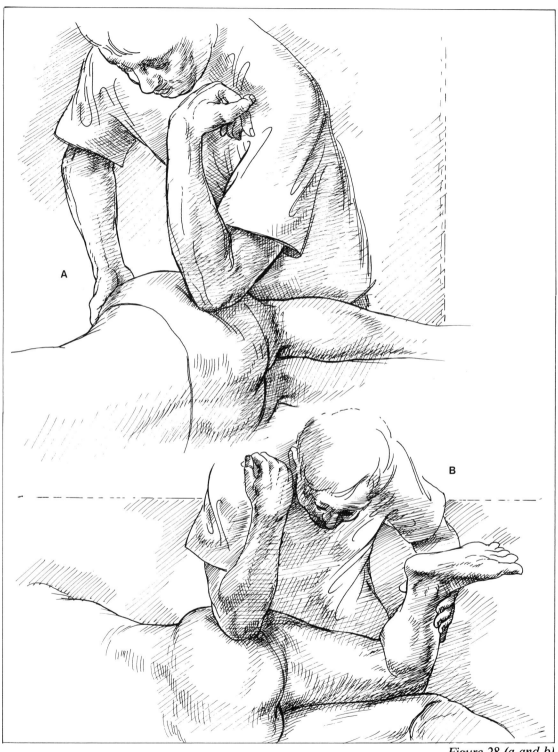

Piriformis techniques.

Figure 28 (a and b)

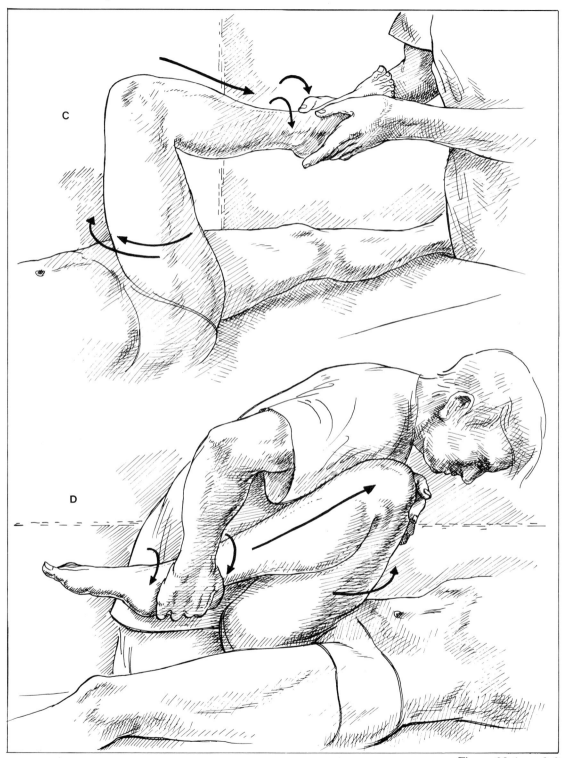

Figure 28 (c and d)

Piriformis techniques.

intercourse. This could also be a basis for impotency in men.

Thumb pressure is sufficient to remedy the problem which might require manipulation but which often yields to the following treatment.

Patient lying on side, affected side uppermost, legs flexed at hip and knees. The operator's elbow is applied to the piriformis tendon and heavy downward pressure is exerted for ten seconds at atime, up to ten times, with a few seconds rest in between. This should relieve symptoms of a traumatic nature where the condition is not of too long standing and where no spinal or sacro-iliac involvement is present. (*See Figure 28a.*)

With Te Poorten's approach to piriformis contracture the patient lies on the non-affected side with the knees flexed and the upper legs perpendicular to the body. The operator places his elbow on the piriformis musculo-tendinous junction and a steady pressure of 20-30 lbs (9-13kg) is applied. With his other hand he abducts the foot so that it will force an internal rotation of the upper leg. The leg is held in the rotated position for periods of up to two minutes. This procedure is repeated two or three times. The patient is then placed in the supine position and the affected leg is tested for freedom of both external and internal rotation. (*See Figures 28b and 28c.*)

The second stage of treatment is performed with the patient in the supine position with both legs extended. The foot of the affected leg is grasped and the leg is flexed at both the knee and the hip. At the same time the foot is turned inward, which forces an external rotation of the upper leg. When the operator causes the patient's leg to be extended, the foot is turned outward, resulting in an internal rotation of the upper leg. During the procedure the patient is instructed to resist the movements; this accomplishes a modified form of isometric activity of the muscles. This treatment method, repeated two or three times, also serves to relieve the contracture of the muscles of external and internal rotation. (*See Figure 28d)*

A number of muscle energy methods are used in normalizing piriformis problems:

1. One such is described in *'The Piriformis Muscle Syndrome', Retzlaff, E.et al, Journal of the American Osteopathic Association*, Vol. 173, June 1974, pp799-807). This involves use of the reciprocal innervation of the piriformis and gluteal muscles of both sides of the body. The patient lies supine, with both legs flexed at both knees and hips. The operator stands at the side of the patient, so that he can apply pressure to the non-affected side with his chest. He palpates the affected piriformis musculo-tendinous junction, posterior to the hip joint, by reaching through and under the patient's flexed legs. At the same time he asks the patient to attempt to abduct the non-affected leg against his body. This results in the non-affected side piriformis muscle contracting. At the same time the reciprocally innervated affected piriformis will note a degree of relaxation in the tense tissues if the procedure is carried out correctly. This should be repeated several times. Each contraction should last from 5 to 10 seconds, and should not involve more than a small degree of effort, initially. The patient should breathe in as the abduction of the non-affected leg is begun, and exhale as the contraction is released. This is known as Berry's procedure, and is based on Sherrington's Law, which demonstrates the simultaneous excitation and inhibition of opposing muscles, which in part states: 'reflexes initiated from points corresponding one with the other, in the two halves of the body, are commonly antagonistic.' (*See Figure 29.*)

Right Piriformis muscle technique using reciprocal inhibition: Patient is supine with both legs flexed. Operator stands so that chest is in contact with knee on non-affected side. Palpating the affected piriformis musculo-tendonous junction, he instructs patient to attempt to abduct the non-affected leg for 5-10 seconds. This is repeated several times until relaxation is noted at point of palpation.

Below Piriformis technique using post isometric relaxation: Operator rotates flexed leg on affected side in order to induce internal rotation of hip. When slack has been taken out the patient is instructed to attempt to return the leg to the upright position, with only moderate effort, thus contracting the piriformis muscle. This attempt is resisted for 5-10 seconds. After exhalation and relaxation the leg should be further rotated to engage the new barrier. Further efforts are made, slightly increasing the effort and duration, if necessary.

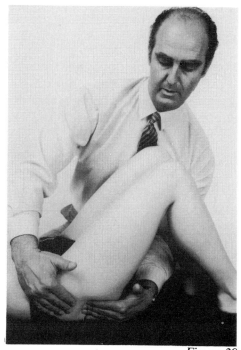

Figure 29

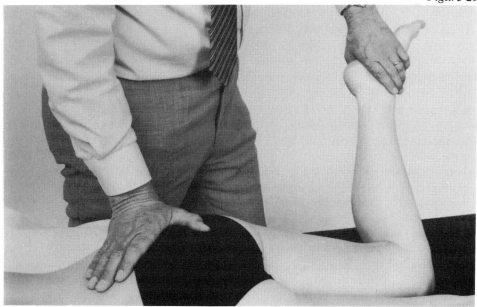

Figure 30

2. Lewit suggests a technique in which the patient is lying prone, with the knee of the affected leg bent at right angles. The operator rotates the leg outwards, so as to induce internal rotation of the hip. The slack is taken out, and the patient is asked to apply counter pressure (attempting to return the leg to a neutral position, and thus externally rotating the hip, and contracting the piriformis). The isometric

contraction, which should not involve more than a slight effort at first, should be maintained for 10 seconds, at which time the patient exhales and lets go simultaneously with the operator. After relaxation for a few seconds, the slack is again taken out by taking the leg further into external rotation (internal rotation of the hip) and the procedure is repeated 3 to 5 times. Self-treatment is possible in the same position. Once the slack has been taken up, the patient raises the lower leg slightly (i.e. returns it towards the midline) and holds this position for 20 seconds or so, before relaxing and allowing it to externally rotate to its maximum, before repeating the procedure a number of times (*see Figure 30*). Gravity is the counterweight in this example. (See Chapter 9 for details of MET methods.)

Stiles' Piriformis Technique (See Figure 31)
3. 'With the patient supine, and the knee on the painful side flexed to 60-70 degrees, face the patient and have him, or her, rest the back of the calf, just above the ankle, on your shoulder. Clasp your hands over the knee to stabilize it, Say to the patient: "Gently push your heel down on my shoulder, and pull your knee towards you." Have him/her push down and pull the knee against your resistance for a few seconds, then relax. The knee should then be extended to its new barrier, by pulling the knee caudad towards you. Repeat the sequence 2 or 3 times. This manoeuvre involves contraction of the quadriceps, the muscle group opposed to piriformis, and reciprocal innervation helps relax the muscle in spasm. Since it also uses muscles that flex the knee (hamstring and posterior muscles of the hip) it inhibits these muscles directly (post isometric relaxation) by stimulating their Golgi receptors. In general these procedures can improve results of straight leg raising tests, when the poor results are due to hamstring or piriformis spasm.'

Iliotibial Band Tensor Fascia Lata Techniques

The iliotibial band, when contracted or pathologically tight, is often misdiagnosed as a sacro-iliac problem. The symptoms associated with its dysfunction may include pain, localized in the region of the medial or posterior superior iliac spine. There may be radiating pain to the anterior, lateral or posterior aspects of the thigh, and also in the iliac fossa, which may suggest visceral disease. The symptoms frequently arise in the sacro-iliac joint, but its dysfunction is the result, in many cases, of tightness in the iliotibial band, the tissues of which may have numerous trigger points present.

One test of a tight iliobitial band is to have the patient lie on the unaffected side, with hip and knee flexed to 90 degrees. The patient is asked to hold the knee down to the table. The other leg, is taken by the operator, who is standing behind the patient. The leg is abducted and extended, to the point where the iliotibial band lies over the greater trochanter. The operator's cephalid hand will be palpating this structure, as the caudad hand raises and extends the suspected limb. The operator slides his cauded hand down so that the leg is supported only at the ankle, thus allowing the knee to fall towards the table. If the iliotibial band is pathologically tightened, then this will not occur, but the leg will remain suspended. The band will palpate as tender under such conditions, as a rule. (*See Figure 32* and refer also to Tests 15 and 16 on page 111.)

Another method is to have the patient side-lying, the side uppermost being the side to be assessed. The lower leg is flexed slightly, and the upper leg also flexed

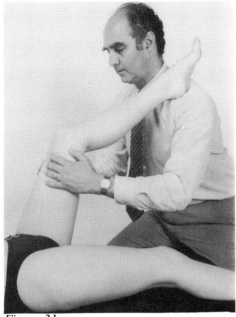 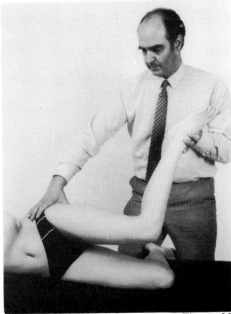

Figure 31   *Figure 32*

Above left Piriformis techniques (Stiles method): Patient is supine with knee on affected side flexed to 60-70° so that the back of the calf rests on the operator's shoulder. The knee is stabilized and the patient asked to push the heel downwards, and to pull the knee towards herself, at the same time, both against resistance, for 5-10 seconds. This contracts the quadriceps which opposes piriformis function, inducing reciprocal inhibition of the piriformis and also PIR of the hamstrings and posterior muscles of the hip.

Above right Test for iliotibial band tightness: Patient sidelying is asked to hold lower knee down to table. The other leg is extended and abducted until iliotibial band is noted to lie over trochanter. The leg is then suspended at the ankle only. The knee on that side should drop to the table. If it fails to do so, then the iliotibial band is restricted and will probably palpate as tender.

and lying slightly forward of the lower leg. The operator rolls the iliotibial band backwards over the trochanter, using the thumbs of both hands. A tight band will allow the foot of that side to move, so that the heel rises from the surfaces, and the leg internally rotates.

Treatment may employ a direct approach, as advocated by Mennell (*Back Pain*,   **Method 1**
Little Brown, 1960) or MET Methods:
    (a) Firstly the patient is placed side-lying, with both legs flexed comfortably. The first contact is with that part of the band distal to the greater trochanter. The *anterior fibres* are stretched first in a manner similar to that which would be used were the hands attempting to snap a stout stick. The fingers are laid over the anterior fibres of the band, distal to the trochanter, just above the knee. The thumbs rest, as a fulcrum, and are placed against the posterior aspect of the anterior fibres,

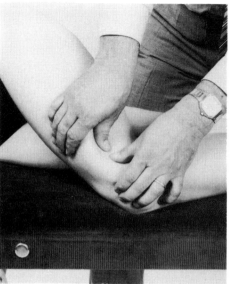

Figure 33

Left The anterior fibres of the iliotibial band are treated by the action of thumbs which are called upon to make a 'snapping' action as though breaking a twig. Pressure on osseous structures should be avoided as these fibres are stretched in this way. The area from the knee to the hip should be covered in this manner.

Right The posterior fibres of the iliotibial band are treated by pressure from the heels of the hands producing alternating thrusting strokes (piston like). Pressure on osseous structures should be avoided. The area from the knee to the trochanter should be covered in this manner.

Far right The tissues over the trochanter are treated by being rolled backwards by thumb pressure, and forwards by pressure with middle fingers.

and the snapping action is achieved by a rapid ulnar deviation of the hands (away from each other). The main force is transmitted through the thumbs, which should stretch the fibres without pressing them against the osseous structures (this would bruise the tissues). A series of movements such as this, starting at the knee and working upwards, is carried out (*see Figure 33*).

(b) The *posterior fibres* are then treated. The heel of each hand is pushed against the fibres alternately. As the heel of one hand pushes against the fibres, the other stabilizes them by grasping the anterior aspect. A series of piston like thrusts are made from above the knee, to the trochanter. Again the thrust must be against the fibres and not against osseous structures (*see Figure 34*).

(c) The region *overlying the trochanter* is treated by rolling it backwards and forwards over the bony prominence. The thumbs are the motive force, being pressed downwards and backwards, to achieve this. The roll is attempting to take the band posteriorly, over the trochanter. In order to roll it forward again, the middle fingers are employed (*see Figure 35*). As it rolls backwards, the heel of the foot on the treated leg should rise from the table (if the band is tight).

(d) The area *above the trochanter* is treated by deep, kneading massage or NMT. This is often easily achieved when the patient is prone, and the tissues are contacted by the fingers of the treating hand, with the operator standing on the side opposite the area being treated. The fingers may be insinuated into the tissues, and a degree of lifting, drag, as well as pressure medialwards, is achieved by the operator leaning backwards and drawing the treating hand towards him. This may be done as part of NMT treatment (see *Figures 40d and 40e). These structures require maintenance stretching, via exercise, if improvement thus achieved is to be held.*

Method 2   This is often more effective than the previous method. It involves either isometric or isolytic contraction.

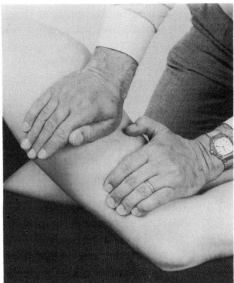 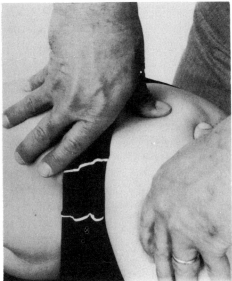

Figure 34 *Figure 35*

Isometric Contraction
In the first instance the patient would lie supine, with the unaffected leg flexed, and the affected leg extended. The operator takes the extended leg into maximum adduction, placing a maximum degree of stretch onto the lateral fibres (the abductors and fascia). In order to achieve this the leg will be brought under the other, flexed, leg. Standing on the side of the unaffected leg, and facing the patient the operator takes out the slack, and asks the patient to make an attempt to abduct the affected leg. This is resisted for ten seconds as the patient inhales. Release coincides with exhalation, and a little more slack is then taken out. The procedure is repeated two or three more times (*see Figure 36*).

Isolytic Contraction
The position is the same as above. Should the above be only partly effective, then, as the patient attempts to abduct the affected leg, (using only a fraction of available strength) the operator overcomes this and forces it further into adduction. This might be uncomfortable, and the patient should be forewarned. This will break down fibrous contractions. Progressively more effort, on the part of the patient, should be introduced on subsequent isotonic eccentric contractions. (See Chapter 9 for explanation of these methods.)

Self-Treatment and Maintenance
The patient lies on the side, on a bed or table, with the affected leg uppermost, and hanging over the edge (lower leg comfortably flexed). The patient may then use post-isometric relaxation, by slightly lifting the hanging leg, 2cm or so, whilst inhaling, and holding this position for a matter of ten seconds or so, before releasing and allowing a greater degree of stretch to take place. This is then repeated several times in order to achieve the maximum available stretch in the tight soft-tissues. The counterforce in this isometric exercise is gravity.

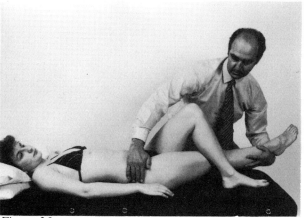

Figure 36

PIR for tight iliotibial band: Supine patient's affected leg is adducted to its maximum position. The patient attempts to abduct the leg, against equal resistance, for about 10 seconds. After release of effort a greater degree of adduction should be introduced and the contraction repeated. If an isolytic effort is required the operator would overcome the effort of the patient to abduct the leg, and would actually force it into greater adduction.

Vapo-Coolant Techniques for Trigger Points

The following method is adapted from the work of Dr's Travell and Mennell.[2] In the first place, one should use a container of vapo-coolant spray with a calibrated nozzle which delivers a moderately fine jet stream. The jet stream should have sufficient force to carry in the air for at least three feet. A mist-like spray is less desirable. See page 177 for details of pressure technique which should precede vapo-coolant technique.

The patient should be comfortably supported to promote muscular relaxation. The container is held about two feet away, in such a manner that the jet stream meets the body surface at an acute angle or at a tangent, not perpendicularly. This lessens the shock of the impact. For the same reason, the stream is sometimes started in air or on the operator's hand and is gradually brought into contact with the skin overlying the trigger point.

The stream is applied in one direction, not back and forth. Each sweep is started at the trigger point and is moved slowly and evenly outward over the reference zone. Probably it is advantageous to spray both trigger and reference areas, since secondary trigger points are likely to have developed within reference zones when pain is very strong. (The direction of movement is also in line with the muscle fibres towards their insertion.)

The optimum speed of movement of the sweep over the skin seems to be about four inches (10cm) per second. Sweeps are repeated in a rhythm of a few seconds on and a few seconds off, until all of the skin trigger and reference areas has been covered once or twice. If aching or 'cold pain' develops, or if the application of the spray sets off a reference of pain, the interval between sweeps is lengthened. Care is taken not to frost or blanch the skin.

During the sweeps, appropriate passive assisted motion should be employed to stretch gently the muscle containing the trigger point. Steady, gentle stretching is usually essential if a satisfactory result is to be achieved. As relaxation occurs, continued stretch should be maintained.

After each series of sweeps, active motion is tested. The patient is asked to move in the directions which were restricted before spraying was begun. An attempt should be made to restore the full range of motion, but always within the limits of pain, since sudden over-stretching increases existing muscle spasm. At the same time precautions are taken not to strain the muscles under treatment, either then or during the next few days.

The treatment is continued in this manner until the trigger points (several are usually present) and their respective pain reference zones have been sprayed. The entire procedure may occupy fifteen or twenty minutes, and cannot be carried out properly if rushed. However, after spraying the first trigger point for a minute or two and testing it for changes in sensitivity to pressure, one can usually predict whether a successful result will be obtained with the technique. Simple exercises which utilize the principle of passive stretch should be outlined to the patient, to be carried out several times daily, after the application of gentle heat (hot packs etc.).

The importance of re-establishing normal motion in conjunction with the use of the vapo-coolant spray is well founded. It may be that the brief interruption by the spray of the stream of pain muscles is not enough and that the input of normal impulses must also be achieved for the successful obliteration of the trigger points to be achieved. MET is also of value in achieving this.

All the methods described in this chapter may be incorporated into general Neuro-muscular Technique treatment.

Technique for Neuro-Lymphatic Reflexes (Chapman's Reflexes) and Index to Illustrations

The reflexes may be treated as part of a general neuro-muscular treatment or on their own in accordance with the recommendations contained in Mitchell's *An Endocrine Interpretation of Chapman's Reflexes*. This advises the treating by light digital pressure of the anterior reflex followed by the corresponding posterior reflex. The anterior point should then be re-examined and if there has been a palpable change, or if sensitivity has diminished, then no more action would be required. If no such change is found then the treatment to the anterior and then the posterior points is again carried out and if still no change is noted then it is assumed that pathology is too great for a rapid change or is irreversible or that there is a musculoskeletal factor maintaining the dysfunction. If this approach is adopted then the grouping of reflexes into systems is a useful method. If one of a group is found to be active then all others in the group should be examined and, if active, treated; for example, the endocrine group comprises: prostate, gonads, broad ligaments, uterus, thyroid and adrenals.

The respiratory group comprises nose, pharynx, eustachion tube, tonsil, larynx, sinus, upper lung, lower lung and bronchi.

The gastro-intestinal group comprises the colon, thyroid, pancreas, duodenum, small intestine and liver. The infections group comprises liver, spleen and the adrenals. The advice therefore is to use reflexes intelligently, treating only what is palpable and sensitive.

Some of the anterior reflexes (the ones which should, in theory, be treated first, lie on the posterior aspect of the body. These include those for haemorrhoids (No. 48) and cerebellar congestion (No. 21) and leucorrhoea (No. 25) and salpingitis (No. 41).

It is suggested that reference be made to the above-mentioned book for more detailed study. The notes following give the reflex by name, number and description of location together with an indication of which drawing illustrates it. It was not found to be possible to incorporate all the drawings onto one picture without creating a confusing series of overlaps. It is suggested that the practitioner learns to search appropriate areas for the type of sensitive tissue changes which are the manifestation of these reflexes and to use the drawings and the following list to become familiar with the patterns and groups of these important aids to healing.

Beryl Arbuckle ('Selected Writings of Beryl Arbuckle, D.O.', *National Osteopathic Institute and Cerebral Palsy Foundation*, 1977) gives practical advice regarding the successful employment of Chapman's reflexes. She urges that the points be not overtreated, giving a timing of anything from 4 to 30 seconds each. She also suggests that after all treatments employing neurolymphatic reflexes, the following routine be followed:

Lymphatic Pump Method 1   Patient prone, operator stands at side of table, half turned towards the head. Patient has pillow under chest, arms over the side. The operator's thumbs are pressed, bilaterally onto the intertransverse spaces, starting at the base of the neck. Pressure is exerted as the patient swings the arms forwards. This swing is repeated each time the thumbs move down one intervertebral space (*see Figure 37*). This will have a stimulating effect on the lymphatic drainage of the body as a whole. (An alternative position for the operator is to stand at head of table, facing caudad.)

Lymphatic Pump Method 2   The patient lies supine, knees and hips flexed. The operator is at the head of the table with hands spread across the patient's chest, below the clavicles, with thumbs

Below left Arbuckle's lymphatic pump techniques: Operator exerts thumb pressure onto intertransverse spaces as prone patient swings arms forward repeatedly as thumbs are moved progressively lower down the spine. This stimulates lymphatic flow and drainage.

Below right Lymphatic pump technique: The operator spreads hands across patient's upper chest, below the clavicles with thumbs resting on sternum. Pressure is exerted downwards and caudad, just sufficient to overcome resistance. The pumping action is performed at a rate which either corresponds with respiration, or up to 150 per minute. Continue for 3-5 minutes. This effectively stimulates lymphatic function and drainage.

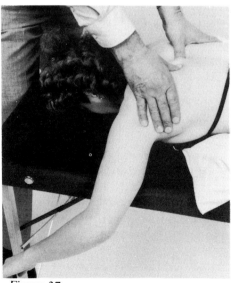

Figure 37

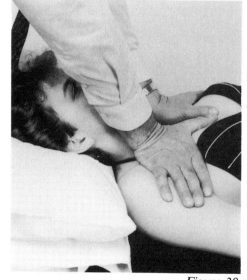

Figure 38

resting next to each other on the sternum, fingers spread laterally. Pressure is introduced by the operator, in a downwards and caudad direction, which is just sufficient to overcome resistance. The patient continues to breathe normally, and does not resist the repetitive pressure of the operator, which should be between a rate which corresponds with the respiratory rate, and 150 per minute. The patient breathes through the mouth, and the pumping action takes over the respiratory function (*see Figure 38*). This should continue for at least three minutes and up to five minutes.

In babies the method can be used with one hand over the sternum, the other under the spine. The effect of this is a dramatic improvement in lymphatic drainage. It is useful in all cases of oedema and infection. It also has a beneficial effect on immune function (*Journal of the American Osteopathic Association*, Vol. 82, No. 1, September 1982).

The use of Chapman's reflexes will provide additional localized drainage, which would support the general drainage and stimulation of lymphatic function, which the methods described above, provide. These methods are particularly useful in children, and their potency in infectious conditions is enormous. None of the procedures described should be painful.

Table 3. Location of Reflexes

Reflex No.	Symptoms or Area	Anterior	Figure	Posterior	Figure
1	Conjunctivitis and retinitis	Upper humerus	39a	Occipital area	39c
2	Nasal problems	Anterior aspect of first rib close to sternum.	39a	Posterior to angle of the jaw on the tip of the transverse process of the first cervical vertebra.	39c
3	Arms (circulation)	Muscular attachments of pectoralis minor to third, fourth and fifth ribs.	39a	Superior angle of scapula and superior third of the medial margin of the scapula.	39c
4	Tonsilitis	Between first and second ribs close to sternum.	39a	Midway between spinous process and tip of transverse process of first cervical vertebra.	39d
5	Thyroid	Second intercostal space close to sternum.	39a	Midway between spinous process and tip of transverse process of second thoracic vertebra.	39c
6	Bronchitis	Second intercostal space close to sternum.	39a	Midway between spinous process and tip of transverse process of second thoracic vertebra.	39d

Reflex No.	Symptoms or Area	Anterior	Figure	Posterior	Figure
7	Oesophagus	As No. 6.	39a	As No. 6	39d
8	Myocarditis	As No. 6.	39a	Between the second and third thoracic transverse processes. Midway between the spinous process and the tip of the transverse process.	39d
9	Upper Lung	Third intercostal space close to the sternum.	39a	As No. 8.	39d
10	Neuritis of upper limb	As No. 9.	39a	Between the third and fourth transverse processes, midway between the spinous process and the tip of the transverse process.	39d
11	Lower Lung	Fourth intercostal space, close to sternum.	39a	Between fourth and fifth transverse processes. Midway between the spinous process and the tip of the transverse process.	39d
12	Small intestines	Eighth, ninth and tenth intercostal spaces close to cartilage.	39a	Eighth, ninth and tenth thoracic intertransverse spaces.	39c
13	Gastric hyper-congestion	Sixth intercostal space to the left of the sternum.	39a	Sixth thoracic-intertransverse space, left side.	39c
14	Gastric hyperacidity	Fifth intercostal space to the left of the sternum	39a	Fifth thoracic intertranverse space, left side.	39e
15	Cystitis	Around the umbilicus and on the pubic symphysis close to the midline.	39a	Upper edge of the transverse processes of the second lumbar vertebra.	39e
16	Kidneys	Slightly superior to and lateral to the umbilicus.	39a	In the interverse space between the twelfth thoracic and the first lumbar vertebra.	39e
17	Atonic constipation	Between the anterior superior spine of the ilium and the trochanter.	39a	Eleventh costal vertebral junction.	39c
18	Abdominal tension	Superior border of the pubic bone.	39a	Tip of the transverse process of the second lumbar vertebra.	39d

Reflex No.	Symptoms or Area	Anterior	Figure	Posterior	Figure
19	Urethra	Inner edge of pubic ramus near superior aspect of symphysis.	39a	Superior aspect of transverse process of second lumbar vertebra.	39e
20	Depuytrens contracture, and arm and shoulder pain	None	—	Anterior aspect of lateral margin of scapulae, inferior to the head of humerus.	39e
21	Cerebral congestion (related to paralysis or paresis).	(On the posterior aspect of the body.) Lateral from the spines of the third, fourth and fifth cervical vertebrae.	39a	Between the transverse processes of the first and second cervical vertebrae.	39d
22	Clitoral irritation and vaginismus	Upper medial aspect of the thigh.	39a	Lateral to the junction of the sacrum and the coccyx.	39d
23	Prostate	Lateral aspect of the thigh from the trochanter to just above the knee. Also lateral to symphysis pubis as in uterine conditions (see No. 43).	39a	Between the posterior superior spine of the ilium and the spinous process of the fifth lumbar vertebra.	39d
24	Spastic constipation or colitis	Within an area of an inch or two wide extending from the trochanter to within an inch of the patella.	39a	From the transverse processes of the second, third and fourth lumbar vertebrae to the crest of the ilium.	39c
25	Leucorrhoea	Lower medial aspect of thigh, slightly posteriorly (on the posterior aspect of the body).	39a & 39c	Between the posterior superior spine of the ilium and the spinous process of the fifth lumbar vertebra.	39d
26	Sciatic neuritis	Anterior and posterior to the tibiofibula junction.	39a	1. On the sacroiliac synchondrosis. 2. Between the ischial tuberosity and the acetabulum. 3. Lateral and posterior aspects of the thigh.	39c
27	Torpid liver (nausea, fullness malaise)	Fifth intercostal space, from the mid-mammillary line to the sternum.	39b	Fifth thoracic intertransverse space on the right side.	39c

Reflex No.	Symptoms or Area	Anterior	Figure	Posterior	Figure
28	Cerebellar congestion (memory and concentration laspses).	Tip of coracoid process of scapula.	39b	Just inferior to the base of the skull on the first cervical vertebra.	39d
29	Otitis media	Upper edge of clavicle where it crosses the first first rib.	39b	Superior aspect of first cervical transverse process (tip).	39c
30	Pharyngitis	Anterior aspect of the first rib close to the sternum.	39b	Midway between the spinous process and the tip of the transverse process of the second cervical vertebra.	39d
31	Laryngitis	Upper surface of the second rib, two or three inches (5-8cm) from the sternum.	39b	Midway between the spinous process and the tip of the second cervical vertebra.	39d
32	Sinusitis	Lateral to the sternum on the superior edge of the second rib in the first intercostal space.	39b	As No. 31.	39d
33	Pyloric stenosis	On the sternum.	39b	Tenth costovertebral junction on the right side.	39e
34	Neurasthenia	All the muscular attachments of pectoralis major on the humerus clavicle, sternum, ribs (especially fourth rib).	39b	Below the superior medial edge of the scapula on the the face of the fourth rib.	39d
35	Wry Neck (Torticollis)	Medial aspect of the upper edge of the humerus.	39b	Transverse processes of the third, fourth, sixth and seventh cervical vertebrae.	39d
36	Splenitis	Seventh intercostal space close to the cartilagenous junction, on the left..	39b	Seventh intertransverse space on the left.	39c
37	Adrenals (allergies, exhaustion, etc.)	Superior and lateral to umbilicus.	39b	In the intertransverse space between the eleventh and twelfth thoracic vertebrae.	39e
38	Mesoappendix	Superior aspect of the twelfth rib, close to the tip, on right.	39b	Lateral aspect of the eleventh intercostal space on the right.	39c
39	Pancreas	Seventh intercostal space on the right, close to the cartilage.	39b	Seventh thoracic intertransverse space on the right.	39e

Reflex No.	Symptoms or Area	Anterior	Figure	Posterior	Figure
40	Liver and gall bladder congestion	Sixth intercostal space, from the mid-mammillary line to the sternum (right side).	39a & 39b	Sixth thoracic intertransverse space, right side.	39e
41	Salpingitis or vesiculitis	Midway between the acetabulum and the sciatic notch (this is on the posterior aspect of the body).	39e	Between the posterior, superior spine of the ilium and the spinous process of the fifth lumbar vertebra.	39d
42	Ovaries	The round ligaments from the superior border of the pubic bone, inferiorly.	39b	between the ninth and tenth intertransverse space and the tenth and eleventh intertransverse space.	39d
43	Uterus	Anterior aspect of the junction of the ramus of the pubis and the ischium.	39b	Between the posterior superior spine of the ilium and the fifth lumbar spinous process.	39d
44	Uterine fibroma	Lateral to the symphysis, extending diagonally inferiorly.	39b	Between the tip of the transverse process of the fifth lumbar vertebra and the crest of the ilium.	39c
45	Rectum	Just inferior to the lesser trochanter.	39b	On the sacrum close to the ilium at the lower end of the iliosacral synchondrosis.	39e
46	Broad ligament (uterine involvement usual).	Lateral aspect of the thigh from the trochanter to just above the knee.	39b	Between the posterior, superior spine of the ilium and the fifth lumbar spinous process.	39d
47	Groin glands (circulation and drainage of legs and pelvic organs).	Lower quarter of the sartorius muscle and its attachment to the tibia.	39b	On the sacrum close to the ilium at the lower end of iliosacral synchondrosis.	39e
48	Haemorrhoids	Just superior to the ischial tuberosity. (These areas are on the posterior surface of the body.)	39d	On the sacrum close to the ilium, at the lower end of the iliosacral synchondrosis.	39d
49	Tongue	Anterior aspect of second rib at the cartilaginous junction with the sternum.	39a	Midway between the spinous process and the tip of the transverse process of the second cervical vertebra.	39d

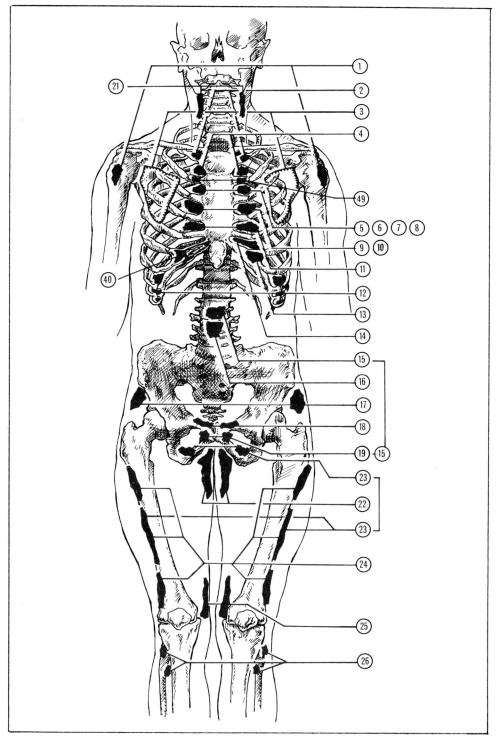

Figure 39a

Chapman's neuro-lymphatic reflexes.

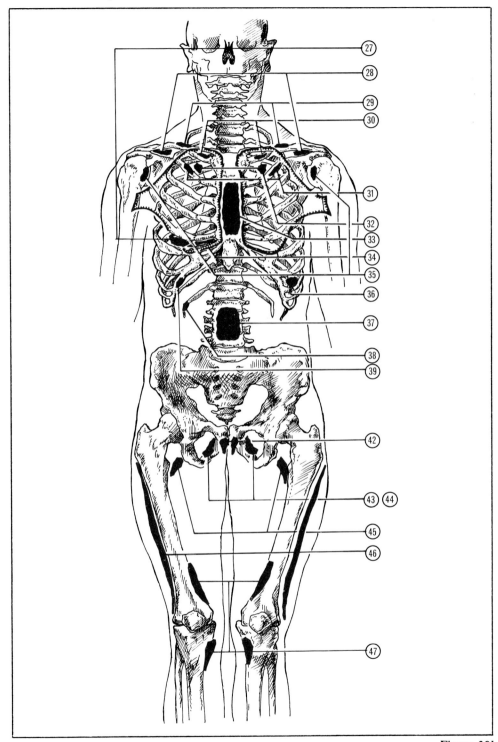

Figure 39b

Chapman's neuro-lymphatic reflexes.

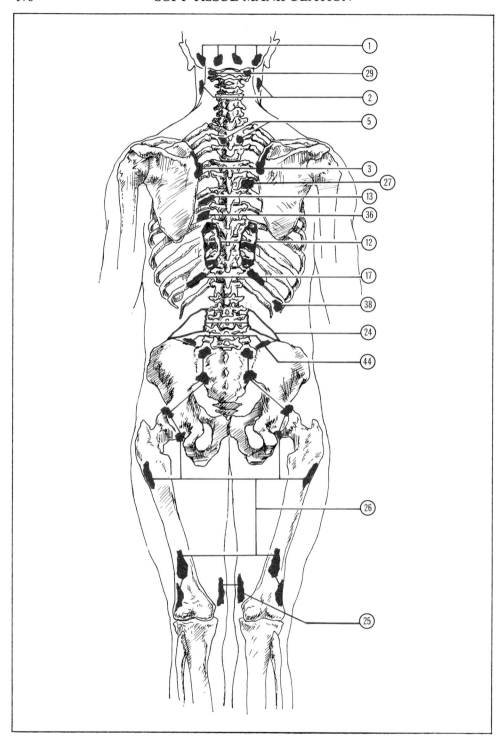

Figure 39c

Chapman's neuro-lymphatic reflexes.

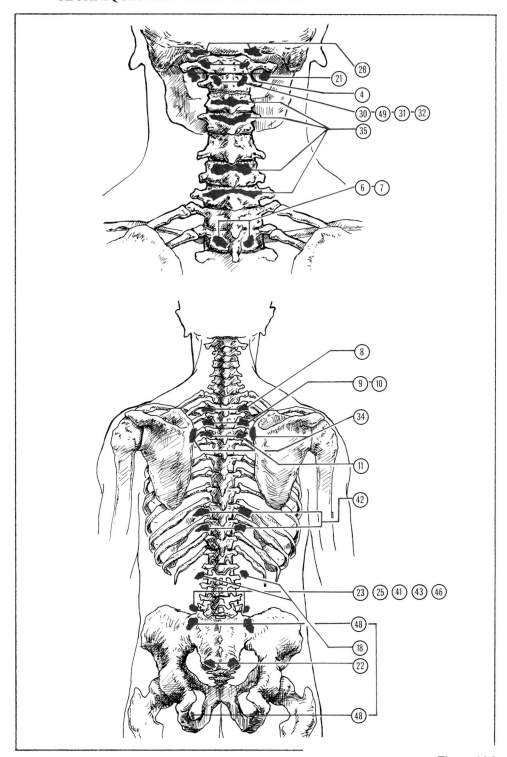

Figure 39d

Chapman's neuro-lymphatic reflexes.

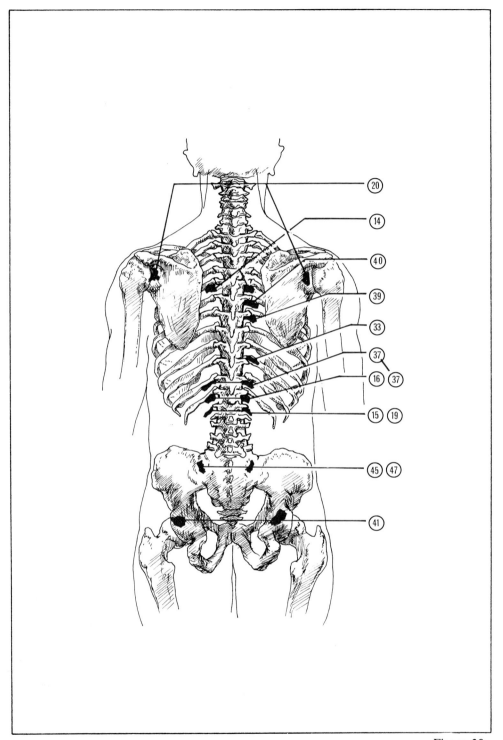

Figure 39e

Chapman's neuro-lymphatic reflexes.

Chapter 6

Basic Spinal
Neuro-muscular Technique

The objectives to which the practitioner's efforts are aimed may include postural reintegration, tension release, pain relief, improvement of joint mobility, reflex stimulation or sedation. There exist a great number of variations to the basic technique as developed by Stanley Lief. Some of these variations will depend upon the particular presenting factors and others upon personal preference on the part of the practitioner. As with all areas of therapy, ideas and techniques have been borrowed from other systems and incorporated into the overall technique. This is valid if these methods fit into the philosophical and practical framework of NMT. Similarities between some aspects of NMT and other manual systems should therefore be anticipated.

What is unique to NMT is its concentration on the soft tissues, not just to give reflex benefit to the body, not just to prepare for other therapeutic methods such as exercise or manipulation, not just to relax and normalize tense fibrotic muscular tissue and not just to enhance lymphatic and general circulation and drainage, but to do all these things and, at the same time, to give the practitioner diagnostic information via the palpating and treating instrument which is usually the hand and, more specifically, the thumb.

The technique can be applied generally or locally and in a variety of positions (sitting, lying etc.). The order in which body areas are dealt with is not regarded as critical in general treatment but is of some consequence in postural reintegration.

The basic spinal NMT treatment and the basic abdominal (and related areas) NMT treatment are the most commonly used and will be our first consideration. The methods described are in essence those of Stanley Lief and Boris Chaitow, both of whom achieved (and in the latter case continue to achieve) a degree of skill in the application of NMT that is unsurpassed. The inclusion of data on reflex areas and effects, together with basic NMT methods, provides the operator with a useful therapeutic tool, the limitations of which will be largely determined by the degree of intelligence and understanding with which it is employed. As Boris Chaitow has written:

> The important thing to remember is that this unique manipulative formula is applicable to *any* part of the body for *any* physical and physiological dysfunction and for both articular and soft tissue lesions.
>
> The learner should begin to develop the art of palpation and sensitivity of fingers by constantly feeling the appropriate areas and assessing any abnormality in tissue

structure for tensions, contractions, adhesions, spasms etc.

It is important to acquire with practice an appreciation of the 'feel' of *normal* tissue so that one is better able to recognize abnormal tissue. Once some level of diagnostic sensitivity with fingers has been achieved, subsequent application of the technique will be much easier to develop. The whole secret is to be able to recognize the 'abnormalities' in the feel of tissue structures. Having become accustomed to understanding the texture and character of 'normal' tissue, the pressure applied by the thumb in general, especially in the spinal structures, should always be firm, but never hurtful or bruising. To this end the pressure should be applied with a 'variable' pressure, i.e. with an appreciation of the texture and character of the tissue structures and according to the feel that sensitive fingers should have developed. The level of the pressure applied should not be consistent because the character and texture of tissue is always variable. These variations can be detected by one's educated 'feel'. The pressure should, therefore, be so applied that the thumb is moved along its path of direction in a way which corresponds to the feel of the tissues.

This variable factor in finger pressure constitutes probably the most important quality an operator of NMT can learn, enabling him to maintain more effective control of pressure, develop a greater sense of diagnostic feel, and be far less likely to bruise the tissue.

Use of Lubricant

The use of a lubricant to facilitate the smooth passage of, for example, the thumb over the surface is an essential aspect of NMT. However, at times the degree of stimulus imparted via the tissues can be enhanced by increasing the tensile strain between the thumb or finger and the skin.

If this effect is required, notably to achieve a rapid vascular response, then no lubricant should be used. Similar reactions will be achieved (with lubricant) where NMT is applied along the intermuscular septa or at the origins and insertions of muscles.

The lubricant used should not allow too slippery a passage of the operating digit. A mixture of two parts rape seed oil to one part lime water provides a suitable degree of lubrication. It should be clear to the operator that underlying tissues being treated should be visualized and, depending upon the presenting symptoms and the area involved, any of a number of procedures may be undertaken as the hand moves from one site to another. There may be superficial stroking in the direction of lymphatic flow, or direct pressure along the line of axis of stress fibres, or deeper alternating 'make and break' stretching and pressure or traction on fascial tissue. At the same time, diagnostic information is being received and this determines the variations in pressure and the direction of force being applied. Such changes must take place without the sudden release or application of force which could irritate the patient and produce violent pains and contraction.

Lief's basic spinal treatment followed the pattern as set out below. The fact that the same pattern is followed at each treatment does not mean that the treatment is necessarily the same. The pattern gives a framework and a useful starting and ending point, but the degree of emphasis applied to the various areas of dysfunction that manifest themselves is a variable factor which makes each treatment different. The areas of dysfunction should be recorded on a case card together with all relevant material and diagnostic findings. The myofascial tissue changes, trigger points and reference zones, areas of sensitivity, restricted motion etc. should all be recorded and referred to at each visit.

Appropriate notes should be made after each visit as to changes in these factors as well as details of the treatment given. To this end a system of 'shorthand' is desirable so that the practitioner can speedily note and decipher the essential elements of a particular visit. A code can be developed to record the patient's observations about the progress made after the previous treatment, e.g. OOX might be used to indicate improvement for the first two weeks after treatment followed by a return of symptoms and XOX might be used to indicate an initial worsening, followed by an improvement and then a deterioration.

To this end the following symbols might be applied: X indicates deterioration; = indicates the same; O indicates improvement. In noting the actual treatment applied the following examples might be instructive. Sp. NMT esp. C1,2 (R). D2,3 (R) + ICS 2,3 and 4(R). LDJ. TFL X2, indicates spinal neuro-muscular technique especially first and second cervical on the right, second and third dorsal on the right, second, third and fourth intercostal spaces on the right, lumbo dorsal junction, tensor fascia lata (both). This would indicate the areas of main fibrotic change or sensitivity. Also to be noted are trigger areas and reflex zones. For example, P° and str. to L/st-mast ★ pt. indicates pressure and stretch technique left sterno-mastoid trigger point.

These examples are meant to encourage the practitioner to keep accurate records. Ideally a universal shorthand would enhance the interchange of information between practitioners. However, what really matters is that the individual understands and refers to his own well-kept records. In this way useful information and patterns of clinical interest can become apparent to the research-minded practitioner. Invariably when, due to pressure of work, there is a lapse of concentration and the notes of a particular treatment are scanty or even missing, the patient will report an interesting development or improvement and the practitioner is left wondering what it was that achieved the change. The development of a personal shorthand to cover all treatment given, whether manipulative, soft tissue, exercise, or any other modality, is an essential aspect of successful case management.

Lief's Basic Spinal Treatment

Lief's basic spinal NMT treatment follows a pattern of placing the patient prone with a medium pillow under the chest, forehead supported by the patient's hands or ideally resting in a split headpiece. The whole spine from occiput to sacrum, including the gluteal area is lightly oiled. The operator should begin by standing half-facing the head of the couch on the left of the patient with his hips level with the mid thoracic area. In order to facilitate the intermittent application of pressure and the transfer of weight via the arm to the exploring and treating thumb, the practitioner should stand with the left foot forward of the right by 12-18 inches (30-45cm), his weight evenly distributed between them, knees slightly flexed.

The first contact is a gliding, light-pressured movement of the medial tip of the right thumb, from the mastoid process along the nuchal line to the external occipital protuberance. This same stroke, or glide, is then repeated with deeper pressure. The movement of the thumb through the tissue is slow, not uniformly slow, but deliberately seeking and feeling for contractions and congestions (to use two words which will be meaningful to any manual therapist). If and when such localized areas are felt the degree of pressure is increased and, in a variably applied manner, this pressure carries the thumb tip across or through the restricting tissue.

It is almost impossible to describe in words what this should feel like to the practitioner let alone the patient. The patient will often report a degree of pain but may say that it 'feels good'. It is a contradiction in terms, but constructive pain is usually felt as a 'nice hurt'.

Practitioner's Posture
The treating arm should not be flexed, since the optimum transmission of weight from the operator's shoulder, through the arm to the thumb tip, is best achieved with a relatively straight arm. This demands that the practitioner ensures that the plinth height is suitable for his own height. Thus, he should not be forced to stand on tip-toe to treat his patient, nor should he have to adopt an unhealthy bent posture. The operator's weight should be evenly spread between his separated feet, both of which are forward facing at this stage. In this way, by slightly altering his own weight distribution from the front to the back foot, and vice-versa, an accurate, controlled degree of pressure can be exerted with minimum arm or hand effort.

The hand itself should not be rigid but in a relaxed state, moulding itself to the contours of the neck or back tissues. To some extent the fingertips stabilize the hand. The thumb's glide is controlled by this so that the actual stroke is achieved by the tip of the extended thumb being brought slowly across the palm towards the fingertips. The fingers during this phase of cervical treatment would be placed on the opposite side of the neck to that being treated. The fingers maintain their

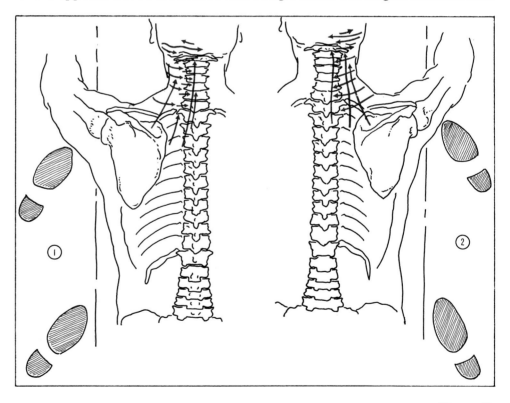

Figure 40a
Neuro-muscular Technique. Illustrating position of operator and lines of application.

position as the thumb performs its therapeutic glide. The illustrations will aid the reader to a better understanding of this description.

Were all the effort to be on the part of the thumb it would soon tire. What has to be learned is that whilst the transverse movement of the thumb is a hand or forearm effort and the relative straightness or rigidity of the last two thumb segments is also a local muscular responsibility, the vast majority of the energy imparted via the thumb results from the practitioner's body position. Increase in pressure can be speedily achieved by simple weight transfer from back towards front foot and a slight 'lean' onto the thumb from the shoulders.

The first two strokes of the right thumb having been completed—one shallow and almost totally diagnostic and the second, deeper, imparting therapeutic effort, the next stroke is half a thumb width caudal to the first. Thus a degree of overlap occurs as these strokes, starting on the belly of the sterno-cleidomastoid, glide across and through the trapezius, splenius capitus and posterior cervical muscles. A progressive series of strokes is applied in this way until the level of the cervico-dorsal junction is reached. Unless serious underlying dysfunction is found it is seldom necessary to repeat the two superimposed strokes at each level of the cervical region.

If underlying fibrotic tissue appears unyielding a third or fourth slow, deep, glide may be necessary. The degree of discomfort engendered in the patient is of some importance. The sensitivity of this region is well known and if pressure is too deep or too long sustained the resistance and tension that may be created can make the treatment counter-productive. It is possible to achieve deep, penetrating pressure, if it is variable in nature and not long held, without undue pain or discomfort. Thus a thinking, intuitive feel for the work is a prerequisite of successful application.

Trigger Point Treatment

Should trigger points be located, as indicated by the reproduction in a target area of an existing pain pattern, then sustained pressure is required for between ten seconds and two minutes. Even this sustained pressure should be slightly variable, i.e. deep pressure for ten seconds followed by a slight easing for a further ten seconds and so on, repeated until the reference pain diminishes or until the maximum time (two minutes) has elapsed. No more than this amount of manual pressure should be applied to a trigger point at any one session.

If, however, this has failed to minimize the referred pain it is often desirable to attempt to further ease the pain by applying ultrasound (pulsed) or a cold application, followed by stretching of the involved muscle, at the same session.

Once the right thumb has completed its series of transverse strokes across the long axis of the cervical musculature, the left hand, which has been resting on the patient's left shoulder, now comes into play. A series of strokes are applied upward from the left of the upper dorsal area towards the base of the skull. The fingers of the left hand rest (and act as a fulcrum) on the front of the shoulder area at the level of the medial aspect of the clavicle. The thumb tip should be angled to allow direct pressure to be exerted against the left lateral aspects of the upper dorsal and the lower cervical spinous processes as it glides cephalid. The subsequent strokes of the thumb should be in the same direction but slightly more laterally placed. The fingers should then be placed on the patient's head at about the temporo-occipital articulation. The left thumb then deals in the same way with the mid and upper cervical soft tissues, finishing with a lateral stroke or two across the insertions on the occiput itself.

In travelling from the nuchal line to the level of the cervico-dorsal junction and back again in a series of overlapping gliding movements, a number of possible trigger points will have been passed. The mid-point of the sterno-mastoid, at the level of the posterior angle of the jaw, can be a source of intense pain which may be felt above the temple in the ear region, below the angle of the jaw (see illustrations in Chapter 3). Similar triggers exist in the splenius capitus, trapzius, posterior cervical and other muscles of the area, all with different target areas. A degree of practice will soon allow these to be speedily located, identified and dealt with.

Posterior Reflex Centres   Also in this area there occur the posterior reflex centres of the neuro-lymphatic type (Chapman's Reflexes), notably those connected with conjunctivitis, cerebellar congestion and ear, nose and throat problems of an inflammatory or congested type, from sinusitus to tonsillitis. Again it is suggested that due study is made of the illustrations in Chapter 5. Treatment of these points is via lightly sustained pressure.

Recall at this point that Gutstein (Chapter 2) found trigger areas in the cervical and upper dorsal region which profoundly affected such diverse conditions as menopausal symptoms, imbalance in skin secretions and excessive perspiration. He stressed the importance of the cervical region and the interscapular area. Among the more important *Tsubo* or acupressure points in the upper cervical area are: Gall Bladder 20, which lies bilaterally in a depression midway between the occipital protuberance and the mastoid at the base of the skull; Bladder 10, which lies bilaterally just lateral to the large bundle of muscular insertions at the occiput; and Triple Heater 17, which lies bilaterally in the depression between the lobe of ear and the mastoid process. These points, if sensitive, should receive a sustained or variable pressure as for the other trigger points. Their influence is felt in a variety of conditions relating to the head, such as migraine, neuralgia, cold symptoms, hyper- and hypo-tension, liver dysfunction etc.

Goodheart mentions levator scapulae 'weakness' as indicating digestive problems and recommends pressure techniques in the cervico-dorsal area and on the medial border of the scapula to help normalize this.

During the treatment special notice should be given to the origins and insertions of the muscles of the area. Where these bony landmarks are palpable by the thumb tip they should be treated by the slow, variably applied pressure technique. Indeed, all bony surfaces within reach of the probing digit should be searched for undue sensitivity and dysfunction. This left cervical area treatment should take no more than two minutes and, in the absence of dysfunction, can be comfortably and successfully dealt with in no more than 90 seconds. Indeed the entire basic spinal NMT treatment can usually be completed in ten to fifteen minutes.

General Treatment Approach   Stanley Lief employed few specific manipulative techniques. His main concern was to attempt to normalize mobility and function (circulation, drainage, nerve function, etc.) and to this end his neuro-muscular treatment was often accompanied by no more than general rotary movements of the cervical and lumbar areas together with a degree of 'springing' or stretching of the dorsal region. Derision on the part of the 'specific' manipulators should be tempered by the fact that this general treatment approach (some would call it 'engine wiping') achieves phenomenal results in terms of improvement in general well being and the alleviation of many specific lesion patterns. Undoubtedly there are specific spinal and joint problems that require an individual approach, however, the correction of the supporting mechanism, via NMT on its own or together with general mobilzing techniques of manipulation, is able to frequently obviate the need for any more detailed technique. Indeed, specific adjusting, which pays no heed to the soft tissue component, is far more likely to fail (in the sense that symptoms speedily return) than the Lief method.

Whichever hand is operating at any given time, the other hand can give assistance by means of gently rocking or stretching tissues to compliment the efforts of the treating hand. Following the treatment of the left side the same procedures are repeated on the right. As the operator changes side it is suggested that one hand maintains light contact with the patient. Indeed it is suggested that once treatment has commenced no breaks in contact be allowed. There is often a noticeable increase in tension in the tissues of the patient if the series of strokes, stretching movements and pressure techniques etc. which make up NMT is interrupted by even a few seconds. A continuity of contact would seem, in itself, to be of therapeutic value, simply as a reassuring and calming measure.

Continuity of Contact

Once both left and right cervical areas have been treated the operator moves to the head of the plinth. Resting the tips of the fingers on the lower, lateral aspect of the neck the thumb tips are placed just lateral to the first dorsal spinal process. A degree of downward (towards the floor) pressure is applied via the thumbs which are then drawn cephalid alongside the lateral margins of the cervical spinous processes. This bilateral stroke culminates at the occiput where a lateral stretch or pull is introduced across the bunched fibres of the muscles inserting into the base of the skull.

The upward stroke should contain an element of pressure towards the spinous process so that the pad of the thumb is pressing downward (towards the floor) whilst the lateral thumb tip is directed towards the centre, attempting to contact the bony contours of the spine, all the time being drawn slowly cephalid to end at the occiput. This combination stroke is repeated two or three times. The fingertips which have been resting on the sterno-mastoid may also be employed at this stage to lift and stretch it posteriorly and laterally. The lateral stretch across the occipital protruberance may be likened to trying to break open a melon. The thumb tips dig deep into the medial fibres of the para-occipital bundle and an outward stretch is instituted, using the leverage of the arms, as though attempting to open out the occiput. The thumbs are then drawn laterally across the fibres of muscular insertion into the skull, in a series of strokes culminating at the occipito-parietal junction.

The fingertips which act as a fulcrum to these movements rest on the mastoid area of the temporal bone. Several strokes are then performed by one thumb or the other running caudad directly over the spinous process from the base of the skull to the upper dorsal area. Pressure should be fairly strong and slow. In the

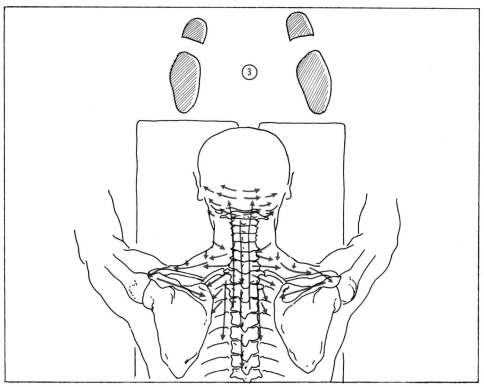

Figure 40b

Neuro-muscular Technique. Illustrating position of operator and lines of application.

same position the left thumb will now be placed on the right, lateral aspect of the first dorsal vertebra and a series of strokes are performed caudad and laterally as well as diagonally towards the scapula.

The fingers are splayed out ahead of the thumb in whichever direction it is travelling so that the force transmitted via the extended arm can be controlled. The fingers act as a fulcrum with the thumb tip being drawn across the palm towards the diagonally opposite point—the tip of the middle or little finger. The thumb should never lead the hand nor be solely 'digging' or pressing without the stabilizing and controlling action of the hand or fingertips also being in operation.

A series of strokes, shallow and then deep, is therefore applied from D1 to about D4 or 5 and outwards towards the scapula and along and across the upper trapezius fibres. The left hand treats the right side, and vice-versa with the non-operative hand resting on the neck or head. Weight transfer to the thumb is achieved by simply leaning forward. The treating arm and thumb should be relatively straight. A 'hooked' thumb in which all the work is done by the distal phalange will become extremely tired and will not achieve the degree of penetration possible via a fairly rigid thumb.

Some operators have hypermobile joints and it is difficult for them to maintain sustained pressure without the thumb giving way and bending back on itself. This is a problem which can only be overcome by attempting to build up the muscular strength of the hand or by using a variation of the above technique, e.g. a knuckle or even the elbow may be used to achieve deep pressure in very tense musculature.

Since it is difficult to apply pressure to the trapezius or sterno-mastoid muscles in such a way as to involve underlying bony structures it is necessary to lightly pinch or squeeze the more sensitive areas of dysfunction to assess trigger points and their related target areas of pain. By using the illustrations in Chapter 3 the location of the trigger points can be predicted and their presence rapidly established. When it is not possible to apply thumb pressure to such a point, a squeezing of the involved muscle area for from ten seconds to two minutes with varying pressure will usually induce a diminution of the referred pain. Once this begins the pressure should be released. If no success is achieved by these means then chilling and stretching should be employed. Several strokes should then be applied directly over the spinous processes caudad to approximately the middorsal area.

Trapezius and Sterno-mastoid Muscles

The operator then moves to the patient's left side standing in the same manner as at the commencement of the treatment but at the level of the patient's waist. With the right hand now resting at the level of the lower dorsal spine the left thumb commences a series of strokes cephalid from the mid-dorsal area. Each stroke covers two or three spinal segments and runs immediately lateral to the spinous process so that the angle of pressure imparted via the medial tip of the thumb is roughly towards the contra-lateral nipple. Again, light and deep strokes are employed and a degree of overlap is allowed on successive strokes.

In this way the first two strokes might run from D8 to D5 followed by two strokes (one light, one deeper) from D6 to D3 and finally two strokes from D4 to D1. Deeper and more sustained pressure should be exerted upon discovering marked congestion or resistance to the gliding, probing thumb. In the dorsal area a second line of upward strokes may be employed to include the spinal border of the scapula as well as one or two searching lateral probes along the inferior spine of the scapula and across the musculature inferior to and inserting into the scapula.

Left Side Treatment

Treatment of the right side may be carried out without necessarily changing position, other than to lean across the patient. However, the shorter practitioner should change sides so that, standing half-facing the head of the patient, the right thumb can perform the strokes discussed above. Apart from trigger points in the lower trapezius fibres others may be sought in levator scapulae, supra and infra spinatus, and subscapularis. Remember that the connective tissue zones affecting the arm, stomach, heart, liver and gall bladder are apparent in the region now being treated. Neuro-lymphatic reflexes relating to the arm, thyroid, lungs, throat and heart occur in the upper dorsal spine including the scapular area.

The intercostal spaces are a rich site of dysfunction. The thumb tip or a fingertip should be run along both surfaces of the rib margin as well as in the intercostal space itself. In this way the fibres of the small muscles involved will be adequately treated. If there is overapproximation of the ribs then a simple stroke along the space may be all that is possible until a degree of normalization has taken place. These intercostal areas are extremely sensitive and care must be taken not to distress the patient.

Right Side Treatment

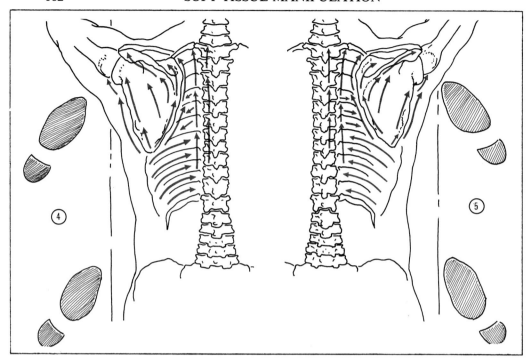

Figure 40c

Neuro-muscular Technique. Illustrating position of operator and lines of application.

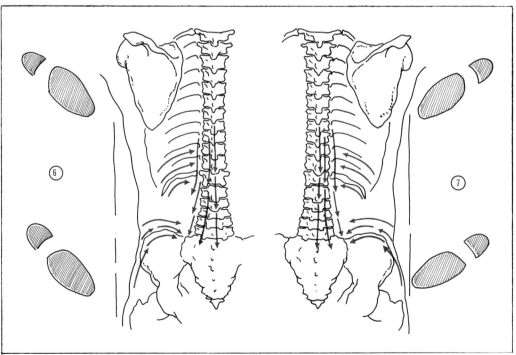

Figure 40d

Neuro-muscular Technique. Illustrating position of operator and lines of application.

The practitioner now half turns so that instead of facing the patient's head he faces the patient's feet. The pattern of strokes is now carried out on the patient's left side by the operator's right hand. A series starting from D8 to D11 followed by D11 to L1, and then L1 to L4 is carried out as before. Two or more gliding strokes with the pressure downwards but angled so that the medial aspect of the thumb is in contact with the lateral margin of the spinous process, are performed at each level. **Change of Position**

The intercostal areas are again treated as described above. The operator steps away from the plinth and glides the thumb along the superior iliac spine from just above the hip to the sacro-iliac joint. Several such strokes may be applied into the heavy musculature above the crest of ilium. The right side application requires the operator to change sides so that facing the patient's waist and half-turned towards the feet, the left hand can deal with the lower dorsal and upper lumbar area and the iliac crest in the manner described above. One or two strokes should then be applied running caudad over the tips of the spinous processes from the mid-dorsal area to the sacrum.

The area we have been describing contains a veritable network of reflex areas and points. The *Tsubo* or acupressure points lying symmetrically on either side of the spine and along the midline have great reflex importance. The so-called 'Bladder' points lie in two lines running parallel with the spine, one level with the medial border of the scapula and the other midway between it and the lateral border of the spinous processes.

Goodheart's work suggests that rhomboid weakness indicates liver problems and that pressure on C7 spinous process and a point on the right of the interspace between the fifth and sixth dorsal spinous process assists its normalization. Latissimus dorsi weakness apparently indicates pancreatic dysfunction. Lateral to seventh and eighth dorsal interspace is the posterior pressure reflex to normalize this. These and other reflexes would appear to derive from Chapman's Reflex theories and are deserving of further study.

In general terms, dysfunction of the erector spinae group of muscles between sixth and twelfth dorsal indicates liver involvement. Similarly fourth, fifth and sixth dorsal area congestion or sensitivity usually involves stomach reflexes and gastric disturbance, whereas D12 and L2 indicates possible kidney dysfunction.

The next treatment position requires the operator to stand at the level of the patient's left hip, half-facing the head of the couch. The left hand and thumb describe a series of cephalid strokes from the sacral apex towards the sacro-iliac area and then laterally along the superior and inferior margins of the iliac crest to the insertion of the tensor fascia lata at the anterior, superior iliac spine. A further series of short strokes of the thumb upwards and laterally in the lumbar area are best described as attempting to stretch and open out from the spine the muscles of the area, notably the sacro-spinal group. **Left Hip Position**

Having treated both left and right sides of the lumbar spine as above the operator uses a series of two-handed gliding manoeuvres in which the hands are spread over the upper gluteal area laterally, the thumb tips are placed at the level of the second sacral foramen with a downward (towards the floor) pressure; they glide cephalid and slowly laterally to pass over and through the fibres of the sacro-iliac joint. This is repeated several times.

Still standing on the left, the operator leans across the patient's upper thigh and engages his right thumb onto the ischial tuberosity. A series of gliding movements are carried out from that point laterally to the hip and caudad towards the gluteal fold. A further series of strokes, always applying deep, probing, but variable pressure is then carried out from the sacral border across the gluteal area to the hip margins. The fingertips during these strokes are splayed out so that they can guide and balance the hand and thumb movement. In these deep muscles the line of the thumb's direction is more towards the tip of the index finger or middle finger rather than to the little fingertip, as it was in the cervical area. In deep, tense gluteal muscle the thumb can be inadequate to the task of prolonged pressure techniques and the elbow may be used to sustain deep pressure for minutes at a time. Care should be taken, however, as the degree of pressure possible by this means is enormous and tissue damage and bruising can result from its careless employment.

The trigger points that may be sought for in the lower lumbar and gluteal areas include those in the following muscle groups: iliocostal, multifidus, longissimus, gluteus medius and gluteus minimus. The connective tissue zones that may be involved include those that involve arterial and venous disturbance to the legs, constipation, liver, gall bladder, heart and bladder.

The neuro-lymphatic reflexes include those that involve the following areas and conditions: the appendix, haemorrhoids, female generative organs, vasiculitis, sciatic nerve, abdominal tension and constipation, prostate, colitis, kidneys, adrenal glands, digestive system, pancreas, liver, spleen and gall bladder.

Having treated the low lumbar area and the gluteals the operator might (if the low back is a problem area) include a series of strokes across the fibres of the tensor

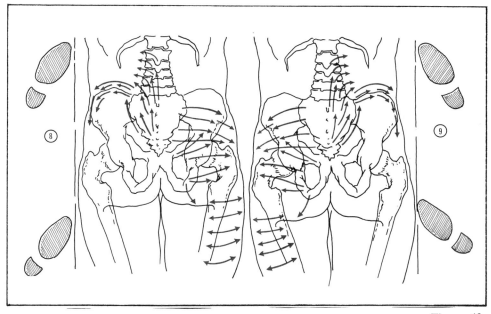

Figure 40e

Neuro-muscular Technique. Illustrating position of operator and lines of application.

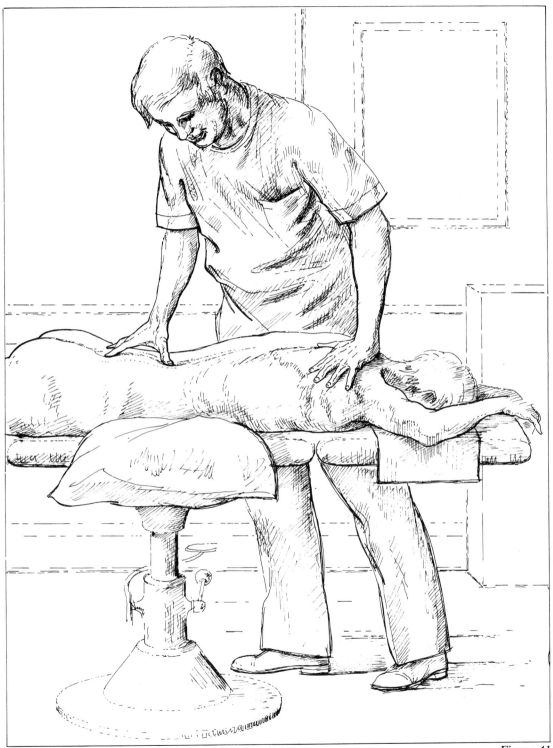

Figure 41

Operator using Neuro-muscular Technique. Note position of feet; straight right arm; right hand position; thumb position. See drawing No. 6 on page 102.

fascia lata from the hip area to the lateral knee area. The tensor fascia lata contains neuro-lymphatic reflexes to the groin glands, the broad, ligaments, spastic constipation and colitis, prostate etc.

Completion of Treatment

This completes the basic spinal NMT treatment apart from any manipulative procedures that might be indicated or thought desirable. Boris Chaitow completes the spinal treatment by standing at the head of the plinth leaning over the patient's upper dorsal area, the palms of both hands totally in contact with the upper lumbar region so that the thenar eminence is resting on the paraspinal musculature and the fingers pointing laterally. The heel of the hand imparts the main contact laterally. A series of gliding strokes is performed with the hands rhythmically alternating with each other so that as the right hand strokes downwards to end its movement on the gluteals the left is being brought back to the lower dorsal area. After it descends the right hand comes back to the start. In this way a series of ten to twenty deep rhythmic strokes are carried out in order to stimulate local circulation and drainage as well as to further relax the patient who may well have tensed during the treatment of the lumbar and gluteal areas.

As stated previously, the basic treatment should take no more than fifteen minutes. The patient should have a sense of release from tension and of well being. This may last for some days. Many feel a sense of tiredness and a great desire to sleep, this should be encouraged. Pain may result in those areas that have borne the main brunt of the pressure techniques. This should be explained to the patient who should be encouraged to note any changes in his condition and to report these at the subsequent visit. The frequency of application of NMT will vary with the condition. In chronic conditions one or two treatments weekly are as much as is ever required. This can be maintained until progress dictates that the interval be lengthened. In acute conditions treatment may be much more frequent, daily if possible until ease is achieved. Of necessity this must depend upon what other modalities are employed.

A simple, precise technique for the alleviation of local and reflex pain, the normalizing and balancing of muscular tone, the restoration of functional harmony and the release of physical and psychic tension is available to all with the patience and intelligence to know what their hands are feeling and to employ the methods developed by Stanley Lief and his followers.

Chapter 7

Basic Abdominal Technique

In treating the abdominal and related areas our attention should focus on specific junctional tissues. These comprise the central tendon and the lateral aspect of the rectal muscle sheaths, the insertion of the recti muscles and external oblique muscles into the ribs, the xiphisternal ligament as well as the lower insertions of the internal and external oblique muscles. The intercostal areas from fifth to twelfth ribs are equally important.

Specific general areas are worthy of consideration in treating conditions affecting particular organs or functions.

Liver dysfunction and portal circulatory dysfunction would call for special attention to the right side intercostal musculature from fifth to twelfth ribs. Especially important are the various muscular insertions into all these ribs.

Gall bladder dysfunction involves the above areas with extra attention to the area of the costal margin, roughly midway between the xiphisternal notch and the lateral rib margins.

Spleen function may be stimulated by attention to the intercostal spaces between the seventh and twelfth ribs on the left side.

Digestive disorders in general will benefit from NMT applied to the central tendon between the recti and directly to the rectal sheaths.

Stomach pain is treated via its reflex area to the left of the xiphisternal notch and to the tendon and rectal sheaths.

Colonic problems and ovarian dysfunction will benefit from reflex NMT application to both iliac fossae as well as to the midline structures.

Dysfunction of the kidneys, ureters and bladder require attention to the inguinal borders of the internal and external oblique insertions, the suprapubic insertions of the recti, the overlying muscles and sheaths of the area and the internal aspects of the upper thigh.

In pelvic congestion relating to gynaecological dysfunction NMT should be applied to the hypogastrium and both iliac fossae. This relieves congestion and stimulates pelvic circulation.

Ileitis and other functional disturbances of the transverse colon and small intestine benefit from NMT applied to the umbilical area.

Prostatic dysfunction will benefit from NMT to the central hypogastric region. Internal drainage massage of the prostate should also be considered.

The above brief indications should be considered in conjunction with other reflex

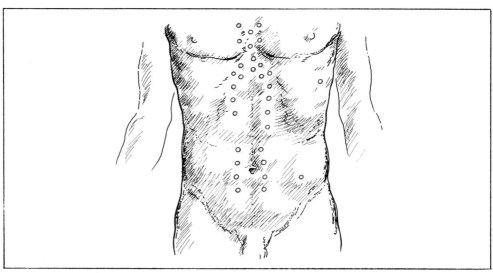

Gutstein's myodysneuric points.

Figure 42a

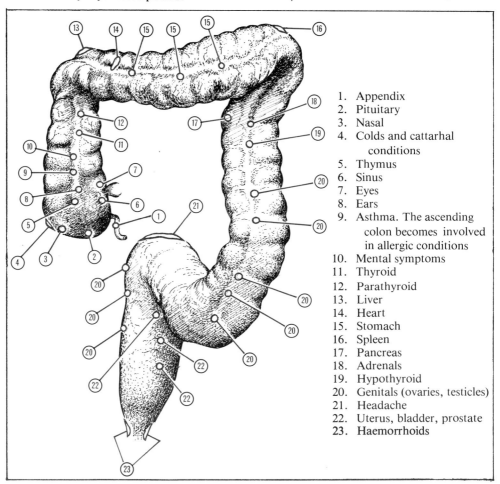

1. Appendix
2. Pituitary
3. Nasal
4. Colds and cattarhal
    conditions
5. Thymus
6. Sinus
7. Eyes
8. Ears
9. Asthma. The ascending
    colon becomes involved
    in allergic conditions
10. Mental symptoms
11. Thyroid
12. Parathyroid
13. Liver
14. Heart
15. Stomach
16. Spleen
17. Pancreas
18. Adrenals
19. Hypothyroid
20. Genitals (ovaries, testicles)
21. Headache
22. Uterus, bladder, prostate
23. Haemorrhoids

Fielder's reflex areas of the large intestine.

Figure 42b

systems and points (see below) as well as to the appropriate spinal areas which would also receive NMT treatment.

Gutstein[1] has noted trigger areas in the sternal, parasternal and epigastric regions and the upper portions of the rectus, all relating to varying degrees of retro-peristalsis. He also noted that colonic dysfunction related to triggers in the mid and lower rectus muscle. These were all predominantly left-sided. Other symptoms which improved or disappeared with the obliteration of these triggers include excessive appetite, poor appetite, flatulence, nervous vomiting, nervous diarrhoea etc. The triggers were always tender spots, easily found by the palpation and situated mainly in the upper, mid and lower portions of the recti muscles, over the lower portion of the sternum and the epigastrium including the xyphoid process and the parasternal regions. The parasternal region corresponds to the insertions of the rectus muscle into the fifth, sixth and seventh ribs (*see Figure 42a*).

Abdominal Reflex Areas

Fielder[2] described a number of reflexes occurring on the large bowel itself. These could be localized by deep palpation and treated by specific release techniques (*see Figure 42b*).

These reflexes palpate as areas of tenderness and may include a degree of swelling and congestion resulting from adhesions, spasticity, diverticuli, chemical or bacterial irritation etc.

In considering the reflexes available in the thoracic and abdominal regions the neuro-lymphatic points of Chapman are also worthy of close attention. To what extent Gutstein's myodysneuric points are interchangeable with Chapman's reflexes or Fielder's reflexes or other systems of reflex study (e.g. acupuncture or Tsubo points and Travell's triggers) and to what extent these involve Mackenzie's work *(see Figure 8)* is a matter for further research. *Suffice it to say that within the soft tissue structures of this region there abound palpable, sensitive, discrete areas of dysfunction which, on a local basis, interfere with or modify functional integrity to a greater or lesser degree, and reflexly are capable of massive interference with normal physiological function on a neural, circulatory and lymphatic level, to the extent of producing or mimicking serious pathological conditions.* Since these areas of dysfunction will often yield to simple, soft tissue manipulative techniques, which are incorporated into Lief's NMT, the value of these techniques becomes apparent. Many of Jones' tender points are noted in the abdominal region. Those strains which occur in a flexed position will usually result in such local dysfunction. This should be borne in mind, and Strain-counterstrain methods used to normalize such dysfunction (Chapter 10). Such strains would require contact of the tender point(s), as well as positioning of the patient in such a manner as to minimize the sensitivity, usually an exaggeration of the flexed position in which the injury occurred.

Bennett's neurovascular points are, in the main, related to the anterior aspect of the body, and may be located during NMT abdominal work. These may relate to Mackenzie's reflex areas.

Mackenzie[3] and others demonstrated a clear relationship between the abdominal wall and the viscera. This and other reflex patterns provide the rationale for NMT application to the abdominal and sternal regions. These reflex patterns vary in individual cases but it is clear that the majority of the organs are able to protect themselves by producing contraction, spasm and hyperaesthesia of the overlying,

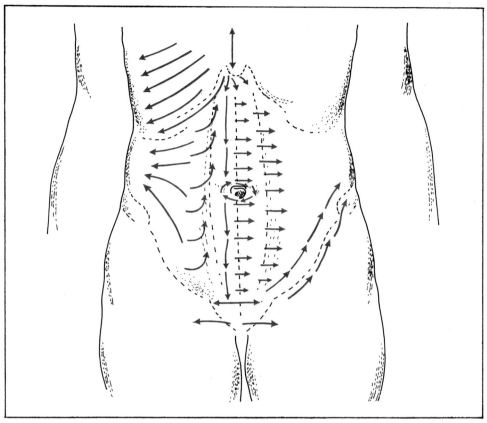

Figure 43

Neuro-muscular general abdominal technique. Lines of application.

reflexly related muscle wall, the myotome. This is often augmented by hyperaesthesia of the overlying skin as well, the dermatome. These reflexes are via the autonomic reflex pathways *(see Figure 8)*.

In treating the abdominal and thoracic regions the patient should be supine with the head supported by a medium-sized pillow and the knees flexed, either with a bolster under them or drawn right up so that the feet approximate the buttocks. Generous application of lubricant should be made to the area being treated.

Intercostal Treatment   The operator positions himself so that he is level with the patient's wrist and a series of strokes are applied with the tip of the thumb along the course of the intercostal spaces from the sternum, laterally. It is important that the insertions of the internal and external muscles receive attention. The margins of the ribs, both inferior and superior aspects, should receive firm gliding pressure from the distal phalanx of the thumb or middle finger. If there is too little space to allow such a degree of differentiated pressure then a simple stroke along the available intercostal space suffices.

The intercostals from the fifth rib to the costal margin are given a series of two or three deep, slow-moving, gliding, sensitive strokes on each side with special reference to points of particular congestion or sensitivity. These areas may benefit from thirty to sixty seconds of sustained or variable pressure techniques. These points will not bear heavy pressure techniques such as may be required in more heavily muscled regions and caution is called for. The operator should bear in mind the various reflex patterns in the region. Gentle probing on the sternum itself may elicit sensitivity in the rudimentary sternalis muscle. If this is found to be sensitive then variable pressure treatment should be applied.

It is not necessary for the operator to change sides during the treatment of the intercostals unless it is found to be more comfortable to do so.

The operator should be facing the patient and be half-turned towards the head with legs apart for an even distribution of weight and with knees flexed to facilitate the transfer of pressure through the arms. Since many of the manoeuvres in the intercostal area and on the abdomen itself involve finger and thumb movements of a lighter nature than those applied through the heavy spinal musculature the elbows need not be kept so straight.

However, when deep pressure is called for, and especially when this is applied via the thumb, the same criterion of weight transference from the shoulder through the thumb applies and the straightish arm is then an advantage for the economic and efficient use of energy.

Having treated the intercostal musculature and connective tissue and used pressure techniques to deal with any trigger points that have been elicited, the operator, using either a deep thumb pressure or a contact with the pads of the fingertips, applies a series of short strokes in a combination of oblique lateral and inferior directions from the xyphoid process.

Rectal Sheath

This is followed by the same contact in a series of deep slow strokes along and under the costal margins. A series of short strokes with fairly deep but not painful pressure is then applied by the thumb, from the midline up to the lateral rectal sheath. This series of strokes starts just inferior to the xyphoid and concludes at the pubic promontory. This series may be repeated on each side several times depending upon the degree of tension, congestion and sensitivity.

A similar pattern of treatment is followed across the lateral border of the rectal sheath. A series of short, deep, slow-moving thumb strokes being applied from just inferior to the costal margin of the rectal sheath until the inguinal ligament is reached. Both sides are treated in this way.

A series of similar strokes is then applied on the one side and then the other laterally from the lateral border of the rectal sheath. These strokes follow the contour of the trunk so that the upper strokes travel in a slightly inferior curve whilst passing laterally and the lower strokes have a superior inclination, as the hand passes laterally. A total of five or six strokes would be adequate to complete these movements and this could be repeated before performing the same movements on the opposite side.

In treating the side on which the operator is standing it may be more comfortable to apply the therapeutic stroke via the flexed finger tips which are drawn towards the operator, or the usual thumb stroke may be used. In treating the opposite side, thumb pressure can more easily be applied, as in spinal technique, with the fingers acting as a fulcrum and the thumb gliding towards them in a series of two- or three-inch long strokes. The sensing of contracted, gangliform areas of dysfunction is more difficult in abdominal work and requires great sensitivity of touch and concentration on the part of the operator.

Symphysis Pubis   Attention should be given to the insertions into, and the soft tissue component of, the pubic bones and the symphysis pubis. A deep but not painful stroke, employing the pad of the thumb, should be applied to the superior aspect of the pubic crest. This should start at the symphysis pubis and move laterally, first in one direction and, after repeating it once or twice, then the other. A similar series, starting at the centre and moving laterally, should then be applied over the anterior aspect of the pubic bone. Great care should be taken not to use undue pressure as the area is sensitive at the best of times and may be acutely so if there is dysfunction associated with the insertions into these structures. A series of deep slow movements is then performed, via the thumb, along the superior and inferior aspects of the inguinal ligament, starting at the pubic bone and running up to and beyond the iliac crest.

The thumbs or fingertips may then be insinuated beneath the lateral rectus border at its lower margins and deep pressure applied towards the midline. The hand or thumb should then slowly move cephalid in short stages whilst maintaining this medial pressure. This lifts the connective tissue from its underlying attachments and helps to normalize localized contractures and fibrous infiltrations.

Umbilicus   A series of strokes should then be applied around the umbilicus. Using thumb or flexed fingertips a number of movements of a stretching nature should be performed in which the non-treating hand stabilizes the tissue at the start of the stroke which firstly runs from approximately one inch superior and lateral to the umbilicus on the right side to the same level on the left side. The non-treating hand then stabilizes the tissues at this end point of the stroke and a further stretching and probing stroke is applied inferiorly to a point about one inch inferior and lateral to the umbilicus on the left side. This area is then stabilized and the stroke is applied to a similar point on the right.

The circle is completed by a further stroke upwards to end at the point at which the series began. This series of movements should have a rhythmical pattern so that as the treating hand reaches the end of its stroke the non-treating hand comes to that point and replaces the contact as a stabilizing pressure whilst the treating hand begins its next movement. A series of three or four such circuits of the umbilicus is performed.

Additional strokes may be applied along the midline and the sheaths of the recti muscles from the costal margins downwards. A soothing culmination to the foregoing ten to fifteen minutes may be applied by a circular clockwise series of movements in which the palm of one hand and heel of the other alternately circle the whole abdominal area. Thus, with the operator standing to the right of the patient, the palm and fingers of the left hand stroke deeply but gently down the left abdominal structures and then across the lower abdomen towards the operator where, using the heel and palm, the right hand takes over the stroke and proceeds up the right side to the costal margin. As this point it changes direction to run across the upper abdomen where the left hand takes over to repeat this pattern several times.

Specific release techniques (see page 142) may be applied during or after this general treatment. Such abdominal treatment can be repeated several times weekly if indicated but normally once a week is adequate until normality is achieved. In chronic conditions of abdominal or pelvic dysfunction the foregoing approach, together with specific release movements and appropriate spinal treatment will have a profound effect on function in the area. With an improvement in circulation and drainage and a reduction in tensions, contractions and reflex activities, the homoeostatic mechanisms of the body will ensure an overall increase in energy and an improvement in the mechanical integrity and biochemical activity of the individual with a consequent lifting of the level of health. Many chronic dysfunctions and problems will simply disappear after a series of NMT abdominal techniques.

[1] Gutstein, R., 'The Role of Abdominal Fibrositis in Functional Indigestion', *Mississippi Valley Medical Journal* (1944), pp. 66-114.
[2] Fielder and Pyott, *The Science and Art of Manipulative Surgery* (American Institute of Manipulative Surgery Inc., 1955).
[3] Mackenzie, Sir James, *Symptoms and Their Interpretation* (London, 1909).

Chapter 8

NMT in Clinical Use

The holistic, total, approach to the problems of man's health is one which looks to the causes of dysfunction and disease and, by removing these, allows the homoeostatic efforts of the body to restore normality. This ideal is not always attainable but remains the aim. Each individual has an optimum degree of biomechanical (structural, postural, functional), biochemical and psychological efficiency that can be realized. It is this optimum that is being aimed for in all therapies that fall into the broad net of holistic healing methods.

NMT takes its place amongst these methods since its objective is to help to restore the structural, functional and postural integrity of the body by removing restrictions and aiding in the normalization of dysfunction. NMT aids the economy and functional ability of the body further by reducing self-perpetuating stress factors such as contractions, spasms and tensions in the soft tissue components of the system. By improving function, removing pain, reducing energy loss, improving posture etc. the effect on psychologically negative states is a positive one.

In itself NMT is only a tool, a useful method or technique which can be of immense use in a variety of conditions. It possesses one further criterion which places it firmly in the holistic armamentary. This being that it does nothing to the body which is harmful to its overall state of health i.e. it has no side-effects. Indeed by normalizing the soft tisues NMT often saves the individual from techniques of a more 'violent' nature which might well produce outward reactions, such as surgery, traction, immobilization etc., and techniques which, whilst not usually harmful, can be painful, such as manipulative joint techniques.

NMT has an immense capability for diagnostic application, and since this can take place at the same time as its therapeutic application it shows economy in the use of time and energy. Since NMT is entirely a manual technique it is not wasteful of resources such as heat, power etc. and is applicable under almost any circumstances or conditions. NMT may be universally applied to any patient of any age suffering from any condition. This is not to say that it will be curative or even of marked value in all conditions. But it will be of some diagnostic and some therapeutic value in every condition and of enormous value in others, since no one is free of some degree of dysfunction, which affects the overall efficiency and economy of the body.

In general terms, NMT may be applied to all cases of musculoskeletal dysfunction and mento-emotional dysfunction with benefit. The basic spinal and basic abdominal techniques are used as diagnostic and therapeutic tools in the majority of cases. The more specific techniques such as psoas, piriformis and abdominal release techniques are used as and when indicated. A general, full body NMT treatment may be applied as part of a programme of postural re-integration.

In specific terms NMT is applied as follows. All conditions of the spine and conditions which involve the arms or legs would receive general spinal technique as well as consideration of local areas, in the limbs affected. Such treatments would be repeated once or twice weekly until a degree of normality had been achieved. As should be obvious, other modalities and techniques would and should be used if called for. NMT combines with anything of a supportive nature which is aimed at the restoration of normal function, such as (in appropriate conditions) ultrasonic therapy, diathermy, manipulation etc.

At the outset the aim of general treatment is to remove the more obvious areas of contraction and stasis. All reflex trigger points should be neutralized by pressure techniques if possible or, if found stubborn, by vapo-coolant or even infiltration methods. As therapy progresses, individual patterns of dysfunction will become clear and more specific NMT would be applied to those spinal, abdominal, intercostal and pelvic areas slow to improve.

Manipulative techniques of a non-specific type are often useful in the normalization of spinal integrity once the initial soft tissue rigidity or dysfunction has been improved. NMT may be applied with infinite gentleness or with robust enthusiasm since it is possible to use the same techniques with a marked difference in the degree of force employed. This enables its application to areas of acute sensitivity as well as in fragile (osteoporotic) and tender areas. As long as the operator is thinking about the task in hand and not applying the techniques in a mechanical, repetitive manner there is no danger of injury or harm.

If treatment is aimed at the removal of symptoms stemming from trigger points, it is essential to normalize all the structures related to the local area of dysfunction. To simply neutralize the trigger that is causing, say, a headache, will produce short-term benefits. If the particular trigger lies in the trapezius muscle then not only must the trigger be normalized and the trapezius treated but the entire cervical and spinal musculature and soft tissues must receive attention. A general rule should be that *no part of the whole should be considered without the whole also being considered.* Thus, even if the spinal areas are receiving the main attention of the therapist on any one visit, the supporting limbs and associated structures should be given some, if only brief, consideration to assess their involvement and possible requirements. The treatments of the back, therefore, calls for the treatment of the front and this calls for the whole to be considered and treated.

General abdominal technique is useful in all cases of digestive and intestinal dysfunction of a non-organic nature. NMT is applicable to all cases of respiratory dysfunction. It is also applicable to all genito-urinary conditions of a non-organic nature. NMT applied to the abdomen will reduce dramatically most tension states of mento-emotional origin. General abdominal technique improves circulatory efficiency through the pelvis and abdominal regions and it improves respiratory function. The reflex points and zones in the spinal area should always be treated prior to thoracic and abdominal technique as indicated.

In a case of spastic constipation, for example, NMT to the lower spinal areas (*see Figure 7a*) and the use of neuro-lymphatic points (*see Figures 39a to 39e*) followed by general abdominal technique would be the pattern recommended. This could be followed by specific abdominal release techniques if areas of marked contractions or 'adhesion' were elicited during the general treatment. Such an approach, combined with general health measures, such as nutritional reform and an exercise and possibly a relaxation programme, will promote a return to normal more speedily than anything else in the author's experience. After all, the body is being given those factors required for normality and since its self-healing tendency is constantly acting, the removal of obstacles (structural, mechanical, dietary) provide the prerequisites for recovery.

In dealing with tension and stress of psychic origin it is as well to recall that the mind will not be calm or relaxed as long as neuro-muscular tensions are present. In applying any form of psychotherapy the use of NMT, applied to the spine and abdomen, will increasingly improve the patient's powers of relaxation. NMT is not seen as an end in itself in this regard, but to be rather as a catalyst to the removal, albeit temporary, of the physical component of a vicious circle. In some cases this physical release of tension, especially when applied to the solar plexus, can produce a sudden emotional release in which the patient may cry and sob. The body becomes a solid mass of tensions and contractions for many individuals. The tensions of life are mirrored by layers of muscular 'armour'. The posture and tensions thus created all carry specific emotional charges and memories and as the physical components are broken down and relaxed so do the emotional memories and feelings associated with their origins come to the surface. NMT applied skillfully to the spine and abdomen becomes a useful tool for the therapist who is attempting to calm the mind of the patient. Tensions thus released do not return unless the causes are still current.

In restoring total structural and postural integrity to the body it is, of course, necessary to apply NMT to all the supporting structures of the body. This would involve the spinal, thoracic and abdominal soft tissues and the limbs, including the feet. NMT and manipulation, where appropriate, will lay the foundations for a return to normal (or to the patient's individual optimum norm). Specific and general exercise, as well as postural re-education, may then follow. It is possible, via such systems as Alexander Technique, to achieve postural and functional normality. It is contended, however, that by the judicious use of NMT and manipulation such re-education becomes much easier and less arduous. It must be easier to learn to use a machine correctly if that machine is capable of functioning correctly!

In attempting to achieve postural and functional normality a fairly long-term view is required. Some workers assert that a series of eight to ten sessions will produce this result. It is the author's experience that whilst the basic ground work can be done in eight to ten treatments, the majority of cases require weekly or fortnightly treatment for 12 to 18 months if they are to achieve optimum improvement. This should be followed by maintenance visits at not less than three monthly intervals.

NMT is universally applicable. It has no side-effects. It combines with all other methods of positive health care. In itself it is capable of improving general function, releasing tension and removing noxious triggers, which may be responsible for myriad symptoms. NMT has limits, but within the framework of its own area of application its only limits lie in the ability of the operator.

One practitioner who has achieved outstanding success in applying NMT to athletic injuries of marked severity is Terry G. Moule D.O. Within the last few years he has restored the former captain of England's soccer team, Gerry Francis, to playing fitness. Surgery to the lumbar spine was the only prospect left for Francis after months of agony under orthopaedic investigation. In desperation Moule was consulted and within a few weeks Francis was playing again. He remains fit and continues to play professional soccer.

A similar return to normality was achieved in the case of the then captain of England's rugby football team, Roger Uttley, whose career appeared to be over after a back injury. Treatment consisting largely of NMT resulted in Uttley returning to the England squad in their successful 1980 season.

An even more startling result of the application of NMT to a spinal injury is that involving the former holder of the world mile and 1500m records Sebastian Coe. He stated in late 1979: 'Last winter I had a back problem. I was having trouble getting a diagnosis, let alone treatment.' Within a few treatments incorporating NMT he was running again and setting world record times. Moule has stated that he is not yet fully satisifed that Coe's back has reached its optimum improvement and he expects greater things still from this fine athlete.

Terry Moule's view of NMT is as follows:

The principle of NMT is that it is of prime importance to treat connective tissue lesions and abnormalities, prior to any manipulative treatment of the bony structures. If more orthodox and less penetrating soft tissue techniques are used, whilst the bony abnormality may be corrected by the application of a specific adjustment, because the soft tissues remain in a similar state to that existing prior to the manipulation, there is a strong likelihood of a recurrence of the lesion. NMT tends to dispense with specific adjustment, for, subsequent to using these specialized soft tissue measures, a generalized mobilization and adjustment will allow the muscular and connective tissues to encourage the bony structures to return to their normal alignment. This may take a little longer to produce relief from discomfort, but in the long run it means that the correction is more permanent and there is less danger of any damage to the muscular and connective tissues from forceful manipulation.

The great advantage of NMT is that it may be applied to any part of the body. It is particularly effective in dealing with problems related to interference with nerve supply; to any form of muscular or connective tissue lesion; to treatment of the abdominal and pelvic organs etc. It is applied mainly by use of the thumb. It may take some years to develop an adequate 'feel' in the hands in general and the thumbs in particular, to effectively diagnose and treat lesions. It is the ability to diagnose through the thumb which is so helpful in the rapid and efficient treatment of all forms of dysfunction. Correctly used it precludes a large number of more conventional techniques and saves a considerable amount of time.

NMT has proved invaluable in the treatment of sports injuries, particularly for the diagnostic reasons outlined above and for the fact that it produces a rapid response as compared to orthodox soft tissue and physiotherapy techniques. With sports injuries one of the major problems is to get the player back in action as soon as possible, particularly where the injury is to a professional sportsman. NMT has been used very effectively on a large number of sportsmen and women following all types of sports.

One of the most common injuries one encounters is hamstring problems. These are particularly prevalent amongst footballers, who in many cases develop the injury through overdevelopment of the quadriceps without adequate attention to the maintenance and mobility (i.e. lengthening and stretching) of the hamstrings at the same time. The normal treatment of hamstring injuries is ultra-sonic and massage. These techniques are not particularly rapid and the resultant loss of overall muscle tone, due to the inability of the leg to be used normally, retards a return to normal function. With NMT a lesion can be accurately and rapidly detected and, by the use of deep thumb manipulation, the soft tissue lesion can be dealt with rapidly and effectively. Where there is muscular fibre damage this can be felt and literally ironed out. The effect of the technique is to stimulate circulation in the area thus encouraging healing. Where there is inflammation and swelling the technique promotes drainage and the restoration of normal tone. With acute lesions the technique is unfortunately painful, but where speed is the prime order in recovery this is a small price to pay.

NMT is also beneficial in the treatment of knee lesions, particularly ligamentous problems and the subsequent inflammation in the joint itself. Correct application of NMT to these lesions will improve drainage from the knee and encourages healing to take place far more rapidly than through orthodox techniques. Where there is knee misalignments or dislocation, reduction of spasm is most important as a prerequisite to satisfactory manipulation of the joint. In many cases injury occurs when the legs become anchored due to studs in the boots. If rotation of the trunk is superimposed onto this static lower limb situation the stress imposed on the knee joint is enormous. The application of NMT prior to attempting correction not only makes the correction less painful but ensures that the result is lasting. NMT is also beneficial in the treatment of prepatellar bursitis, and any synovial inflammatory problems.

A problem which plagues many sportsmen, particularly footballers, basketball players and volleyball players, is pain in the groin and down the inside of the leg. This is commonly treated as a sacroiliac or a lumbar problem when, in many cases, it is due to a lesion of the symphysis-pubis. There are a number of techniques for dealing with problems of this joint but none so dramatically successful as the application of NMT.

The technique's effectiveness in producing long-term benefits is perhaps best underlined by the results with sportsmen such as Roger Uttley and Gerry Francis, who had both received short-term benefit from manipulative treatment. The application of NMT, without any change in the manipulative techniques being employed, except to make them less specific, produced long-term improvement which allowed a return to active participation in their respective sports. In both cases the main problem was an imbalance in muscle tone with excessive tension causing persistence of the joint dysfunction. The removal of these soft tissue factors restored balance and encouraged the body to return to normal function, as it always tries to do.

In summary, the benefits of NMT in general use are (1) that it is a technique which removes causes rather than dealing with symptoms. (2) It removes the necessity for the bulk of specific manipulation, instead it encourages the body to normalize itself. (3) It is applicable to any part of the body. From the specific sports injury point of view the main advantage of NMT is that it provides (1) a more rapid recovery rate and (2) a more permanent one.

My own experience confirms the validity of Terry Moule's comments. NMT apart from all the myriad applications discussed in earlier chapters, is the finest soft tissue system for helping to normalize acute and chronic injuries. In the past 30 years I have used these methods on tens of thousands of patients. In many cases sporting and theatrical performers have been restored to normal in a short space of time. Where the 'show must go on' — and in present terms this applies to athletic and sporting performance just as much as to theatrical performance — time is vital. NMT and the various methods that may accompany it, such as ultrasonics, manipulation, hydrotherapy, exercise, cryotherapy etc. have been successful time after time. I have found NMT invaluable in dealing with acute injuries affecting such personalities as Richard Burton (acute torticollis during the filming of *Look Back in Anger*), James Booth (acute low back during the West End run of *Fings Ai'nt What They Used To Be*), Christopher Neame (neck injury sustained in fall from balcony during *Romeo and Juliet*), Bryan Forbes (neck strain during filming of *League of Gentlemen*), Harry Andrews (fell off horse during filming of *Devil's Disciple*).

All of these were able to resume work within one day of the injury. In all cases no proper treatment facilities were available. Conditions ranged from the dressing room for James Booth to the lush grass of Tring Park for Harry Andrews. No equipment was available other than my hands and no treatment was used other than NMT and gentle mobilization. The economy, versatility and effectiveness of NMT has proved equally useful on countless occasions.

The successful use of NMT calls for the applied thought of the practitioner. The body responds rapidly to the help this technique offers. Its limitations are almost always related to the limitations of the practitioner. Its success is in direct proportion to the dedication and intelligence with which it is applied.

Chapter 9

Muscle Energy Techniques

A revolution is taking place in manipulative therapy. This involves a movement away from the most commonly used, high velocity/low amplitude thrusts (characteristic for most chiropractic and much osteopathic manipulation) towards gentle methods which take far more account of the soft tissue component. One such major area of therapy is that which may be termed muscle-energy technique, although there are a variety of other terms used to describe aspects of it. Terminology is sometimes confusing, and we should attempt to ensure that descriptions are apt and accurate. These methods employ variations on a basic theme, which primarily involves the use of the patient's muscular effort in one of a number of ways, in association with the therapist's efforts, which may match, and thus counteract, the effort of the patient (isometric contraction); or overcome the effort of the patient, thus moving the area, joint etc., in the direction opposite to that in which the patient is attempting to move it (isotonic eccentric contraction); or partially match the effort of the patient, thus allowing, although slightly retarding, the patient's effort (isotonic concentric contraction).

These variations may be used in a number of ways, which alter the degree of effort used by both patient and operator, as well as the duration and direction of such efforts, and the number of times the procedure is performed. The essence of the method is that it uses the energy of the patient, which may be employed in one or other of the manners described above. A major consideration, apart from degree of effort, duration and frequency of use, is that the direction in which the effort is made may be varied, so that the operator's force is directed towards overcoming the restrictive barrier, or just the opposite, in which the operator's counter-effort is away from the barrier. In the case of a shortened muscle, or group of muscles, the decision is required as to whether to direct the patient to attempt to stretch the shortened muscle (or group) or to attempt to contract it further, both against resistance.

There are a variety of guidelines as to which choice(s) should be made. Paul Williams MD, in his major book *The Lumbo-sacral Spine* (McGraw Hill, 1965) states a basic truism, which is often neglected by the professions which deal with musculoskeletal dysfunction. He says: 'The health of any joint is dependent upon a balance in the strength of its opposing muscles. If for any reason a flexor group loses part, or all of its function, its opposing extensor group will draw the joint into a hyperextended position, with abnormal stress on the joint margins. This situation exists in the lumbar spine of modern man.'

Lack of attention to the muscular component of joints in general, and spinal joints in particular, results in frequent inappropriate treatment of the joints thus affected. Correct understanding of the role of the supporting musculature would frequently lead to normalization of these tissues, without the need for heroic manipulative efforts. MET and NMT focus attention on these structures, and offer the opportunity to correct both the weakened musculature, and the shortened, often fibrotic, antagonists.

Careful examination of tissues in the area of discomfort or pain, whether spinal or otherwise, almost always reveals the presence of tense musculature. Normalization of this is frequently all that is required to produce, not only symptomatic relief, but also functional normality. MET is the product of a variety of schools in that its origins may be found in orthopaedic and physiotherapy literature, as well as osteopathic work. The current interest in these methods crosses all such political and therapeutic barriers. MET, as presented in this book, owes most of its development to osteopathic medicine.

The osteopathic profession's credit for most of the recent development of these methods is fair, inasmuch as many applications and refinements have sprung from that school of medicine. However, earlier work of a similar, if simpler, type was employed by physiotherapists who, among other terms, described a more limited version as *'proprioceptive neuromuscular facilitation'* (PNF). This method tended to stress the importance of rotational components in the function of joints and muscles, and used this aspect in the resisted (isometric) exercise. A term now much used, in regard to more recent developments of these methods, is that of *post-isometric relaxation* (PIR). This relates to the effect of subsequent relaxation, experienced by a muscle, or group of muscles, after brief periods, during which an isometric contraction is performed.

Thus we have the terms proprioceptive neuromuscular facilitation, or post isometric relaxation, representing variations on this theme. A further aspect of the complex of effects, noted in such manoeuvres, is that of *reciprocal inhibition*. When a muscle is isometrically contracted, its antagonist will be inhibited, and will relax immediately following this. Thus the antagonist of a shortened muscle, or group of muscles, may be isometrically contracted, in order to achieve a degree of ease and additional movement in the shortened tissues. This is plainly not post isometric relaxation but another phenomenon. Other terms which have been applied to methods such as these, include *'hold-relax'* technique, *'contract relax'* technique, and there is the more recent arrival, which has a distinctly American ring, *myokinesis*.

Lewit and Simons ('Myofascial Pain: relief by post isometric relaxation', *Archives of Physical Medical Rehabilitation,* Vol 65 August 1984, pp452-6) state that, whilst reciprocal inhibition is a factor in some forms of therapy, related to post-isometric relaxation techniques, it is not a factor in PIR itself. They point out that: 'The effectiveness of contract-relax and rhythmic stabilization, for increasing range of motion, is said to depend to some extent upon the neurophysiological principle of reciprocal inhibition: voluntary activation of the agonist (the shortened muscle receiving therapy) promoted inhibition of this antagonist, and vice versa. Persistence of the reciprocal inhibition effect could logically be a significant factor in rhythmic stabilization, when both require voluntary contraction of the antagonist to the muscle under treatment. However, since contraction of the antagonist is avoided in post-isometric relaxation, reciprocal inhibition is not likely to be a factor. It is more likely that the stretch equalizes the lengths of the sarcomeres throughout each muscle fibre, thus normalizing the function of the contractile elements in the muscle.'

Where pain of an acute or chronic nature precludes easy employment of the muscles involved, the use of the antagonists is patently of value. Thus MET incorporates both post-isometric relaxation, and reciprocal inhibition methods, as well as aspects unique to itself, such as isokinetic techniques, described later in this section.

It is the intention in this book to use the term 'muscle energy technique' (MET), and this is seen as a complementary method to the other forms of soft tissue manipulation also described in this text. NMT and MET can be used together, or separately, and will be noted in practice to have an almost synergistic effect, in that MET is found to work more effectively after the application of NMT, and vice versa.

A number of researchers have reported on the usefulness of MET in the treatment of trigger points, and this must be seen as an excellent method of achieving the ultimate objective in treating these myofascial states, which is the restoration of a situation where the muscle in which the trigger lies is capable once more of achieving its full resting length, with no evidence of shortening. In this way MET can replace, or combine with, the methods of trigger point treatment discussed in Chapter 5 (chilling, stretching, etc.).

The terms used in MET require clear definition and emphasis:

● An *isometric contraction* is one in which a muscle, or group of muscles, or a joint, or region of the body, is called upon to contract, or move in a particular direction, and in which that effort is matched by the operator's effort, so that no movement is allowed to take place.
● An *isotonic contraction* is one in which movement does take place, in that the counterforce offered by the operator is either less than that of the patient, or is greater. In the first example there would be an approximation of the origin and insertion of the muscle(s) involved, as the effort exerted by the patient more than matches that of the operator. This has a tonic effect on the muscle(s) and is called a *concentric isotonic contraction*. This method is useful in toning weakened musculature.

   Should the second isotonic alternative be employed, the origin and insertion of the muscles involved would not approximate, but would in fact get further apart, due to the greater effort of the operator's counterforce overcoming the muscular effort. This is described as an *eccentric isotonic contraction* and is also called, in some works, an *isolytic contraction*. This manoeuvre is useful in cases where there is present, in the soft tissues, a degree of fibrotic change. The effect is to stretch and alter these tissues, thus allowing an improvement in elasticity and circulation.

It is sometimes easier to describe these variations simply in terms of whether the operator's force is the same as, less than, or greater than that of the patient. In any given case there is going to exist a degree of limitation in movement, in one direction or another, which may involve purely soft-tissue components of the area, or actual joint restriction (in such cases there is bound to be some involvement of soft tissues). The operator will establish, by palpation and by mobility assessments (motion palpation), the direction of maximum 'bind' or restriction. This is felt as a definite point of limitation in one or more directions. In many instances the muscle(s) will be shortened and incapable of stretching and relaxing. Should the isometric, or isotonic contraction, which the patient is asked to perform, be one in which the contraction of the muscles or movement of the joint is away from the barrier or point of bind, whilst the operator is using force in the direction which goes towards, or through that barrier, then this form of treatment involves what is called a *direct action*. Should the opposite apply, in which the patient is attempting to take the area, joint, muscle, towards the barrier, and the operator is resisting, then this is an *indirect* maneouvre.

As with so much in manipulative terminology, there is disagreement even in this apparently simple matter of which method should be termed 'direct' and which 'indirect'. Grieve (*Mobilisation of the Spine,* Churchill Livingstone, 1985, pp 190) describes the variations thus: 'Direct action techniques in which the patient attempts to produce movement towards, into or across a motion barrier; and indirect techniques, in which the patient attempts to produce motion away from the motion barrier, i.e. the movement limitation is attacked indirectly.'

On the other hand, Goodridge ('Muscle Energy Technique: Definition, explanation, methods of procedure,' *Journal of the American Osteopathic Association,* Vol 81, Dec 1981, No. 4 pp 249-54) states, having previously illustrated and described a technique where the patient's effort was directed away from the barrier of restriction: 'The aforementioned illustrations used the direct method. With the indirect method the component is moved by the operator away from the restrictive barrier.' If the operator is moving away from the barrier, then the patient is moving towards it, and in Goodridge's terminology (i.e. osteopathic) this is an indirect approach. In Grieve's terminology (physiotherapy) this is a direct approach. Plainly these views are contradictory.

David Heiling DO, of the Philadelphia College of Osteopathic Medicine, has a solution to this. Noting that muscle energy techniques always involve two opposing forces, the patient's and the operator's, he feels that it is judicious to indicate which force is being used to characterize a given technique. Thus an *operator-direct method* is also equally accurately described as a *patient-indirect method*. He feels that operator-direct methods (in which the patient is using muscles usually already in spasm or shortened) are more appropriate to managing chronic conditions, rather than acute ones, in which the muscles which are being asked to contract could have oedema or muscle damage, and could go further into spasm. Operator-direct methods are particularly suitable for rehabilitation, where muscle shortening and clot organization have occurred. Patient direct techniques are more suitable to acute conditions, where the antagonists to the shortened muscles are called on to contract.

Before considering the various alternatives which exist, as to degree of effort, time involved, and frequency of employment, we should look at some of the mechanisms involved in these procedures. Karel Lewit MD (*Manipulative Therapy in Rehabilitation of the Locomotor System*, Butterworth, 1985) discussing the methods, states that medullary inhibition is not capable of explaining their effectiveness. He considers that the excellent results obtained may relate to: (1) during resistance of minimal force, only a very few fibres are active, the others being inhibited while, (2) during relaxation (in which the shortened musculature is taken gently to its new limit) the stretch reflex is avoided, a reflex which is brought about even by passive and non-painful stretch.

He concludes that this method demonstrates the close connection between tension and pain, and between relaxation and analgesia. His method of using muscle energy technique (which he terms post-isometric relaxation) is to take the shortened muscle to a position in which it attains its maximum pain-free length, without stretching. The slack is taken up in the same manner as in joint mobilization. Having reached the extreme position the patient is asked to resist with a MINIMUM of force, and to breathe in. This resistance is held for about ten seconds, during which the operator attempts to push the muscle in a direction which would stretch it, were resistance not present. The degree of effort, in Lewit's method, is minimal. The patient may be instructed to think in terms of using ten, or twenty, per cent of their available strength. Never is the manoeuvre allowed to develop into a contest of strength, between the operator and patient. After ten seconds, or so, the operator and the patient cease all effort, and the operator senses that relaxation has indeed taken place. The patient may then be instructed to breathe in and out deeply, and on exhalation the operator should be able to take the previously restricted muscle, painlessly, further towards its normal resting position, without resistance. The slack is again taken up, and the procedure repeated. The period between isometric contraction efforts may last as long as ten seconds, during which the spontaneous relaxation of the muscle is used to advantage by gently taking it towards its new barrier. If no improvement is noted, then the subsequent isometric effort may be lengthened to as much as half a minute. It is not usually necessary to ask for increased effort, although this variable may be used to effect in some cases. If isometric relaxation has been forthcoming then the following contraction may be of the same, or shorter, duration. Repetition may be performed three to five times. It is desirable to continue for as long as results continue to be forthcoming. When no more relaxation appears to be obtainable, at that session, then it is time to cease. Lewit uses interesting combinations of activity to coincide with isometric exercises of this sort. Not only are efforts timed to coincide with inspiration, and relaxation with exhalation, but various eye movements are used to facilitate the direction of desired movement of the joint, body part, or muscle. Thus the patient is asked to look to one side, away from the direction of desired relaxation, during the active phase of contraction, and towards the direction of relaxation when this phase is operating.

These methods are based on research which indicates, for example, that flexion is enhanced by the patient looking downwards, and extension by looking upwards. Similarly, side-bending is facilitated by looking towards the side involved. These ideas are easily proved, by self-experiment. An attempt to flex the spine, whilst maintaining the eyes in an upwards looking position, will be found to be less successful than looking downwards at that time. These eye-direction aids are also useful in manipulation of the joints. Lewit suggests, as do many others, that trigger points and 'fibrocytic' changes in muscle will often disappear after MET contraction methods. He further suggests that referred local pain points, resulting from problems elsewhere, will also disappear more effectively than where local anaesthesia or needling (acupuncture) methods are employed. Such points may be equated with Jones' 'tender' points (see Chapter 10).

Poor results from use of these methods may relate to an inability to localize muscular effort sufficiently, for, unless local muscle tension is produced in the precise region of the soft tissue dysfunction, then the method will fail. Also, of course, underlying pathological changes may have taken place in joints or elsewhere, which make this of short-term value only, since such changes will ensure recurrence of muscular spasms, sometimes almost immediately. Identification of the tight muscles, in any complex postural problem, is sometimes less simple than it seems.

Marvin Solit, a disciple of Ida Rolf, describes one common error ('A study in Structural Dynamics', *1963 Year Book of Osteopathy*): 'As one looks at a patient's protruding abdomen, one might think that the abdominal muscles are weak, and that treatment should be geared towards strengthening them. By palpating the abdomen, however, one would not feel flabby, atonic muscles which would be the evidence of weakness; rather, the muscles are tight, bunched and shortened. This should not be surprising because here is an example of muscle working overtime maintaining body equilibrium. In addition these muscles are supporting the sagging viscera, which normally would be supported by their individual ligaments. As the abdominal muscles are freed and lengthened, there is a general elevation of the rib cage, which in turn elevates the head and neck.'

Attention to tightening and hardening these supposedly weak muscles via exercise, observes Solit, results in no improvement in posture, or in reduction in the 'pot-bellied' appearance. Rather the effect is a further depressing of the thoracic structures, since the attachments of the abdominal muscles, superiorly, are largely onto the relatively mobile, and unstable, bones of the rib cage. Shortening these muscles simply achieves a degree of pull on these structures, towards the stable pelvic attachments below. The approach, adopted by Rolfing, is to free and loosen these overworked, and only apparently weakened, tissues. This allows for a return to some degree of normality, freeing the tethered thoracic structures, and thus correcting the postural imbalance. Attention to the shortened, tight, musculature, is the primary aim. Exercise is not suitable at the outset, until this primary goal is achieved.

Lewit discusses the element of muscular stretch required in MET, and maintains that this factor does not always seem to be essential. In some areas self-treatment, by use of gravity as the resistance factor is effective, and in such cases there is sometimes no element of stretch involved of the muscles in question. Stretching of muscles, during MET, according to Lewit, is only required when contracture due to fibrotic change has occurred, not if there is simply a disturbance in function. He quotes trials in which 351 painful muscle groups, or muscle attachments, were treated by MET (Post isometric relaxation) in 244 patients. Analgesia was achieved in 330 cases, immediately, and there was no effect in only 21. These are remarkable results by any standards.

J. Bourbillon, in his book *Spinal Manipulation* (3rd edition), Heinemann, London, 1982) states that shortening of muscle seems to be a self-perpetuating phenomenon, which results from an over-reaction of the gamma-neurone system. It seems that the muscle is incapable of returning to a normal resting length as long as this continues. Whilst the effective length of the muscle is thus shortened, it is nevertheless capable of shortening further. The pain factor seems related to its inability thereafter, to be restored to its anatomically desirable length. The conclusion is that much joint restriction is a result of muscular tightness and shortening. The opposite may also apply, where damage to the soft or hard tissues of a joint is a factor. In such cases the periarticular and osteophytic changes, all too apparent in degenerative conditions, are the major limiting factor in joint restrictions. In both situations, however, MET may be useful, although more so where muscle shortening is the primary factor.

The restriction which takes place as a result of tight, shortened, muscles, is usually accompanied by some degree of lengthening, and weakening, of the antagonists. A wide variety of possible permutation exists, in any given condition, involving muscular shortening, which may be initiating, or be secondary to, joint dysfunction, combined with weakness of antagonists. A combination of isometric and isotonic methods can effectively be employed to lengthen and stretch the shortened groups, and to strengthen and shorten the weak, overlong muscles.

There exists a common tendency, amongst some schools of therapy, to encourage the strengthening of weakened muscle groups, in order to normalize postural and functional problems. Vladimir Janda expresses well the reasons why this approach is literally putting the cart before the horse: 'In pathogenesis, as well as in treatment of muscle imbalance and back problems, tight muscles play a more important, and perhaps even primary, role in comparison to weak muscles.' (*The Neurobiological Mechanisms in Manipulative Therapy,* Ed. Irvin Korr, Plenum Press, 1978). He continues with the following most important observation: 'Clinical experience, and especially therapeutic results, support the assumption that (according to Sherrington's law of reciprocal innervation) tight muscles act in an inhibitory way on their antagonists. Therefore, it does not seem reasonable to start with strengthening of the weakened muscles, as most exercise programmes do. It has been clinically proved that it is better to stretch tight muscles first. It is not exceptional that, after stretching of the tight muscles, the strength of the weakened antagonists improves spontaneously, sometimes immediately, sometimes within a few days, without any additional treatment.'

Here then is a sound, well reasoned, clinical and scientific observation, which directs our attention and efforts towards the stretching and normalizing of those tissues which have shortened and tightened. MET is superbly designed to assist in this endeavour, especially if combined with the unique diagnostic and therapeutic effects of NMT. This is the route we should encourage, in soft tissue manipulation, with the knowledge that MET also provides an excellent method for assisting in the toning of weak musculature, should this still be required, after the stretching of the shortened antagonists.

It is clear from the evidence of many researchers that the localization of forces is the critical factor in the success, or otherwise, of MET. The degree of effort which should be used in contraction of muscles, is a point which is debated. The importance of specifically involving the appropriate muscles, in a manner which directs them to contract directly towards, or away from, the restrictive barrier is, however, not debated. The accurate localization of forces depends very much on the skill of the operator. Being able to sense accurately the degree and point of resistance is an acquired skill, involving the proprioceptive perception of movement and any resistance to this. By easing a joint, or area, towards its barrier, and knowing when to call for an isotonic or isometric effort, and whether to yield to, or overcome, that effort (in the isotonic manoeuvres) provides the operator with a varied number of therapeutic tools.

Aspects of the physiology of muscles and tendons are worthy of a degree of review, insofar as MET and its effects are concerned. The tone of muscle is largely the job of the Golgi tendon organs. These detect the load applied to the tendon, via muscular contraction. Reflex effects, in the appropriate muscles, are the result of this information being passed from the Golgi tendon organ back along the cord. The reflex is an inhibitory one, and thus differs from the muscle spindle stretch reflex. Sandler describes some of the processes involved ('Physiology of Soft Tissue Massage', *British Osteopathic Journal,* January 1983): 'When the tension on the muscles, and hence the tendon, becomes extreme, the inhibitory effect from the tendon organ can be so great that there is sudden relaxation of the entire muscle under stretch. This effect is called the lengthening reaction, and is probably a protective reaction to the force which, if unprotected, can tear the tendon from its bony attachments. Since the Golgi tendon organs, unlike the (muscle) spindles, are in series with the muscle fibres, they are stimulated by both passive and active contractions of the muscles.'

Pointing out that muscles can either contract with constant length and varied tone (isometrically), or with constant tone and varied length (isotonically) he continues: 'In the same way as the gamma efferent system operates as a feedback to control the length of muscle fibres, the tendon reflex serves as a reflex to control the muscle tone.'

The relevance of this to soft tissue massage is explained thus: 'In terms of longitudinal soft tissue massage, these organs are very interesting indeed, and it is perhaps the reason why articulation of a joint, passively, to stretch the tendons that pass over the joint, is often as effective as relaxing the soft tissues as direct massage of the muscles themselves. Indeed, in some cases, where the muscle is actively in spasm, and is likely to object to being pummelled directly, articulation, muscle energy technique, or functional balance techniques, that make use of the tendon organ reflexes, can be most effective.' The use of this in therapy is obvious Sandler explains part of the effect of massage on muscle as follows: 'The (muscle) spindle and its reflex connections constitute a feedback device which can operate to maintain constant muscle length, as in posture; if the muscle is stretched the spindle discharges increase, but if the muscle is shortened, without a change in the rate of gamma discharge, then the spindle discharge will decrease, and the muscle will relax.'

He believes that massage techniques cause a decrease in the sensitivity of the gamma efferent, and thus increase the length of the muscle fibres, rather than a further shortening of them; this produces the desired relaxation of the muscle. Via a combination of NMT and MET, we thus have the ability to influence both the muscle spindles, and also the Golgi tendon organs.

No single individual deserves credit for MET, but its inception into osteopathic work must be credited to F. L. Mitchell Snr in 1958. Since then his son, and many others, have evolved a highly sophisticated system of manipulative methods. Among these are Edward Stiles DO, who has described a number of valuable techniques (*Patient Care,* 15 May 1984, pp16-97 and 15 August 1984, pp117-164.) Dr Stiles describes a number of methods, most of which involve operator direct manoeuvres, in which the post-isometric relaxation factor is dominant. These techniques, he believes, exert a build-up of tension in the already contracted muscles, which causes the Golgi receptor system to begin reporting the increased tension, in relation to surrounding muscles, thus reflexly inhibiting spasm. Stressing that manipulation is not the answer to everything, he elaborates on the theme of the wide application which it does have. He states: 'Basic science data suggests the musculoskeletal system plays an important role in the function of other systems. Research indicates that segmentally related somatic and visceral structures, may affect one another directly, via viscerosomatic and somaticovisceral reflex pathways. Somatic dysfunction may increase energy demands, and it can affect a wide variety of bodily processes; vasomotor control, nerve impulse patterns (in facilitation), axionic flow of neurotrophic proteins, venous and lymphatic circulation and ventilation. The impact of somatic dysfunction on various combinations of these functions may be associated with myriad symptoms and signs. A possibility which could account for some of the observed clinical effects of manipulation.' Stiles employs muscle energy methods on about 80 per cent of his patients, and functional techniques (see page 231) on 15 to 20 per cent. He uses high velocity thrusts on very few cases. The most useful manipulative tool available is, he maintains, muscle energy technique.

Stiles, as with most of the other practitioners using muscle energy methods, stresses the importance of accurate, precise, structural diagnosis. By careful motion palpation, determination is made as to restricted joints or areas, and which of their motions is limited. Precise, detailed localization is required if there is to be accuracy in determining the direction in which the patient is to direct their forces, so that the specific restricted barrier can be engaged. It is possible to actually create hypermobility in neighbouring segments, rather than normalizing the restricted segment, by innappropriate use of these methods. For example, if a particular restriction is present in a lumbar vertebrae (say limitation in gapping of the L4-L5, left side facets, on flexion.) Should a general attempt, not localized to this segment, be used, which involved the joints above and below the restricted segment, hypermobility of these joints could result thus leading to an incorrect assumption that overall mobility had been improved. The local restriction would remain, however.

Precise Location of Forces: Example of Lumbar Dysfunction

In order to localize the effort at this segment, the patient would require to be positioned, so as to engage the barrier in that joint. One hand would gently palpate the facets of L4-L5, whilst the seated patient was guided into a flexed and side bent position, which precisely engaged the barrier of motion. At that point there would be an instruction for the patient to attempt to return to an upright position, whilst the operator's force would be directed towards restraining any movement at all. This would be maintained for 3 to 5 seconds (Stile's method) with no more than perhaps 20 per cent of the patient's strength being employed in the effort (and synchronized to breathing, as mentioned above). After this, when all efforts had ceased, the barrier would normally be found to have retreated, so that greater flexion and side bending could be achieved, without effort, before re-engaging the barrier. Repetition would continue several times, until the maximum degree of motion had been obtained. The exact opposite method could also be employed, in which, having engaged the barrier, the patient attempted to move through it, whilst being restrained. This would bring into play reciprocal inhibition of the contracted muscles, which might be involved in, though not necessarily causing, the inability of the joint to gap normally.

By using the antagonists, instead of the affected muscles, less pain would be produced, were this an acute problem. This, and other methods involving spinal structures, will be described in greater detail later. This is merely an attempt to illustrate the importance of correct structural diagnosis, prior to use of these methods. Localization of restrictions, and identification of muscular contractions and fibrotic changes, is a matter of careful palpation, and the use of basic NMT in this quest is recommended.

The essence of muscle energy methods is the harnessing of the patient's muscle power. The next prerequisite is the application of counterforce in a predetermined manner. In isometric methods this counterforce must be unyielding. No test of strength must ever be attempted. Thus the patient should never be asked to 'try as hard as he can' to move in this or that direction. It is important before commencing that this, and the rest of the procedure, be carefully explained, so that a clear idea is obtained by the patient as to his role. The direction, limited degree of effort, and duration, must be clear, as must the associated instruction regarding breathing patterns, and eye movements (if any).

Preparing Joints for Manipulation Using MET

The value of using muscle energy methods is varied. It has applications which are aimed at normalizing soft tissue structures, such as shortened or tense muscles, with no direct implications as to the joints associated with these. It can be used to help to normalize joint mobility, via its applicability to the soft tissues, which may be the major obstacle to free movement. It may be employed to help to reduce the fibrotic changes in chronic soft-tissue problems, and also to tone weakened, lengthened, structures, which may be present in the antagonists of shortened soft tissues. It may also be employed in a *pre-manipulative mode*. In this instance the conventional manipulative procedure is approached, as it would normally be, whether this involves leverage or a thrust technique. The operator can then, having positioned himself and the patient appropriately for the adjustment (manipulative effort), ask the patient to 'push back' against this position. The operator will have engaged the barrier, and will have taken out the slack that was available in the soft tissues of the joint(s), in order to achieve this position. The resistance, or pushing back, against this position which is held by the operator, involves a patient-indirect, isometric, contraction, which would have the effect of contracting the shortened muscles. After holding this effort for several seconds, both operator and patient would simultaneously release their efforts, in a slow deliberate manner. This can be repeated several times, with the additional slack being taken out after appropriate relaxation by the patient.

Having engaged the barrier a number of times, the operator would decide when adequate release of restraining tissues had taken place and would then make the adjustment as normal. Laurie Hartman (*Handbook of Osteopathic Technique*, Hutchinson, 1985), states that: 'if the patient is in the absolute optimum position for a particular thrust technique during one of these repetitions (of MET), the joint in question will be felt to release. Even if this has not occurred, when retesting the movement range there is often a considerable increase in range and quality of play'.

He suggests that the operator use the temporary rebound reflex relaxation in the muscles, which will have followed the isometric contraction, to perform the technique. This will allow successful completion of the adjustment with minimal force. This refractory period of relaxation lasts for a few seconds and is valuable in all cases, but especially where the patient is tense or resistant to a manipulative effort.

Whenever force is applied, by the patient, in a particular direction, and when it is time to release that effort, the instruction must be to do so gradually. Any quick effort is self-defeating. The coinciding of the forces at the outset (patient and operator) as well as at release is important. The operator must be careful to use enough, but not too much, effort, and to ease off at the same time as the patient. Where weak muscles are being toned, via isotonic methods, the operator allows the concentric contraction of the muscles, as the patient attempts to move in a manner which employs the hypotonic structures. There are several methods possible. Such exercises always involve an operator's force which is less than that applied by the patient. The subsequent isotonic concentric contraction of the weakened muscles allows approximation of the origins and insertions to be achieved under some degree of control by the operator. In such cases the efforts are usually suggested as being of short duration, ultimately employing maximal effort on the part of the patient.

Strengthening Joint Complex with MET

The major variation on this method of simple isotonic contraction is to use what has been called *isokinetic contraction* (also known as *progressive resisted exercise*). In this the patient, starting with a weak effort, but rapidly progressing to a maximal contraction of the affected muscle(s), introduces a degree of resistance to the operator's effort to put the joint, or area, through a full range of motion. The use of isokinetic contraction is reported to be a most effective method of building strength, and to be superior to high repetition, lower resistance exercises. (*J. American Osteopathic Association*, Vol. 79 No. 11, July 1980, pp689). It is also felt that a limited range of motion, with good muscle tone, is preferable (to the patient) to normal range with limited power. Thus the strengthening of weak musculature in areas of permanent limitation of mobility is seen as an important contribution in which isokinetic contractions may assist.

Isokinetic contractions not only strengthen the fibres which are involved, but have a training effect which enables them to operate in a more co-ordinated manner. There is often a very rapid increase in strength. Because of neuro-muscular recruitment, there is a progressively stronger muscular effort as this method is repeated. Contractions, and accompanying mobilization of the region, should take no more than four seconds, at each contraction, in order to achieve maximum benefit with as little fatiguing as possible, of either the patient or the operator. Prolonged contractions should be avoided. The simple and safest applications of isokinetic methods involve small joints, such as those in the extremities. Spinal joints may be more difficult to mobilize whilst muscular resistance is being fully applied. The options in achieving increased strength, via these methods, therefore involves a choice between a partially resisted isotonic contraction or the overcoming of such a contraction, at the same time as the full range of movement is being introduced. Both of these options should involve maximum contraction of the muscles by the patient. Home treatment of such conditions is possible, via self-treatment, as in other MET methods.

Note: Both isotonic concentric and eccentric contractions, will take place during the isokinetic movement of a joint.

Reduction of Fibrotic Changes with MET

The other application of isotonic contraction is that in which the direct contraction is resisted and overcome by the operator. This has been termed *isolytic contraction*, in that it involves the stretching, and sometimes the breaking down, of fibrotic tissue present in the affected muscles. Adhesions of this type are broken down by the application of force by the operator which is just greater than that of the patient. This procedure can be uncomfortable, and the patient should be advised of this, as well as the need for them to apply only sufficient effort to ensure that they remain comfortable. Limited degrees of effort are therefore called for at the outset of isolytic contractions. This is an eccentric contraction, in that the origins and insertions of the muscles involved will become further separated, despite the patient's effort to approximate them.

In order to achieve the greatest degree of stretch, in the condition of myofascial fibrosis for example, it is necessary for the largest number of fibres possible to be involved in the isotonic contraction. Thus there is a contradiction, in that in order to achieve this large involvement, the degree of contraction should be a maximal one, and yet this is likely to produce pain, which is contra-indicated.

By combining MET and NMT, some degree of this problem is likely to be solved. NMT, applied to a region containing fibrotic change, will allow for subsequent use of MET, in an isolytic (or any other) phase, with less discomfort. The patient should be instructed to use about 20 per cent of possible strength on the first contraction, which is resisted and overcome by the operator, in a contraction lasting 3 to 4 seconds. This is then repeated, but with an increased degree of effort on the part of the patient (assuming the first effort was relatively painless). This continuing increase in the amount of force employed in the contracting musculature may be continued until, hopefully, a maximum contraction effort is possible, again to be overcome by the operator. In some muscles, of course, this may provide a heroic degree of effort on the part of the operator, and alternative methods are therefore desirable. NMT would seem to offer such an alternative. The isolytic manoeuvre should have as its ultimate aim a fully relaxed muscle. This will not always be possible.

Lest we forget, the process of ageing is a major reason for the changes which may be found in soft tissues, and which would benefit from isolytic contraction as part of MET treatment. NMT is also of course effective in dealing with such changes, which as well as resulting from ageing are a likely result of strain or trauma.

An article in *The Journal of the Royal Society for Medicine* (Vol. 76, December 1983, 'Connective Tissues: The natural fibre reinforced composite material') discusses connective tissue changes, and asks pertinent questions: 'Ageing effects the function of connective tissue more obviously than almost any organ system. Collagen fibrils thicken, and the amounts of soluble polymer decrease. The connective tissue cells tend to decline in number, and die off. Cartilages become less elastic, and their complement of proteoglycans changes both quantitatively and qualitatively. The interesting question is how many of these processes are normal, that contribute blindly and automatically, beyond the point at which they are useful? Does prevention of ageing, in connective tissues, simply imply inhibition of crosslinking in collagen fibrils, and a slight stimulation of the production of chondroiten sulphate proteoglycan?'

The effects of NMT and MET, both directly on these tissues as well as on the circulation and drainage of the affected structures, indicates that the ageing process can be retarded. This is a well established phenomenon, and is capable of influencing long-term health and mobility. Destruction of collagen fibrils is a serious matter. Although they may be replaced in the process of healing, scar tissue formation is common, and this makes repair inferior to the original tissues, both in functional and structural terms. Isolytic contraction has the ability to break down tight, shortened, tissues. The replacement of these with superior material will depend, to a large extent, on the subsequent use of the area (exercise, etc.) as well as the nutritive status of the individual. Collagen is dependent on adequate vitamin C, and a plentiful supply of amino-acids, such as proline, hydroxyproline and argenine. Protection of collagen status is dependent upon adequate presence of such antioxidant compounds as glutathione perixodase, which prevents free radical damage of such tissues. Manipulation, aimed at the restoration of a degree of normality in connective tissues, should take careful account of nutritional requirements.

It should always be borne in mind that when a muscle or muscle group is shortened in this manner, the antagonists are likely to be hypotonic, and it is advisable for these to receive attention subsequently, via isokinetic or other means (not necessarily at the same treatment session).

Spasm Release with MET

The most useful MET methods are those which achieve release of spasm and tension in muscles (or groups of muscles) or of joints. Any restriction should benefit, to some extent, from such an approach, although some will be more successfully treated by these means than others. If proprioceptive and palpatory skills are adequate, then the operator may gently feel the way towards the maximum degree of movement available in any particular muscle or joint. In some cases this will involve restriction in only one direction. For example, in the case of tension or fibrotic changes in the adductors of the upper leg.

The patient, in a prone position, may be assessed by the operator, who would gently abduct the limb to the point of 'bind'. Having engaged this barrier, the isometric effort on the part of the patient would be either to contract the adductors, which are shortened, whilst the operator resists this; or the opposite, involving contraction of the abductors, whilst resistance is again applied to prevent any movement. The first would be an operator-direct approach, hoping for subsequent post-isometric relaxation of the tight muscles. The second method would be a patient-direct approach, in which the contraction of the abductors was trying to pull the tight muscles past their barrier of resistance. This would rely on reciprocal inhibition for its effects. Were the muscles considered suitably fibrotic, then an isolytic (isotonic eccentric) contraction could be employed, in which the adductors, were contracted, with the effort being more than matched by the operator, who would progressively abduct the limb, thus stretching the contracting fibres, and

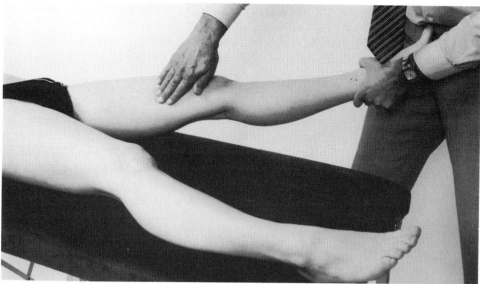

Figure 44

Assessment and treatment of tight adductors: The operator has abducted the supine patient's limb to the point of 'bind'. Having engaged this barrier the patient is asked to contract either the adductors or the abductors against isometric resistance. This would produce either post isometric relaxation (PIR) or reciprocal inhibition in the muscles of the inner thigh, depending upon the choice.

hopefully achieving a degree of destruction of some of the fibrous element.

A further alternative, in this example, would be the use of isokinetic mobilizing of the area, or isotonic concentric contraction, applied to the abductors, in order to tone these, presuming them to be weak as a result of their antagonists, the adductors, being shortened and tight.

The variations possible can be seen to be multiple, and the skill of the practitioner would be in the selection, and combination, of such manoeuvres.

The initial skill, however, is in the identification of the restriction. In this example, the abduction of one extremity would be found to be less free than the other, or they may both be found to be limited, in relation to what might be anticipated. This would be a relatively simple assessment. However, in the case of a spinal joint, there are many variables possible. Thus, although a particular spinal region or joint may be limited in flexion, for example, it would probably also be limited in one or other direction of, say, side-bending and/or rotation. All the restrictions should be identified, and these may be dealt with individually or together. Thus flexion could be introduced, to the current limit available, and then the patient instructed to minimally apply pressure against the restraining hand(s) of the operator, which would be preventing an effort to extend the area. After several efforts of this sort, each time engaging the new limit of flexion, it might be considered opportune to attempt to improve one or other of the associated limitations, side-bending, rotation, etc. On the other hand, the compound restriction could be engaged from the outset. In such a case the area would be so positioned as to be flexed and rotated, or side-bent and rotated, and this position held (detailed guidance as to the precise hold would depend on the structures involved) whilst the patient was instructed to attempt to de-rotate and to bring the area into an upright position, extending it and neutralizing the side-bending, all against unyielding resistance.

In this way the complex of muscles involved in the restriction(s), would be contracting, and multiple releases of tension, spasm and contraction could occur simultaneously. The area would then be again taken to its barrier, in these various directions, and the process repeated. As a complete reversal of this, the patient could be asked, once the barrier had been engaged in one or more of the directions of limitation, to attempt to force the area through the barrier, whilst the operator resisted. This latter method would involve the antagonists of the shortened muscles, and would therefore be relying on reciprocal inhibition of these in order to subsequently achieve greater ranges of movement.

Torticollis and MET

Such methods are more applicable to an acute situation, thus avoiding involvement, in the contraction process, of the irritated muscles themselves. In a case of torticollis, for example, where the patient presents with a side-bent neck, were this to involve shortened musculature (spasm) on the right, any attempt by the patient to involve further contraction of these muscles, as would be the case were the operator-direct approach involved (operator pushing to the left, to attempt to overcome the barrier, whilst the patient counterpushed to the right, using the affected muscles) would be likely to be painful. The use of the antagonists, in which the patient tried to engage the barrier, whilst the operator resisted, would therefore be more desirable, in such a situation, and be less likely to increase the already existing spasm.

A less acute situation would call for the operator direct approach. Torticollis would also benefit from NMT, trigger point treatment, and frequently from spinal adjustment, if this is necessary.

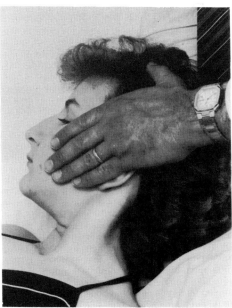

Torticollis: The patient has torticollis, with restriction of rotation to the left (the muscles on the right side of the neck are in spasm). The operator isometrically resists the patient's effort to pass through the restrictive barrier, as she attempts to turn to the left, using the non-affected muscles. Reciprocal inhibition is therefore produced in the muscles in spasm. This is a patient-direct effort, and in an acute situation would be less uncomfortable than an attempt to resist an operator-direct attempt, to turn the head through the barrier.

Figure 45

Identification of the restriction is critical, and this can only be achieved via the development of the skills required to assess joint mechanics, combined with a sound anatomical grasp. Assessment, via motion palpation, is called for. If forces are misdirected then results will be poor, and may exacerbate the problem. Localization of the point of restriction, in joint problems, is the major determining factor, as to success or otherwise, of MET (and all manipulation). Goodridge states: 'Monitoring of force is more important than intensity of force. Localization depends on the operator's palpatory proprioceptive perception of movement (or resistance to movement) at or about the specific articulation.' He continues: 'Monitoring and confining forces to the muscle group, or level of somatic dysfunction involved, are important in achieving desirable changes. Poor results are most often due to improperly localized forces, usually too strong.'

Lewit and Simon suggest that the contraction should be held for ten seconds or so, in the initial isometric effort. This is a gentle degree of effort, in their application of MET. Stiles suggests a 3 to 5 seconds contraction, and this too involves only a percentage of the available strength of the patient (in isometric contractions).

Self-Treatment Lewit is keen to involve patients in home treatment, using MET. He describes this aspect thus: 'Receptive patients are taught how to apply this treatment to themselves, as autotherapy, in a home programme. They passively stretched the tight muscle with their own hand. This hand next provided counter pressure to voluntary contraction of the tight muscle (during inhalation) and then held the muscle from shortening, during the relaxation phase. Finally, it supplied the increment in range of motion (during exhalation) by taking up any slack that had developed.'

Self-treatment methods are not suitable to all regions (or to all patients) but there are a large number of areas which lend themselves to such methods. Use of gravity, as a counter pressure source, is often possible in self-treatment. For example, in order to stretch quadratus lumborum, the patient stands, legs apart and sidebending, in order to impose a degree of stretch to the shortened muscle. By inhaling and *slightly* pushing the trunk towards an upright position, against the weight of the trunk, which gravity is pulling towards the floor, and then releasing the breath at the same time as trying to bend further towards the side, a greater degree of movement will have been achieved.

Lewit suggests, in such a movement, that the counter-movement against gravity be accompanied by movement of the eyes upwards, and the attempt to bend further to the side, by looking downward. These eye movements facilitate the effects. Several attempts, by the patient, to induce greater freedom of movement, in any restricted direction, should achieve good results, by means of such simple measures.

The principles of MET are now hopefully clear, and the methods seen to be applicable to a large range of problems. Rehabilitation, as well as first-aid, and some degree of normalization of both acute and chronic soft-tissue and joint problems, are all possible, given correct application. Combined with NMT, this offers the practitioner the chance of achieving safe and effective therapeutic intervention.

It is not the intention of this book to provide an entire range of muscle-energy

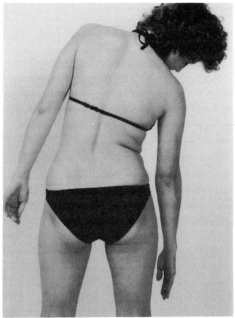 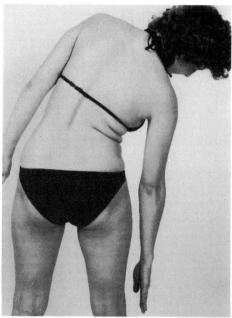

Figure 46   *Figure 47*

PIR Self-treatment of quadratus lumborum: The patient stands, feet apart, and sidebends so that maximum stretch is imposed upon the shortened musculature. Using breathing patterns described in the text she then comes slightly towards the upright position (position 1). On subsequent exhalation and relaxation she then allows the body to sidebend further to the side (position 2) and repeats the exercise several times more. Gravity is supplying the counterforce when she comes slightly upright.

applications. Specific examples will be found in various sections in Chapter 5, which deal with psoas muscle spasm (or contraction) piriformis contraction, temperomandibular joint dysfunction, and tensor fascia lata (ilio-tibial band) shortening. In this chapter we have already seen examples of possible MET application (spasm, muscle weakness, muscular infiltration with fibrous tissue etc.) as well as guidelines for the use of particular aspects of MET, in torticollis and lumbar vertebral dysfunction. These examples should provide competent practitioners with basic guidelines, via which they can vary the content of any MET methods which they may choose to use, to meet the particular requirements present in any given case. Below we provide several more examples, which are derived from the work of Dr Edward G. Stiles D.O., Dr Karel Lewit MD, Dr John Goodridge D.O. and Gregory Grieve F.C.S.P. (Physiotherapist). These are meant to expand the awareness of the reader as to options and variations in MET use, and not to provide a comprehensive list of all possible applications, since that would require a textbook on its own. It should by now be clear that MET may be employed as part of *any approach* to soft tissue, or joint dysfunction.

Dr Stiles's Methods in Cervical Problems (*Patient Care*, (15 August 1984)

To test for dysfunction in the upper cervical region, the patient lies supine. The operator flexes the neck slightly, with one hand, whilst the other cradles the neck. Flexion of this small degree, stabilizes the cervical area below C2, so that evaluation of atlanto-axial rotation may be carried out. The region C1 and C2 is usually responsible for half the gross rotation of the neck. With the neck flexed, it is then passively rotated to both left and right. If the range is greater on one side, then this is indicative of a probable restrictive barrier, which may be amenable to MET. If rotation to the left is normally about 85 degrees, but in this instance it is restricted, then palpation of muscle tissues at the level of the facets of C2 (just below the level of joint dysfunction) should indicate contraction or tension locally on the right. This may or may not be tender, but the likelihood is that it will be so if there is dysfunction. (Pain is often more noticeable at the level of any hypermobile joint rather than where the actual restriction is noted. This may be ascertained by palpation and motion palpation, feeling the tissues as the joint is moved).

If dysfunction is suspected at the atlanto-axial joint, then C2 is stabilized, in order to isolate C1 for treatment. A fingertip is placed on the left transverse process of C2, so that it cannot turn left when the patient's head is turned left. The operator's second finger, of the left hand (which is cradling the neck in flexion) is rested as a barrier to prevent left rotation of C2, and the head is then taken gently into left rotation. C1 and the head move, and C2 remains fixed. The barrier is engaged when C2 starts to move. This will be felt by the palpating finger. The slack is removed, and at that point the patient is asked to turn the head gently to the right, away from the barrier. The operator's right hand should be resting on the right side of the patient's head, to prevent this right rotation. The patient's force is exerted against the operator's and this is maintained for a few seconds (4 to 10). Patient and operator release their efforts at the same time, and the operator then attempts to take the head further to the left, without force, to engage the new barrier. This is repeated two or three times. This monitoring and stabilizing pressure on C2 is minimal, since the patient's effort is not a strong one (this must be stressed to the patient). The patient is using the muscles which are in spasm, or contracted (preventing rotation left) and, according to Dr Stiles, 'the exertion builds up tension in the contracted muscles; the Golgi receptor system starts reporting the increased tension in relation to surrounding muscles, and spasm is reflexly inhibited.' This is an operator-direct approach, involving post-isometric relaxation.

Dr Stiles's Comments regarding Whiplash Injury and MET

In such conditions X-ray pictures are often normal, as are neurological examinations. Pain is nevertheless present, often of major proportions. Careful examination should show some segments which are not capable of achieving a full range of movement. These would normally correlate with palpable tissue change and sensitivity. More often than not there is a restriction in which a vertebrae is caught in flexion (forward bending). Less commonly extension fixations may be noted. Each vertebrae should be tested to note its ability to flex, extend, side-bend and rotate. MET is applied to whatever specific restrictions are found, as in the example above.

Wherever a restriction is noted, in any particular direction, MET should be used. For example, if C3-4 facets close properly as the neck is side-bent to the left, a characteristic physiological 'springing' will be noted as the barrier is reached. If on the right, however, there is dysfunction as the neck is side-bent to that side, the facets will not be felt so close, and a pathological barrier will be noted, which is characterized by a lack of 'give', or increased resistance. This restriction may be expressed in two ways. The *positional diagnosis* would be that the segment is flexed and side-bent to the left (and therefore rotated left). The *functional diagnosis* would be that the joint will not extend, side-bend, or rotate to the right. With the patient in the same position as was used in diagnosis (supine, neck slightly flexed). The operator's right middle fingers would be placed over the right pillars of C3-4, and the neck taken to the maximum position of side-bending rotation to the right, engaging the barrier. The left hand is placed over the patient's left parietal and temporal areas. With this hand offering counterforce, the patient is invited to side-bend and rotate to the left, for a few seconds. This employs the muscles which are shortened, and which are preventing the joint from easily side-bending and rotating to the right. Post-isometric relaxation of these will follow, and the neck should be taken to its new barrier, and the same procedure repeated 2 or 3 times. An alternative would be for the patient to engage the barrier whilst the operator resisted.

General Procedure Using MET for Cervical Restriction

Prior to any testing Stiles suggests a general manoeuvre, in which the patient is sitting upright. The operator stands behind, and holds the head in the midline, with both hands stabilizing it, and possibly employing his chest to prevent neck extension. The patient is told to try (gently) to flex, extend, rotate and side-bend the neck, in all directions, alternately. No particular sequence is necessary, as long as all directions are engaged, five or six times. Each muscle group should undergo slight contraction, against unyielding force. This relaxes the tissues in a general manner. Traumatized muscles will relax without much pain, via this method.

Acromio-clavicular (AC) Dysfunction

Stiles suggests beginning evaluation of AC dysfunction at the scapula, the mechanics of which closely relate to AC function. The patient sits erect and the spines of both scapula are palpated by the operator, standing behind. The hands are moved medially, until the medial borders of the scapulae are identified, at the level of the spine. Using the palpating fingers as landmarks, the levels are checked to see whether they are the same. Inequality suggests AC dysfunction. The side of dysfunction remains to be assessed. Each is tested separately. To test the right side AC joint, the operator is behind the patient, with the left hand palpating over the joint. The right hand holds the patient's right elbow. The arm is lifted in a plane, 45 degrees from the saggital and frontal planes. As the arm approaches 90 degrees elevation the AC joint should be carefully palpated for hinge movement, between the acromion and the clavicle. In normal movement, with no restriction, the palpating hand should move slightly cauded, as the arm is abducted beyond 90 degrees. If the AC is restricted the palpating hand will move cephalad, and little or no action will be noted at the joint itself, as the arm goes beyond 90 degrees.

   Muscle energy technique is employed with the arm held, as for testing above. If the scapula on the side of dysfunction is higher than that on the normal side, then the humerus is placed in external rotation, which takes the scapula caudad against the barrier. If, however, the scapula on the side of the AC dysfunction is already lower than the scapula on the normal side, then the arm is internally

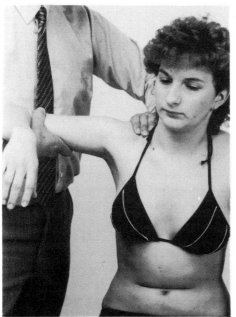

Acromio-clavicular dysfunction: Having assessed the nature of the dysfunction, the operator is stabilizing the acromio-clavicular joint and has externally rotated the humerus in order to take the scapula caudad against the restriction barrier (see text for alternatives). An isometric contraction is introduced as the patient attempts to direct the right elbow towards the floor, with less than full strength, against unmoving resistance, for 5-10 seconds. The procedure is repeated several times until maximum release is obtained.

Figure 48

rotated, taking the scapula cephalad against the barrier. The left hand (we assume this to be a right-sided problem) stabilizes the distal end of the clavicle, with caudad pressure being applied by the left thumb being placed over the upper aspect of the scapula, and the first finger of the left hand over the distal aspect of the clavicle. The combined rotation of the arm, as appropriate, and the downward pressure exerted by the left hand, provides an unyielding counterforce. The arm will have been raised until the first sign of inappropriate movement at the AC joint was noted. This is the barrier, and at this point the various stabilizing holds (internal or external arm rotation, etc.) are introduced. An unyielding counter-pressure is applied at the point of the patient's elbow, and the patient is asked to try to take that elbow towards the floor with less than full strength. After a few seconds the patient and operator relax, and the arm is once more taken towards the barrier. Again greater internal, or external, rotation are introduced, to take the scapula higher or lower, as appropriate. The isometric contraction is again called for, and the procedure repeated several times. It is worth recalling that many practitioners advise respiratory accompaniment to the efforts described, with inhalation accompanying effort, and exhalation accompanying relaxation and the engagement of the new barrier. The procedure is repeated until no further improvement is noted in terms of range of motion.

MET Exercise for Beginners

John Goodridge D.O. ('MET Definition, explanation, methods of procedure' *JAOA*, Vol. 81, No. 4, P249) describes a simple method for beginning to become familiar with MET.

> 1. After grasping the supine patient's foot and ankle, in order to abduct the lower limb, the operator closes his eyes during the abduction, and feels, in his own body, from his hand through his forearm, into his upper arm, the beginning of a sense of resistance.

2. He stops when he feels it, opens his eyes, and notes how many degrees in an arc, the patient's limb has travelled.

3. He compares the arc with the arc produced on the opposite side. In treatment, for example, if the abducted right femur reaches resistance sooner than the left, then restriction of abduction exists. To remove this restriction, the patient's limb is positioned in that arc of movement, where resistance is first perceived, and at this point the physician employs a MET to lessen the sense of resistance, and increase the range of movement.

When a left-right assymetry in range of movement exists, that assymetry may be due to either a hypertonic or hypotonic condition. Differentiation is made by testing for strength, comparing left and right muscle groups. If findings suggest weakness is the cause of assymetry in range of motion the antagonists will probably be found to be contracted, and these should receive first attention, using MET. Subsequent assessment may show that hypotonic muscles require toning and this may be achieved using isotonic contractions. The following steps are used to strengthen weakened tissues in all areas.

1. The operator positions the limb, or area, so that the muscle group will be at resting length, and thus will develop the strongest contraction.

Strengthening Weak Muscles

2. The operator explains the direction of movement required, as well as the intensity and duration of that effort. The patient contracts the muscle with the objective of moving the part through a complete range, quickly (about 2 seconds).

3. The operator offers counterforce, which is less than that of the patient's contraction, and maintains this throughout the contraction. This is repeated several times, with a progressive increase in operator's counterforce (the patient's efforts in the strengthening mode is always maximal).

Were the objective to lengthen shortened adductors, on the right, several methods could be used. The patient could contract the right *abductors,* against equal operator counterforce, in order to relax the adductors by *reciprocal inhibition;* or the patient could contract the right *adductors* against equal operator counterforce, in order to achieve *post-isometric relaxation;* or the patient could contract the right *adductors* whilst the operator offered greater counterforce, thus overcoming the isotonic contraction *(eccentric-isotonic, or isolytic, contraction).*

Lengthening Shortened Muscles

In all these examples the shortened muscles would have been taken to their pain free limit of stretch before commencing the contraction. Goodridge explains that the last two methods (post-isometric relaxation and isolytic method) would increase the tension in the tendons of the muscles, and this would stimulate the efferent firing of the Golgi bodies, and cause muscle fibres to relax and lengthen. Lewit and Simon's ('Myofascial Pain: Relief by post-isometric relaxation', *Arch. Phys. Med. Rehabil.* Vol. 65, August 1984) discuss several methods whereby MET may be employed, either by the operator or as self-treatment.

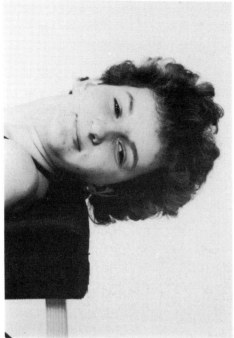 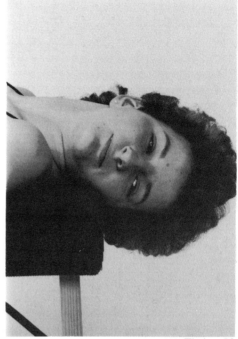

Figure 49   *Figure 50*

Sternomastoid self-treatment: The head of the patient is rotated away from the side of shortening or tenderness so that the head is slightly over the edge of the couch. Maximum comfortable stretch is introduced, with gravity imposing the counterforce. The head is then raised slightly (*Figure 49*) and this is held for 5-10 seconds. As the breath is released and the muscle relaxed, the tight musculature of the neck will release slightly and the head should then be taken to its furthest degree of stretch (*Figure 50*) before the isometric contraction is repeated with gravity again acting as the counterforce. In self-treatment, the relaxation phase, after the isometric contraction, should last at least as long as the contraction.

Sternomastoid Tenderness or Contraction

The head of the patient is rotated away from the side of shortening, or tenderness, in the sternomastoid, to impose maximal comfortable stretch. The patient is lying supine, with the head hanging over the edge of the table, head rotated away from the side of the contracted muscle. This produces gravitational counterforce on the stretched muscle, causing tension on the sternal head of the muscles. The patient attempts to lift the head, with minimal force, whilst the operator supplies counterforce, for five to ten seconds. After relaxation the head is further rotated and retroflexed to the new tolerable barrier. This is repeated several times.

Self-treatment can be applied by the patient, in this position, using hand pressure and/or gravity, against which minimal effort is used to raise the head, and to rotate it towards the midline. After such an effort the muscles are relaxed to allow full stretch, before repetition (*see Figure 49*).

Extensors of the Wrist

The patient sits facing the operator who bends the elbow and supports this in one hand, whilst the other hand flexes the patient's wrist and fingers, which are facing

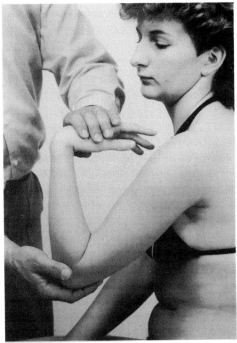 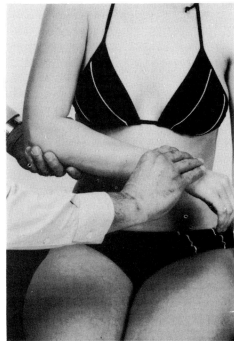

Figure 51   *Figure 52*

Treatment of dysfunction of extensors of the wrist: The wrist is flexed as illustrated, and with minimal force the patient is asked to extend the fingers against resistance for 5-10 seconds. The flexion of the fingers and wrist is repeated and the contraction performed again until maximum release is obtained. This condition may accompany a painful lateral epicondyle. If this is so then the patient attempts to supinate the pronated forearm against resistance (Note left arm illustrated for extensor dysfunction, right arm for epicondyle tenderness).

the patient. This flexed position is held, whilst the patient is requested to extend the fingers, with minimal force, against the counterforce of the operator. During relaxation, after five seconds or so, the operator flexes the fingers as far as they will comfortably go, before the contraction is repeated. Flexion of both wrist and fingers will be limited if the *extensors are tight.*

This may accompany restricted ability to supinate the forearm, in a condition involving a *painful lateral epicondyle.* MET should also be applied to the pronated forearm, which involves resistance of a patient's attempt to supinate (*see Figures 51 and 52*).

Painful medial humeral epicondyle accompanies tension in the *flexors* of the wrist. With elbow flexed, the wrist in maximal dorsi-flexion, and pronation exaggerated by pressure on the ulnar side of the palm, a resisted effort to supinate the hand is made. Pronation and dorsi-flexion are again taken to the limit, and the procedure repeated three or four times (*see Figure 53*). All these methods are capable of adaptation to self-treatment, by means of the patient applying the counterpressure.

An example is given below in which stretching of muscles is avoided, and their tensing is used instead, e.g. *coccygeal tenderness.*

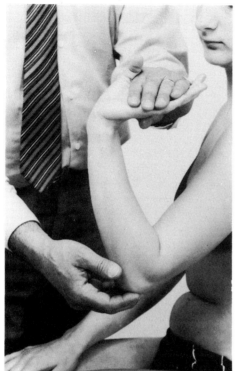

Left Treatment of painful medial epicondyle of elbow: This condition usually accompanies tension of the flexors of the wrist. The wrist is positioned as illustrated, the maximal dorsiflexion of the wrist and pronation exaggerated. Pressure is placed on the ulnar side of the palm and an effort made by the patient, against resistance, to supinate the hand. After this pronation and dorsiflexion are again taken to the pain-free limit, before repeating the isometric contraction.

Below Coccygeal tenderness: The glutei and levator ani are contracted for 5-10 seconds and then released repetitively. The operator monitors this, or self-treatment may be introduced, with the patient monitoring the contraction with her own hands. With self-treatment a contraction of some 20 seconds, and an equal rest place is suggested. The counterpressure in this type of contraction is provided by the muscles themselves.

Figure 53

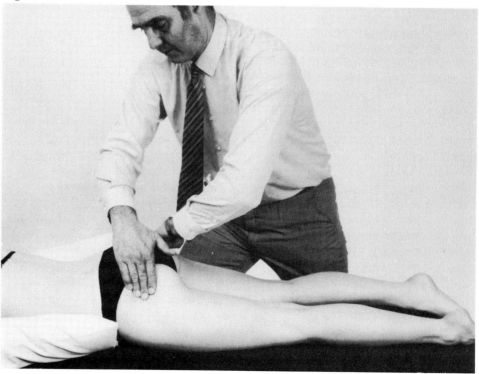

Figure 54

If there is involvement of gluteus maximus, or levator ani, then it is often sufficient to apply the operator's hands to the mass of the glutei, telling the patient to contract the muscles slightly, and then to relax. The feeling of strong muscle tonus progressively decreases with successive cycles, without any stretching needed (*see Figure 54*).

Self-Treatment

When self-treatment is used, stretching is also not always needed. Gravity may provide the counterforce, as in the sternomastoid contraction above. In such cases (i.e. no counterforce apart from gravity) the relaxation phase should last as long as the contraction phase (at least 20 seconds according to Lewit and Simon). They point out that the gravity counterforce is continued during both the contraction and the relaxation phase. Deep inhalation, followed by exhalation, is important in self-treatment, as in MET applied by the practitioner.

Painful Long Biceps Tendon: MET

Lewit describes this method: The patient sits in front of the operator, with the affected arm behind the back, the dorsal aspect of that hand passing beyond the buttock on the opposite side. The therapist grasps this hand, bringing it into pronation, to take up the slack. The patient is instructed to attempt to take the hand into supination. This is resisted for about ten seconds, by the operator, and the relaxation phase is used to take it further into pronation, with simultaneous extension of the elbow. Three to five repetitions are undertaken. Self-treatment is possible with the patient applying counterpressure, with the other hand.

Gravity Induced Post-Isometric Relaxation of Quadratus Lumborum (Self-Treatment)

The patient stands, legs apart, bending sideways. The patient inhales and slightly raises trunk (a few centimetres) at the same time as looking ceilingward (with the eyes only). On exhalation the side-bend is allowed to slowly go as far as it can, whilst the patient looks towards the floor. This is repeated a number of times. Eye positions influence the tendency to flex, and side-bend (eyes look down) and extend (eyes look up). (*See Figures 46 and 47.*)

Lumbosacral Ligament Pain

Increased tension is usually noted on the side which palpates as tender. Adduction of the leg on that side is usually restricted. The patient is supine, the operator stands on the side opposite the painful side. The leg is flexed at knee and hip, and brought to a position of greatest adduction, with the operator holding the knee. The adduction of the flexed leg, and the degree of hip flexion, should be taken to the point of the most pronounced pain. (This may correspond to sites of iliolumbar or sacro-iliac ligaments). The position of greatest resistance is normally the position of greatest sensitivity. At this point the patient is asked to attempt abduction and extension of the hip, against operator counterforce. Only a slight effort should be initiated at first. This is held during inhalation, for ten seconds or so. During relaxation, accompanied by exhalation, adduction is increased. This might cause some pain. This is repeated 3-5 times, each time starting from the new barrier of resistance.

Grieve describes a low back approach, using MET, which closely resembles that described by Goodridge. The following is a brief summary.

Low Back Dysfunction and MET

The example is of a spine which is capable of full flexion, but in which palpable left side-bending, and left rotation, fixation exists, in the lumbar spine. The patient sits on a stool, feet apart and flat on the floor. The left arm hangs between the patient's knees. The operator stands at the patient's left side, with his left leg straddling the patient's left leg. The operator reaches across, and holds the patient's right shoulder, whilst the right hand palpates the vertebral interspace between the spinous processes immediately below the vertebrae which is restricted in maximum left rotation.

The patient is asked to slump forwards, until the segment under inspection is most prominent, posteriorly. At this point the operator presses his left pectoral area against the patient's left shoulder and, with the patient still flexed, the spine is side-bent by the operator, without resistance, so that the patient's right hand approximates the floor. The operator then rotates the patient to the right, until maximum tension is felt to build at the segment being palpated. This is the barrier. (*See Figure 55.*)

At this time the first MET procedure is brought into play. The patient is asked to attempt to reach the floor with their right hand, and this is resisted by the operator. This may last for 5 to 10 seconds, after which the patient relaxes (exhaling). The operator increases the side-bending and rotation to the right, before increasing the degree of flexion. This is the new barrier, and the procedure of attempting to increase these directions of spinal movement (side-bending and rotation to the right, and flexion) is repeated, against resistance, a further 3 to 4 times. These movements all involve reciprocal inhibition of the shortened muscle fibres, which are holding the restricted area in left side-bending and left rotation. The antagonists are being contracted isometrically, to induce relaxation of these structures. (*See Figure 56.*)

After this the patient, who is flexed and rotated, and side-bent to the right, attempts to push against the operator's chest, with the left shoulder (i.e. attempts to rotate left and side-bend left, as well as to extend). This is maintained for a few seconds before relaxation, re-engagement of the barrier, and repetition. This contraction involves those structures which have shortened, and so the isometric contraction produces post-isometric relaxation in them. The slack is again taken out, by taking the patient further into right side-bending, rotation and flexion. Grieve then suggests that the patient be asked to perform a series of stretching movements to the floor, first with the left hand and then with the right hand, before being brought into an upright position by the operator, against slight resistance of the patient. The condition is then reassessed. The operator's position alters, after the isometric effort to the left, so that he now stands behind the patient, guiding the rotation and side-bending and extension, with a hand on each shoulder. Grieve uses both reciprocal inhibition, and post isometric relaxation, in this manoeuvre. (*See Figure 57.*)

Goodridge describes two basic MET procedures to achieve the same end. The same pattern of dysfunction is assumed. Goodridge states: 'If the left transverse process of L5 is more posterior, when the patient is flexed, one postulates that the left caudad facet did not move anteriorly and superiorly along the left cephalad facet of S1, as did the right caudad facet. The movement to resolve the non-movement is postulated to have minute movements in the directions of flexion, lateral flexion (side-bending) to the right and rotation to the right, restricted. It

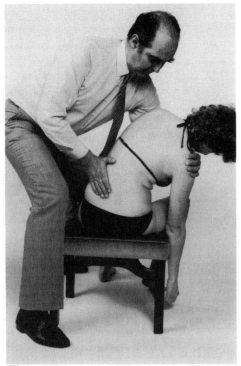

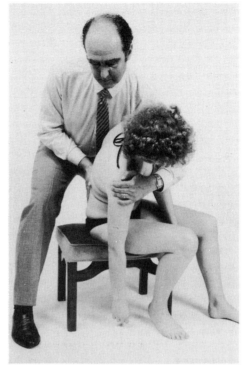

Figure 55

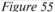

Above Low Back Dysfunction (full flexion ability assumed, with restriction in sidebending and rotation to the right noted): Operator palpates vertebral interspace as the patient sequentially flexes, sidebends and rotates to the right until maximum tension is elicited, and most prominent posterior excursion obtained, of segment under treatment.

Above right The patient is instructed to attempt to reach towards the floor with the right hand, against resistance from the operator, for 5-10 seconds, during inhalation. After a relaxation of all efforts, and exhalation, the patient is taken further towards the barrier, and the procedure is repeated. This effort involves reciprocal inhibition of fibres on the left of the spine, which are involved in the restriction, and which prevent free movement to the right.

Right The patient is asked to push against the chest of the operator with the left shoulder and to simultaneously attempt to derotate and extend the spine. This is resisted isometrically. Repetition of this induces PIR of the contracted fibres.

Figure 56

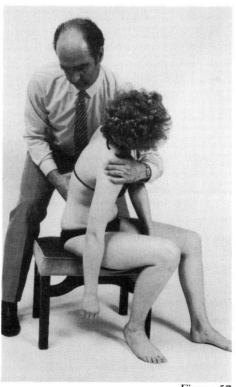

Figure 57

is further postulated, or conceptualized, that the non-moving side is restrained by hypertonicity (or shortening) of some muscle fibres. Therefore, the operator devises a muscle energy procedure to decrease the tone of (or to lengthen) the affected fibres.'

The position, as described by Grieve above, is adopted. Patient seated, left hand hanging between thighs, operator at his left, patient's right hand lateral to his right hip and pointing to the floor. The operator's right hand monitors either L5 spinous or transverse process. The patient's left shoulder is contacted against the operator's left axillary fold, and upper chest. The operator's left hand is in contact with the patient's right shoulder. The patient slouches to flex lumbar spine, so that apex of posterior convexity is located at L5-S1 articulation. Operator induces first right-side-bending, and then right rotation (patient's right hand reaches to the floor) and localizes movement at L5. The patient is then asked to move in one or more directions, singly or in combination with each other. These would involve left side-bending, rotation left, and/or extension, all against operator's counterforces.

The patient is, in all of these, contracting muscles on the left side of the spine, but is not changing the distance between the origin and insertion in muscles on either side of the spine. This achieves post-isometric relaxation, and subsequent contractions would be initiated after appropriate taking up of slack and engagement of the new barrier. An alternative to this is that, having attained the position of flexion, right side-bending and right rotation localized at the joint in question, the patient is asked to move both shoulders in a translation to the left, against resistance from the operator's chest and left anterior axillary fold. Neither of the shoulders should rise or fall, from the line of translation, during the effort. Whilst the patient is attempting to move in this manner the operator palpates the degree of increased right side-bending which it induces, at L5-S1. As the patient eases off from this contraction, as described, the operator is able to increase right rotation and side-bending until, once again, restraint is noted.

The objective of this alternative method is the same as the previous example, but the movement involves, according to Goodridge, a concentric-isotonic procedure, because it allows right lateral flexion of the thoracolumbar spine, during the effort.

Some MET methods are very simple, others involve conceptualization of multiple movements, and the localization of forces to achieve their ends. The principles remain the same, and can be applied to any muscle or joint dysfunction since the degree of effort, duration of effort and muscles utilized, provide unlimited variables, which can be tailored to meet all needs.

Sequential Assessment of Tight Muscles and Appropriate M.E. Treatments

Janda (see page 207) informs us that postural muscles have a tendency to shorten, not only under pathological conditions but often under normal circumstances. It is interesting to learn that 85 per cent of the walking cycle is spent on one leg and that this is the most common postural position for man. Those muscles which enable this position to be satisfactorily adopted (one-legged standing) are genetically older; they have different physiological, and probably biochemical, qualities compared with phasic muscles which normally weaken and exhibit signs of inhibition in response to stress or pathology.

Most of the problems of the musculoskeletal system involve pain related to aspects of muscle shortening. Where weakness (lack of tone) is apparently a major element

Muscle Energy Technique: Summary of Variations

Type of Contraction	Indications	Modus Operandi	Forces	Duration	Repetitions
Isometric patient-direct.	Relaxing muscular spasm or contraction. Mobilizing restricted joints. Preparing joint for manipulation.	Affected muscle not employed. Antagonists used, therefore shortened muscles relax via reciprocal inhibition. Patient is attempting to push through the barrier of restriction.	Operator's and patient's forces are matched. Initial effort involves approximately 20% of patient's strength; slow increase to no more than 50% on subsequent contractions. Increase of duration often more effective than increase in force.	4 to 10 seconds initially, increasing to up to 30 seconds in subsequent contractions, if greater effect required.	3 to 5 times.
Isometric operator-direct.	Relaxing muscular spasm or contraction. Mobilizing restricted joints. Preparing joint for manipulation.	Affected muscles used, therefore shortened muscles relax via post-isometric relaxation. Operator is attempting to go through barrier of restriction.	Operator's and patient's forces are matched. Initial effort involves approximately 20% of patient's strength; slow increase to no more than 50% on subsequent contractions. Increase of duration often more effective than increase in force.	4 to 10 seconds initially, increasing to up to 30 seconds in subsequent contractions, if greater effect required.	3 to 5 times.

Muscle Energy Technique: Summary of Variations

Type of Contraction	Indications	Modus Operandi	Forces	Duration	Repetitions
Isotonic concentric.	Toning weakened musculature.	Contracting muscle is allowed to do so, with some resistance from operator.	Patient's force is greater than operator resistance. Patient uses maximal effort available, but force is built slowly not via sudden effort.	3 to 4 seconds.	5 to 7 times.
Isotonic eccentric (isolytic).	Stretching tight fibrotic musculature.	Contracted muscle is prevented from doing so, via superior operator effort. Origin and insertion do not approximate. Muscle is taken to, or as close as possible to, full physiological resting length.	Operator's force is greater than patient's. Less than maximal patient's force employed at first. Subsequent contractions build towards this, if pain not excessive.	2 to 4 seconds.	3 to 5 times if pain not excessive.
Isokinetic (isotonic and isometric contractions).	Toning weakened musculature. Building strength in all muscles involved in particular joint function. Training effect on muscle fibres.	Patient resists with moderate effort at first, progressing to maximal effort subsequently, as operator puts joint through its full range of movements.	Operator's force overcomes patient's effort to prevent movement. First mobilization involves moderate force, progressing to full force subsequently.	Up to 4 seconds.	2 to 4 times.

it will often be found that antagonists to these are shortened, reciprocally inhibiting their tone, and that prior to any effort to strengthen weak muscles, short ones should be dealt with by appropriate means (MET, NMT etc.) after which spontaneous toning occurs in the previously flaccid muscles. If tone is still inadequate then, and only then, should exercise and/or isotonic procedures be brought in.

We must learn to assess short, tight muscles in a standardized manner. Janda suggests:

> To obtain a reliable evaluation the starting position, method of fixation and direction of movement must be observed carefully. The prime mover must not be exposed to external pressure. If possible the force exerted on the tested muscle must not work over two joints. The examiner performs at an even speed a slow movement that brakes slowly at the end of the range. To keep the stretch and the muscle irritability about equal the movement must not be jerky. Pressure or pull must always act in the required direction of movement. Muscle shortening can only be correctly evaluated if the joint range is not decreased as in a bony limitation or joint restriction.

It is in shortened muscles, as a rule, that reflex activity is noted. This takes the form of local dysfunction variously named as trigger points, tender points, zones of irritability, neurovascular and neurolymphatic reflexes etc. (See chapters 2 and 3). Localizing these is possible via normal palpatory methods or as part of neuromuscular diagnostic treatment.

Identification and treatment of tight muscles may also be systematically carried out as described below.

1. *Assessment of tight gastrocnemius*

Patient is supine with feet extending over edge of couch. For right leg examination operator's left hand grasps Achilles tendon just above heel, with no pressure on tendons. The heel lies in the palm of the hand, fingers curving round it. The right hand is placed so that the fingers rest on the dorsum of the foot (these must rest all the time, not apply a pulling stretch) with the thumb on the sole, lying along the medial margin. This position is important as mistakes may involve placing the thumb too near the centre of the sole of the foot. Stretch is introduced by a pull on the heel with the left hand, whilst the right hand maintains the upward pressure via the thumb (along its entire length). The heel of the right hand prevents sideways movement of the foot.

A range should be achieved which takes the foot to a 90 degree angle to the leg.

The leg must remain resting on the couch all the while and the right hand holding the heel must be placed so that it is an extension of the leg, not allowing an upward (ceilingward) pull when stretch is introduced.

2. An alternative method is to have the patient seated on the couch, legs outstretched, and to have him/her bend towards the toes with arms extended. If toe touching is possible, *but toes are plantar-flexed,* then there is probably shortness of the gastrocnemius-soleus muscles.

3. *Assessment of tight soleus*

Method No. 1 assesses gastrocnemius and soleus. To assess only the soleus the same procedure is adopted with the knee passively flexed (over a cushion, for example).

4. If the patient is asked to squat, trunk slightly flexed, feet apart, so that the buttocks rest between the legs, it should be possible to go fully into this position with the heels flat on the floor. If not, and the heels rise from the floor as the squat is performed, soleus is shortened.

Treatment of shortened gastrocnemius and/or soleus

The exact position is adopted as in test No. 1 above. The operator takes out all the slack available by stretching the heel downwards with the left hand whilst exerting pressure upwards along the medial margin of the foot with the right hand. The patient then attempts, using only about 20 per cent of his/her strength and whilst holding the breath, to push against this mild degree of stretch for 7 to 10 seconds (attempting plantar flexion of the ankle, not curling the toes). This resisted contraction of the tight muscles is released slowly by both patient and operator, and the stretch is then carried to its new barrier, with no force at all. This is repeated several times until no further gain is achieved. At this point the patient is asked to introduce an attempt to reverse the forces previously applied, so that he/she attempts to dorsiflex the foot, at the ankle, against resisted effort. This employs the antagonists of the tight muscles. When the isometric contraction has been performed the new barrier is engaged by the operator gently taking the foot to its new limit of dorsiflexion without undue effort.

5. Assessment of shortness in flexors of the hip

Patient is supine with buttocks at end of couch, coccyx almost over the edge. The leg not being assessed is flexed as far as it is possible in order to tilt the pelvis posteriorly to flatten the lumbar curve against the couch. This leg is held (by patient and operator) in order to maintain (lock) this position of the pelvis. The leg to be tested should lie so that the upper leg is horizontal to the surface of the couch with the lower leg hanging down freely. If the thigh cannot lie horizontal to the couch then it indicates a shortened iliopsoas muscle. Additional downward pressure on the distal thigh applied by the operator, should allow for extension at the hip, if it does not then the iliopsoas is very much shortened.

If the lower leg cannot flex completely to hang vertically in this position, then there is a probable shortening of rectus femoris. If additional downward pressure on the lower third of the femur of the tested leg results in compensatory extension of the lower leg, at the knee, then rectus femoris is very short.

If both hip and knee are flexed as above (thigh unable to lie horizontal to surface of couch and lower leg unable to hang vertically) then both iliopsoas and rectus femoris are shortened.

If there is a marked lateral deviation of the patella and a deep hollow noted on the outer thigh, then tensor fascia lata is probably shortened. If additional pressure is applied on the lower third of the thigh of the tested leg, to take it slightly more into adduction, and this increases the hollow in the outer thigh over the iliotibial band, then the tensor fascia lata is very short.

6. The prone patient lies with both legs outstretched. If the iliopsoas is shortened then the hip remains in flexion. Passive flexion at the knee may result in a compensatory increase in spinal lordosis and increased flexion at the hip, indicating rectus femoris shortening.

7. The patient is sidelying, tested side uppermost. Lower leg is flexed comfortably.

Upper leg is allowed to hang behind the body so that foot can drop over back edge of couch. Leg should be able to drop into adduction whilst body maintains contact along its length without arching. If leg fails to drop when pelvis is fixed there is shortening of tensor fascia lata and iliotibial band.

8. The patient is sidelying, tested leg uppermost. Lower leg is flexed and held to the couch. Upper leg is flexed at hip and knee and is abducted and extended by the operator whose hand holds this leg at the ankle thus allowing the knee to fall into adduction, towards the couch. It will not do so if there is shortening of the iliotibial band, even if the patient is totally relaxed.

Treatment of shortened iliopsoas
The patient lies as in the test position (No. 5 above). See Figure 19 on page 132. See pages 132-137 for various psoas muscle techniques.

Treatment of shortened rectus femoris
The patient is prone with a cushion under the abdomen to reverse a tendency to increased lumbar lordosis. The affected leg is flexed at the knee and the operator stabilizes the thigh of this side by a downward controlling pressure below the ischial tuberosity. Holding the lower leg just above the ankle the operator takes the lower leg into maximum comfortable flexion and then asks the patient, with appropriate breathing as described above, to attempt to straighten the leg. It is imperative that increased lordosis does not occur. This resisted contraction is held for 7-10 seconds and then released, after which the leg is flexed further, thus stretching the rectus femoris. Repeat until no further gain is achieved. Antagonists should not be employed as cramp may occur.

Or the patient is prone, as above, affected leg flexed at knee and extended at hip with operator stabilizing the trunk of the patient with one hand, whilst the other hand cradles the knee of the affected leg. The patient's foot rests at the operator's shoulder level. The patient is asked to press down against the shoulder with the ankle, with appropriate breathing, for 10 seconds or so, and with less than full strength. After release the hip is extended further (avoid lordosis if possible) and further flexion of the lower leg is introduced, to reach the new barrier of restriction. The procedure is then repeated.

Treatment of shortened tensor-fascia lata
This condition is often associated with recurrent 'sacro-iliac' problems as well as pain felt in the region of the trochanter. Specialized soft tissue methods are described on pages 156-158. In addition Muscle Energy methods may be used as described on page 159 (illustrated in Figure 36, page 160). Self-treatment is described on page 159.

Assessment of shortened hamstrings (biceps femoris, semitendinosus and semimembranosis)

9. The patient is supine with legs outstretched. In order to assess tightness in the left leg hamstrings, the right leg must be fixed to the couch by a downward pressure applied above the knee, avoiding the patella by the operator's cephalid hand. The operator is standing at the side of the leg to be tested facing the couch. The lower leg is grasped with his/her caudad hand, keeping the knee of that leg in extension

and resting the heel of that leg in the bend of the elbow, to prevent lateral rotation of the leg.

Range of movement should allow elevation of the leg to about 80 degrees.

10. If the hip flexors are shortened, as assessed using the methods above, and causing a forward tilt of the pelvis and stretch of the hamstrings, a modification of No. 9 is required.

The patient is supine with the leg not to be tested flexed at the hip with the sole of the foot on the couch. This tilts the pelvis backwards and allows the lumbar curve to remain flat against the couch. All other aspects of No. 9 above are repeated. Or, use the assessment described on pages 110 and 111 and illustrated on pages 112 and 113.

Treatment of shortened hamstrings

Position as in No. 9, or No. 10 (if hip flexors are very short), above. The resisted isometric contraction is introduced once the painfree limit of stretch is achieved, with the patient attempting to push the leg down against resistance for 7 to 10 seconds with appropriate breathing. On release the procedure is repeated until no further gain is achieved in degree of stretch.

In order to employ the antagonists of the hamstrings, the quadriceps, a simple reversal of direction may be used, in which the patient attempts to raise the extended leg against resistance.

Or, the supine patient flexes the affected hip fully. The knee is extended as far as possible, with the back of the lower leg resting on the shoulder of the operator who stands facing cephalward. If this involves the right leg of the patient then the operator's left hand will rest on the anterior aspect of patient's shin. The operator's right hand stabilizes the patient's extended unaffected leg against the couch. The patient is asked to attempt to straighten the lower leg (i.e. extend the knee) employing 20 per cent of the strength in the quadriceps. This is resisted by the operator for 7 to 10 seconds. The leg is extended at the knee to its new limit after relaxation and the procedure is repeated.

Or, in this same position the patient attempts to flex the knee (causing downward pressure against the operator's shoulder, with the back of the lower leg) thus employing the hamstrings themselves isometrically for 7 to 10 seconds (with appropriate breathing). After relaxation the muscles are stretched further towards their new barrier.

This last method can also be described as the operator attempting to straighten the leg (extend the knee further) against the resistance of the patient.

Combination of forces

In order to produce a combined contraction effectively, there could be an instruction to the patient to pull upwards (cephalid) with the flexed upper leg whilst pushing downward toward the floor with the lower leg. This effectively contracts both the quadriceps and the hamstrings, thus inducing both post-isometric relaxation and reciprocal inhibition which facilitates subsequent stretching out of tight hamstrings.

Testing for tightness of adductors of the thigh (pectinius, adductor brevis, magnus and longus, semimembrinosus, semitendinosis and gracilis)

11. Supine patient places leg to be tested so that operator (standing lateral to the

leg, facing cephalid) can rest the foot of the straight leg in the crook of his/her couchside elbow. Non-tested leg is placed in slight abduction with foot over the edge of the end of the couch. Operator's couchside hand rests on the anterolateral aspect of the tibia, maintaining downward pressure to ensure constant extension of the lower leg. The other hand is in contact with the lateral thigh distal to the trochanter. Lateral rotation of the foot is prevented by its position against the operator's upper arm.

The pelvis and untested leg should remain in position throughout and be fixed if possible.

Abduction is introduced to its maximum. When limit is reached the knee is flexed and further abduction attempted.

Abduction should be possible to about 40 degrees. If there is no increase in abduction when the knee is flexed then it is assumed that pectinius and the adductors are shortened. Comparison of the two legs is desirable to assess which is capable of greater abduction.

If range of movement is greater with the knee extended than with the knee flexed then gracilis and biceps femoris are probably shortened.

Treatment of shortened adductors
Patient supine with affected side hip flexed, foot resting on couch. External rotation of the hip is introduced to allow maximum abduction of knee. This is stabilized by the operator to resist an attempt by the patient to adduct the knee. After appropriate isometric contraction the leg is taken into greater abduction.

Or, the straight leg of the supine patient (close to edge of couch) is abducted and extended to its pain free limit, and the operator, after taking out the slack, uses appropriate resistance to prevent adduction isometrically or isolytically. Repeat several times until no further gain is achieved (see Figure 44 on page 214).

To employ antagonists the abducted leg should be brought closer to the midline rather than attempting contraction of the lateral thigh muscles whilst the leg is fully abducted. Cramp could ensue in such a position. Having brought the leg into relative abduction the operator can then resist an attempt (20 per cent of strength only) to abduct the leg.

Testing for shortness of piriformis
When short, the supine patient will display external rotation of the leg on the side of shortness as well as a shorter leg on that side.

12. Patient is supine with tested leg flexed at hip and knee. Operator maintains pressure along long axis of flexed leg, at the knee, to fix pelvis. This leg if flexed, adducted and medially rotated using a contact on the medial aspect of the lower leg. Adduction and medial rotation will be limited and uncomfortable at the end of the range if piriformis is short.

Direct palpation of piriformis is usually not possible, but if it is shortened then its fibres will be palpable on direct pressure, patient prone and contact into the region of the sciatic notch.

Treatment of shortened piriformis
Direct inhibitory pressure is useful as desribed and illustrated on pages 150 to 156.

13. *Assessment of shortness in quadratus lumborum.*
See page 225 for description and page 217 for illustration.

Treatment of shortened quadratus lumborum
See Figure 46 and 47 on page 217.

14. *Assessment of shortness in paravertebral muscles*
The patient is seated on couch, legs extended, pelvis vertical. Flexion is introduced in order to approximate forehead to knees. An even curve should be observed and a distance of about 4 inches from the knees achieved by the forehead. No knee flexion should occur and the movement should be a spinal one, not involving pelvic tilting (see pages 110 to 113).

15. The patient sits at edge of couch, knees flexed and lower legs hanging over edge. Hamstrings are thus relaxed. Forward bending is introduced so that forehead approximates the knees. Pelvis is fixed. If bending of trunk is greater in this position than in No. 14 above, then there is probably tilting of the pelvis and shortened hamstring involvement. During these assessments, areas of shortening in the spinal muscles may be observed, for example on forward bending a lordosis may be maintained in the lumbar spine, or flexion may be very limited even without such lordosis. There may be obvious overstretching of the upper back and relative tightness of the lower back.

16. *Assessment of thoraco-lumbar dysfunction*
This important transition region is the only one in the spine in which two mobile structures meet and dysfunction results in alteration of the quality of motion between these structures (upper and lower trunk-dorsal and lumbar spines). In dysfunction there is often a degree of spasm or tightness in the muscles which stabilizes the region, notably: psoas, erector spinae of the thoraco-lumbar region, often quadratus lumborum and rectus abdominus.

Symptomatic diagnosis of muscle involvement is possible as follows: Psoas involvement usually triggers abdominal pain if severe and produces flexion of the hip and the typical antalgesic posture of lumbago. Erector spinae involvement produces low back pain at its caudal end of attachment and interscapular pain at its thoracic attachment (as far up as the mid thoracic level).

Quadratus lumborum involvement causes lumbar pain and pain at the attachment of the iliac crest and lower ribs.

Rectus abdominus contraction may mimic abdominal pain and result in pain at the attachments at the pubic symphesis and the xyphoid process, as well as forward bending of the trunk and restricted ability to extend the spine.

There is seldom pain at the site of the lesion in thoraco-lumbar dysfunction.

Assessment is by direct palpation of the various muscles for contraction and sensitivity.

17. Screening involves having the patient straddle the couch in a slightly flexed posture (slight kyphosis). Rotation in either direction enables segmental impairment to be observed as the spinous processes are monitored. Restriction of rotation is the most common characteristic of this dysfunction.

M.E. treatment of thoraco-lumbar dysfunction
Psoas and/or quadratus lumborum may be treated as above.

M.E. treatment of erector spinae muscle
The patient sits with back to operator on treatment couch, legs hanging over side and hands clasped behind the neck. Operator places knee on the couch close to the patient, side towards which sidebending and rotation will be introduced. Operator passes hand in front of axilla on side to which patient is to be rotated, across front of patient's neck, to rest on the shoulder opposite. The patient is drawn into anteflexion, sidebending and rotation over the operator's knee. The operator's free hand monitors the area of spasm and ensures that the various forces localize at the point of maximum contraction. When the patient has been taken to the comfortable limit of stretch he/she is asked to look (eyes only) towards the direction from which rotation has been made, whilst holding the breath for 7-10 seconds. This will cause an increase in contraction of the muscles which have shortened. The patient is then asked to release the breath and to look towards the direction in which sidebending/rotation has been introduced. The operator takes the patient further in all the directions of restriction, towards the new barrier. This whole process is repeated several times. Finally the patient may be asked to breathe in and to gently attempt to rotate further against resistance, whilst holding the breath for 7-10 seconds. This involves contradiction of the antagonists. After relaxation the new barrier is again approached. (See pages 226 to 228 for description of similar methods for low back conditions.)

M.E. treatment of rectus abdominus
The patient lies at end of couch so that buttocks are almost clear of the edge. One leg is resting on a stool. The leg on the side to be treated is held in the air by the patient, introducing contraction of the rectus on that side. This involves gravity induced isometric contraction (the muscle effort is matched by a pull from gravity.) This is held for 7-10 seconds whilst the breath is held, and then released to allow a stretch of the muscle, as the leg is pulled by gravity slowly towards the floor. Repetition is performed several times, and then the other side is treated in the same manner. Operator resistance may be introduced against an attempt to lift the leg, as an alternative to the gravity method.

NOTE: Not all the muscles involved in thoraco-lumbar dysfunction pattern described above may need treatment since when one or other is treated appropriately the others tend to normalize. Underlying causes must also always receive attention.

Further muscle energy treatment of tight back muscles
NMT and other soft tissue methods may be used as well as muscle energy methods, such as:

The patient stands in front of operator who locks both arms across patient's abdomen. Operator stabilizes his/her position by spreading legs apart with one well in front of the other, front one at least level with feet of patient.

The patient is asked to bend forward over the operator's arms which resist the movement. Gravity assists the patient's effort against the operator's resistance. The effort employs the abdominal muscles isometrically, thus inducing subsequent relaxation of dorsal musculature via reciprocal inhibition.

18. *Assessment of shortness in pectoralis major*
The patient supine, lying with arms alongside the body and side to be tested near

the edge of the couch. The tested arm is held at the mid-humeral level and is moved passively from the starting position upward and outward with the palm facing the ceiling. The upper arm should reach the horizontal plane and, with additional pressure, be able to increase its range of movement. It is possible in this position to palpate for tightened areas in the muscle. The upper arm will not reach the horizontal plane if there is such shortening. The location of the shortening is discovered by palpation. The thorax should be stabilized during the raising of the arm so that no twisting of the thorax occurs or increase in lordosis is noted, during the effort. The forearm should not be used to control the arm but the humerus. Assessment of subclavicular portion of pectoralis involves abduction at 90 degrees from the body. The tendon of pectoralis at the sternum should then be palpated and should not be found to be tense even at maximum abduction of the arm.

Treatment of shortened pectoralis
The position of testing is adopted and the operator resists the patient's attempt to adduct and flex arm at shoulder for 7 to 10 seconds, using appropriate breathing patterns. Subsequent increases of degree of abduction and extension is achieved. Monitoring of the shortened tissues is desirable to ensure that they take part in the isometric contraction.

Lower parts of pectoralis if shortened will limit elevation of the arm, and appropriate positions should be ensured to bring the shortened fibres into involvement in the isometric contraction.

19. Assessment of shortened trapezius (upper)
The sitting patient's neck is side-flexed without flexion, extension or rotation, whilst the opposite shoulder is stabilized from above. The range is compared on each side, and palpation discovers location of shortened fibres. If sitting is not possible then, in a supine position, the same procedure is carried out with the ear being approximated to the shoulder.

Treatment of shortened upper trapezius
The patient is supine, and takes head away from side of shortness, sidebending towards opposite shoulder. The operator fixes shoulder on affected side, from above, and takes out slack. The patient is asked to look towards the side of shortness (eyes only) whilst holding the breath. This eye movement will tighten the shortened muscles. The operator resists the tendency for the muscle to contract. After appropriate relaxation the head is taken further into sidebending, thus stretching the shortened muscle. The patient may also be asked to lift the shoulder against resistance with slight force as a means of bringing into play other fibres.

Self-treatment is possible with the patient holding the head in position of maximum pain-free sidebending, whilst the hand of the affected side grasps the side of the couch thus fixing the shoulder. Eye movement is used towards the affected side as a means of introducing contraction of the shortened muscles which are restrained from producing movement by the patient's position, as described. After relaxation greater stretch is achieved. Repeat several times.

20. Assessment of shortened levator scapulae
The patient is supine, lying with arms alongside body. The arm on the side to be tested is flexed above the head, and abducted towards the head, elbow flexed to approximately 90 degrees, so that the palm of that hand is facing ceilingward and

lies behind the patient's neck/upper back. The operator steadies the head with one hand and the shoulder on the side being assessed with the other by caudad pressure on the elevated and abducted elbow. Maximum flexion of the cervical spine is introduced, together with rotation and sidebending away from the side being assessed. If the levator scapulae is shortened then the range of movement is decreased and the insertion on the scapulae is painful on palpation. Shortness of this muscle often results in pain on the spinous process of C2 and the upper border of the scapula.

Treatment of shortened levator scapulae
The patient is supine with head near end of couch, and elbow of flexed arm above the head. The operator exerts pressure on scapula by applying pressure caudally on elbow, which lies against his/her thigh. The head is lifted and bent away from the affected side until resistance is noted. The slack is taken out and the patient is asked to look towards the affected side whilst a deep breath is taken and held. Operator resists the tendency this has to turn the head in that direction. On exhalation and relaxation of the muscles the eyes are turned towards the opposite side from the shortness, and the operator slightly increases the degree of extension and sidebending to the new barrier of resistance. During the isometric contraction the patient may also be asked to introduce upward pressure via the elbow against which the operator's thigh is exerting downward pressure.

The examples given above should not be seen as definitive. There are many other methods of Muscle Energy employing the same principles. The key to success is identification of shortened fibres and introduction of painless muscle energy procedures to ensure the release of the tightness which prevents normal function.

Students and practitioners are asked to spend time learning identification of shortened muscles via assessments such as those described in these notes as well as via soft tissue palpation using NMT or other methods.

Chapter 10

Strain-Counterstrain
(Tender Point) Technique

The work of Lawrence Jones D.C., has been touched on elsewhere. This pioneering researcher into methods which address the pains and dysfunctions of the body, has developed a method of treatment of joint and soft-tissue dysfunction of supreme gentleness. He has given the name 'Strain-Counterstrain' to the method and, insofar as it impinges upon aspects of the work described previously, in relation to various localized soft-tissue changes (myofascial triggers, Chapman's neurolymphatic reflexes, etc.) we will examine some of his ideas and methods.

His concepts derive, in part, from his conclusions regarding the role of muscles in somatic dysfunction and pain processes. He points out that it has long been thought that, in a situation of mechanical restriction of motion, the associated tense, and often painful musculature, is in this condition because of its vain attempt to overcome the supposed restriction in articular motion. His concept sees the situation differently. In a balanced state the muscles supporting a joint will be feeding a flow of information, derived from the various sensory structures in these muscles and their tendons, relating to the tone of the muscles.

Should a severe overstretching of a joint occur, some muscles will be impelled to send messages as to their overstretched situation, from both their primary and secondary nerve endings. Some muscles, relatively unaffected by the strained position, would be shortened rather than stretched, and are unstressed. They would send a minimum of impulse to the CNS. The reaction of the body to this stressed situation varies with the time available to it. Should a deliberate response be forthcoming, allowing the stretched muscles a slow return to normal, then resolution of the problem takes place and joint mobility is restored. This happens only if a slow return to neutral position is achieved. All too often, however, the situation is one of almost panic response, as the body makes a rapid attempt to restore the position of the overstretched muscle. The result is a reflex overcontraction which occurs not in the muscle(s) which have been stretched, *but in those which were shortened, i.e. the unstrained antagonist(s).* The resulting spasm in these causes the fixation of the joint, and prevents any attempt to return it to normal. The position in which this fixation takes place is not the extreme in which the overstretching of the muscles first occurred, but lies between that extreme position, and the neutral position of the joint. Any attempt to force this towards its anatomically correct position, will be strongly resisted by the shortened fibres.

It is, however, not difficult to take the joint further towards the position in which the strain occurred, thus shortening the fibres, already in spasm, even further.

By taking the joint as close to the position in which the original strain took place, we find an interesting phenomenon. This is that the pain in the area seems to resolve and, if this position is held for a period (Jones suggests 90 seconds), then the spasm in the shortened tissues will resolve. It is then possible to return the joint to its normal resting position, *as long as this is done extremely slowly.* The muscles which had been over-stretched might remain sensitive for some days, but for all practical consideration the joint will be normal again.

Jones believes that the sudden stretch, which took place in the muscles, which subsequently remained shortened, at the moment when the panic reaction took place, resulted in the spindles of the muscle reporting to the CNS that it was being strained, even before it had reached its resting length. We will look at these thoughts again later in this section. Many low back problems are consistant with this scenario. The individual is bending, perhaps lifting, and an off-guard movement, or a sneeze, results in excessive strain, which becomes manifest as a problem only at the moment of the attempt to return to neutral, often via a sudden movement. No pain is felt whilst bending, only at the instant of reversing that position. This is the moment at which the muscles, antagonistic to those which have stretched, over-react, and are therefore placed in spasm. Whether or not this precise sequence is involved, Jones has found that by carefully positioning the joint, whether this be a small extremity joint, or a spinal region, into a position of neutral (which is frequently an exaggeration of the distorted position in which the body is holding the area) a resolution of the spasm described takes place.

A further finding of Jones is that almost all joint problems have associated with them areas of tenderness. These can be palpated, and when the joint is suitably positioned to ease the spasm this results in the tenderness in these points diminishing. He dubs these points 'tender' points. Describing his methods he states: 'Finding the myofascial tender point, and the correct position of release, will probably take a few minutes at first. Watching a skilled physician find a tender point, in a few seconds, and a position of release in a few seconds more, may give a false impression of simplicity to the neophyte.'

It may take longer than a few minutes initially. Once found, the tense tender point is palpated with just less than sufficient pressure to cause pain in normal tissue. The pain sensitivity should be apparent to both the physician, and the patient. By careful guiding of the joint, and constant palpation, a monitoring of progress towards the ideal neutral position is possible. Both muscle tension and the patient's report of either increasing, or diminishing, pain in the palpated point, will guide the operator to the position where eventually there is a feeling of relative ease in the soft tissues. An absence of 'bind' and also, most importantly, the patient's report that pain has markedly diminished are the desired indicators.

Jones states: 'The point of maximum relaxation accompanied by an abrupt increase in joint mobility, within a very small arc, is the mobile point.' This term designates the ideal position of comfort to the patient. After holding this for one and a half minutes, the operator slowly returns the area to its neutral position.

What are the tender points? Jones equates them with trigger points and Chapman's reflexes. This cannot be strictly accurate, although a degree of overlap in all these points is of course possible. There are differences in the nature, if not

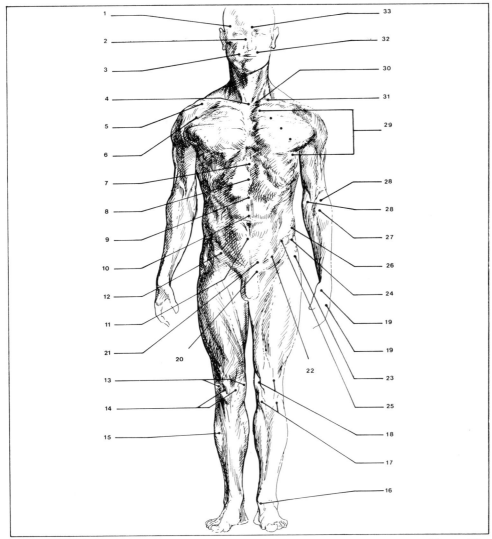

Figure 58a

Location of Tender Points

Note: These points are not fixed, they will vary within the region indicated, depending upon the specific mechanics involved in the trauma or strain which has occurred in the tissues or regions mentioned.

1. Squamosal
2. Nasal
3. Masseter-tempero-mandibular
4. Anterior 1st thoracic
5. Anterior acromio-clavicular
6. Latissimus dorsi
7. Anterior 7th thoracic
8. Anterior 8th thoracic
9. Anterior 9th thoracic
10. Anterior 10th thoracic
11. Anterior 11th thoracic
12. Anterior 2nd lumbar
13. Medial and lateral meniscus
14. Medial and lateral extension strain of meniscus
15. Tibialis anticus, medial ankle
16. Flexion strain of ankle
17. Medial and lateral hamstrings
18. Medial and lateral patella
19. Thumb and fingers
20. Low ilium, flare out
21. Anterior fifth lumber
22. Low ilium

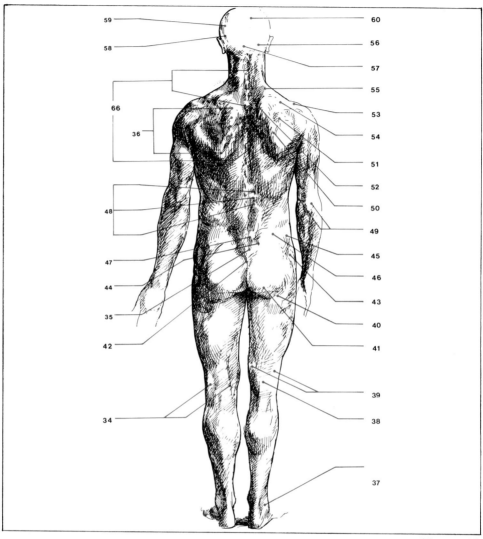

Figure 58b

23. Anterior lateral trochanter
24. Anterior 1st Lumbar
25. Iliacus
26. Anterior 12th thoracic
27. Radial head
28. Medial and lateral coronoid
29. Depressed upper ribs
30. Anterior 8th cervical
31. Anterior 7th cervical
32. Infra-orbital nerve
33. Supra-orbital nerve
34. Extension strain of ankle
    (tender point on gastrocnemius)
35. High flare out sacro-iliac
36. Elevated upper ribs
    (tender points on angles of ribs)

37. Lateral ankle strain
38. Posterior cruciate ligament strain
39. Anterior cruciate ligament strain
40. Posterior medial trochanter
41. Posterior medial trochanter
42. Coccyx or sacro-iliac (high flare out)
43. Posterior lateral trochanter
44. Lower pole 5th lumbar
45. 4th lumbar
46. 3rd lumbar
47. Upper pole 5th lumbar
48. Upper lumbars
49. Medial and lateral olecrenon
50. 3rd thoracic and shoulder strain or pain
51. Lateral second thoracic; shoulder strain or pain
52. Medial 2nd thoracic; shoulder

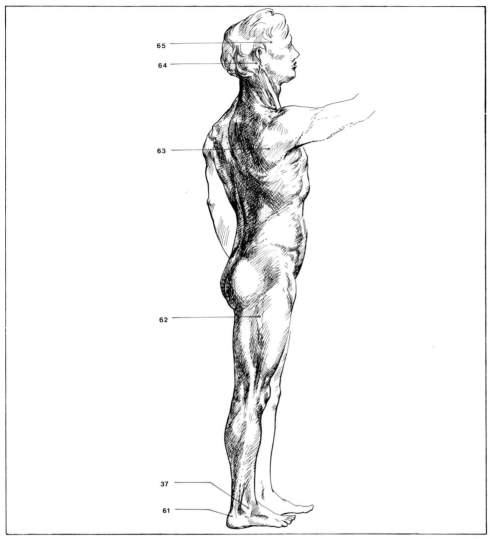

Figure 58c

53. Posterior acromio-clavicular	60. Right lambdoid
54. Supraspinatus	61. Lateral calcaneus
55. Elevated 1st rib	62. Lateral trochanter
56. Posterior 1st cervical	63. Subscapularis
57. Inion	64. Postero-auricular
58. Left occipito-mastoid	65. Squamosal
59. Sphenobasilar	66. Inter-vertebral extension dysfunction

Points are illustrated on one side of the body only but most are potentially present bilaterally. Many other areas are associated with the tender point phenomenon, depending upon the particular stress or strain imposed upon the joint(s) in question. Points on the cranium are named for the region in which they are found and not for the joint to which they relate. Relief of pain in a tender point, by the careful positioning of the body area, indicates efficacy or otherwise of the measure.

Most tender points on the anterior body surface relate to flexion (forward bending) strains and most on the posterior aspect of the body relate to extension (backward bending) strains.

in the feel, of these different points (see chart on pages 234 and 235). Myofascial trigger points will refer sensitivity, pain, or other symptoms, to a target area when pressed. This is not the case with Chapman's reflex points (neurolymphatic points) which are found in pairs. Such anterior and posterior neurolymphatic points, whilst palpating as tender are not specifically related to joint dysfunction, as are Jones' tender points (and quite frequently as are trigger points). Acupuncture points are usually located just beneath the skin, according to Jones, whereas his 'tender' points are located deeper in muscle, tendon, ligament or fascia. This seems to be an oversimplification of acupuncture points, which are located at some depth, in many instances, and which require penetration of the needle to reach structures in the tendons, ligaments, etc. at times.

It is worth considering that, in acupuncture, there exists a phenomenon known as the 'spontaneously sensitive point'. This arises in response to trauma, or joint dysfunction, and is regarded, for the duration of its existence, as an 'honorary' acupuncture point. As is generally known the points of acupuncture, which receive treatment via needling, heat, pressure, lasers, etc. are clearly defined and mapped. Only these spontaneously arising points, associated with joint problems, are exceptions to this, and become available to treatment for the duration of their sensitivity. In the text of my book *Acupuncture Treatment of Pain* (Thorsons, 1976) I make the following comment: 'Local tender points in an area of discomfort, may be considered as spontaneous acupuncture points. The Chinese term these Ah Shi points, and use them in the same way as classical points, when treating painful conditions.' Thus, it would seem, that Jones' points are in many ways the same, if not identical to Ah Shi points. These are described as first having been utilized in the treatment of pain during the Tang dynasty (618-907). The physician Sun Szu-miao is credited with advancing the idea that tender spots could serve as acupuncture points, in addition to the established ones (*An Outline of Chinese Acupuncture,* Foreign Language Press, Peking, 1975). He is quoted as referring to them and stating: 'Puncture wherever there is tenderness.'

Lawrence Jones seems, therefore, to have discovered a further use for tender points, apart from puncturing them. Maintaining a sufficient degree of pressure on such a point allows the patient to be able to report on its diminishing nature, as the joint is positioned appropriately. It becomes a monitor and guide for the practitioner. The disappearance, or at least marked diminution, of pain, noted on pressure, after holding the joint in the position of ease for the prescribed period, is instant evidence as to the success of the procedure. The holding of this pressure, during the 90-second period recommended by Jones, leads to a further question, one which Jones acknowledges as being asked of him. This is whether the pressure on the tender point is not in itself therapeutic.

He describes the nature of both the question and answer in his book *Strain-Counterstrain* (American Academy of Osteopathy, 1981): 'The question is asked whether the repeated probing of the tender point is therapeutic, as in acupressure, or Rolfing techniques [Author's note: or as in NMT]. It is not intentionally therapeutic, but is used solely for diagnosis and evidence of accuracy of treatment.' This answer could be thought of as being equivocal for it does not address the possibility of a therapeutic end-result from the use of pressure on the tender point, but states only what the *intention* of such pressure is.

It may be assumed that some therapeutic effect does derive from sustained inhibitory pressure on such a spontaneously arising tender point, for several reasons. In the use of acupuncture there is clear evidence of a pain-reducing effect, from the use of pressure on acupuncture points. Since acupuncture authorities, both in China and the West include these points (spontaneously tender points seem to be in every way the same as traditional Ah Shi points) as being suitable for needling, *or pressure techniques*, the avoidance of a clear answer on this point by Jones may be taken to indicate that he has not really addressed himself to this possibility. That his method had other mechanisms, which achieve release of pain and spasm in injured joints, is not disputed. The total effect of Strain-counterstrain would seen to derive from a combination of the positioning of the joint in a neutral position, and the pressure on the tender point. The positioning is similar, but not identical, to that described in what is termed 'functional' technique, by Harold Hoover. Hoover's methods involved the positioning of a joint with a limited range of motion, in what he called a 'dynamic neutral' position. He sought a position in which there was a balance of tensions, fairly near the anatomical neutral position of the joint. Jones also aims at a position of ease, but he relates more to the identical position in which the original strain occurred. By combining this position, in which the shortened muscle(s) are able to release themselves (see below for a more detailed description of the supposed mechanisms), as well as applying pressure which, despite his doubts, appears to almost certainly involve a therapeutic effect, Jones has been able to produce dramatic improvements in severe and painful conditions.

Jones came to a number of conclusions as a result of his work, which may be summarized thus:

The pain in joint dysfunction is related very much to the position in which the joint is placed. Varying from acute pain in some positions, to a pain free position which would be almost directly opposite the position of maximum pain. The dysfunction in a joint, which has been strained, is the result of something which occurs in response to the strain, a reaction to it. The palpable evidence of this is found by searching not in the tissues which were placed under strain, *but by seeking in the antagonists of these overstretched tissues.* These painful structures were not stretched at the time of the injury, but were in fact shortened, and have remained so. *In these shortened tissues the tender points will be found.*

Jones describes the use of the points thus:

Jones' Technique

A physician skilled in palpation techniques will perceive tenseness and/or oedema as well as tenderness. The tenderness, often a few times greater than that for normal tissue, is for the beginner the most valuable sign. He maintains his palpating finger over the tender point, to monitor expected changes in tenderness. With the other hand he positions the patient into a posture of comfort and relaxation. He may proceed successfully, just by questioning the patient, as he probes intermittently, while moving towards the position. If he is correct, the patient can report diminished tenderness in the tender area. By intermittent deep palpation he monitors the tender point, seeking the ideal position at which there is at least a two-thirds reduction in tenderness. (This degree of stimulus is at least the equivalent of that given in the acupressure or Tsubo techniques, of similar tender points, and must have therapeutic implications.)

The key to successful normalization, via these methods, is the discovery of the position of maximum ease of the joint, in which the tender point becomes less so. Most importantly, the subsequent return to the neutral resting position, after the maintenance of the joint in this position of ease for 90 seconds, is very slowly accomplished. Without this slow re-positioning, the likelihood exists of a sudden return to a shortened state of the previously disturbed structures. Joints affected in this way behave in an irrational manner, in that they do the converse of what a relaxed, normal, joint would do. When a strained joint is placed in a position which exaggerates its deformity, it feels more comfortable, which is not what a normal joint does, Jones explains the mechanics of this as follows:

'The structures of the body responsible for reporting the positional states of joints are the proprioceptive nerve endings. Everything we have learned about joint dysfunction points to them as the major site of beginning the disorder. What could go wrong with proprioceptive nerve endings?' Jones answers, and elaborates, by identifying a crucial difference between the role of the muscle spindles themselves, and that of the primary (annulospiral) proprioceptive nerve endings. Both discharge messages, more or less in proportion to the length of the muscle fibres, but the annulospiral endings have a unique role in that they also report in proportion to the *rate* at which stretch is occurring. Muscle spindles report on the lengths of the muscle, at any particular moment, with the primary endings reporting both current length and the speed with which change in length is occurring. From this information the CNS is able to assess the anticipated future behaviour of the area. If a joint is in the process of being stretched, in a particular direction, the antagonists to those tissues being stretched are shortened, and the proprioceptor input of these, reports little or no change. Because of the stretched antagonists, the short muscles will also be reciprocally inhibited and relaxed, at the same time. If there should occur, at such a moment, an emergency, and the protective attempt to strengthen the joint would place a rapid degree, and rate, of stretch on the shortened relaxed musculature, the messages deriving from the proprioceptive nerve endings would, under such crisis conditions, probably indicate strain long before the muscle had reached its full length.

Jones continues his reasoning thus: 'Once begun, this inappropriate message of strain, when there is none, cannot be turned off by the body. One would think that the CNS, through a reduced outflow of gamma motor neurons, would relax intrafusal fibres enough to restore the primary proprioceptive rate of firing. Korr offers the hypothesis that the CNS, seeking a response from the hypershortened and silent primary endings, begins an extraordinary outflow which, followed by an unusually fast stretching, results in gamma gain that the body is unable to reduce to normal.'

Since the position during Jones' therapeutic methods is the same as that of the original strain, the shortened muscles are re-positioned in such a manner as to allow the dysfunctioning proprioceptors to cease their activity. Korr's explanation is: 'The shortened spindle nevertheless continues to fire, despite the slackening of the main muscle, and the CNS is gradually able to turn down the gamma discharge and, in turn, enables the muscles to return to 'easy neutral', at its resting length. In effect, the physician has led the patient through a repetition of the lesioning process with, however, two essential differences. First it is done in slow motion, with gentle muscular forces, and second there have been no surprises for the CNS; the spindle has continued to report throughout.' ('Proprioceptors and somatic dysfunction', *The Journal of the American Osteopathic Association,* Vol. 74, March 1975, pp638-50).

Here, then, is the thinking behind the methods of Strain-counterstrain. From the viewpoint of those employing soft-tissue manipulation, these offer an excellent method of aid in normalization of strained, painful, areas and joints. Its emphasis on the muscle spindles is in contrast to the emphasis on the Golgi tendon bodies, which MET methods employ. Thus, different methods and mechanisms are involved, and different tissues are used to achieve therapeutic benefits. The methods of Strain-counterstrain and MET are not in any way contradictory, and there is every chance that, in order to achieve maximum benefits, both methods should be employed at the same session of treatment, since they do not seem in any way to have conflicting elements one to the other.

The effects of MET would enhance the ultimate use of Strain-counterstrain, and should therefore be used initially, together with any appropriate NMT, in either a diagnostic or therapeutic mode. NMT is useful in identifying soft-tissue dysfunction. Once identified, differential diagnosis is required. Should the area of soft-tissue change be identified as a trigger point, by virtue of its referring pain or other symptoms, elsewhere, then appropriate treatment might incorporate pressure, stretch and chilling, or MET methods. Should the sensitive myofascial area be related to a joint which had been restricted or painful, then it may be assessed for the characteristics of Jones' tender points. If on continued palpation of such a point, it became markedly less sensitive, when the joint was placed in a position which might be an exaggeration of its position of distortion, then the appropriate treatment could follow a sequence of NMT, applied to these structures, (with emphasis on the origins and insertions of the muscles, tendons, ligaments etc.) followed by MET to achieve maximum ease in the tight, shortened, musculature, followed by the positioning methods as described by Jones.

In this way a progression of therapy would have been used, each preceding method aiding the following one. NMT would be used partially diagnostically and partially therapeutically. MET is sometimes all that is required thereafter, and sometimes is the preceding method to Strain-counterstrain, which finally allows the fibres of the shortened muscles to relax, and to restore joint normality.

Jones has identified a number of conditions which are related to predictable tender points. From experience he has concluded that when tender points are found on the anterior surface of the body they are (with a few exceptions) indicative of the associated joint requiring a degree of forward-bending during its treatment. This also of course indicates that the joint was probably initially injured in a forward-bending position. Thus information as to the original injury position helps to direct the search for the tender points to the likeliest aspect of the body. The exception to this rule is that the tender point related to the 4th cervical vertebrae, when injured in flexion, is not treated with the neck in flexion, but side-bending and rotation, away from the side affected.

Tender points, found on the posterior aspect of the body, indicate joint dysfunction which calls for some degree of backward-bending in the treatment. There are also exceptions to this rule, notably involving the piriformis muscle, and the 3rd and 5th cervical vertebrae. These exceptions involve a degree of flexion on treatment.

The illustrations on pages 234 and 235 will guide the reader to the most common tender point positions, as noted by Jones. No specific descriptions as to technique are given, since, as indicated, the positioning of the joint will depend upon the nature of the injury which befell it. Proprioceptive skills, and the use of careful palpation, will enable the required technique to be acquired. Reading of Jones' book is suggested for greater detail and understanding.

The following examples are for general guidance only and are taken from Strain-counterstrain by Lawrence Jones.

Treatment for Forward-Bending Joint Dysfunction from 9th Thoracic to 1st Lumbar Levels

'This one procedure is usually effective for any of this group. To permit the supine spine to flex at the thoracolumbar region, a table capable of being raised at one end is desirable. A flat table may be used if a large pillow is placed under the patient's hips, raising them enough to permit flexion to reach the desired level of the spine. With the patient supine, the physician raises the patient's knees and places his own thigh below those of the patient. By applying cephalad pressure on the patient's thighs, he produces marked flexion of the patient's thoracolumbar spine. Usually, the best results come from rotation of the knees moderately towards the side of tenderness. These joint dysfunctions account for many low-back pains

Treatment for forward bending strain from 9th thoracic to 1st lumbar level: The patient is placed supine in flexion, using a cushion for the upper back and flexing the knees and hips, which are rotated towards the side of dysfunction. The operator's cephalid hand palpates the tender point. He continues to position the patient until this no longer palpates as tender. This position is held for 90 seconds after which a slow return is made to a neutral position. A flexion strain would produce a tender point anteriorly and calls for a flexed position for release to occur.

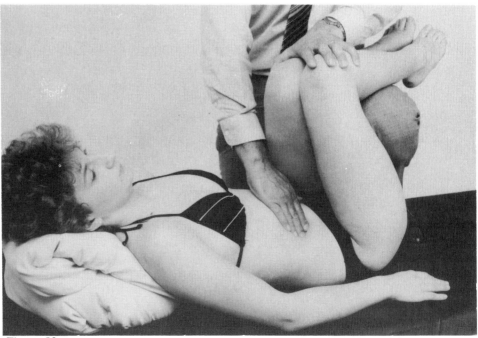

Figure 59

that are not associated with tenderness of the vertebrae posteriorly. The pain is referred from the anterior dysfunction, into the low lumbar, sacral and gluteal areas. Treatment directed to the posterior pain sites of these dysfunctions, rather than to the origins of the pain, has been disappointing.' The position involves marked flexion through the joint as well as appropriate side-bending and rotation consequent upon which will be the dimunition of sensitivity in the tender points contacted on the anterior body surface. Once this is noted to occur the position is held for a minute and a half. The tender point will be found on the abdominal midline, or slightly to one side, and should be palpated during this manoeuvre. (*See Figure 59.*)

The patient is prone. 'The head is supported by the doctor's left hand holding the chin. The operator's left forearm is held along the right side of the patient's head for better support. The right hand monitors tender points on the right side of the spinous processes. The forces applied are mostly extension, with slight side-bending and rotation left.'

'The tender points of the posterior thorax are located interspinally, paraspinally and at the rib angles, when there exist extension dysfunctions of intervertebral

Prone Position Treatment of Lower Posterocervical and Upper Posterior First and Second Thoracic Joints

Treatment for lower postero-cervical and upper posterior 1st and 2nd thoracic joint strain: The prone patient's head is supported in operator's right hand. The left hand monitors tender point located on the left side, spinous process. Forces are introduced by extension of the head, sidebending and rotation to the left. When the tender point is reported as being pain-free or much reduced in sensitivity, the position is held for 90 seconds, before a slow return is made to neutral. (Note hand positions are reversed in text above.)

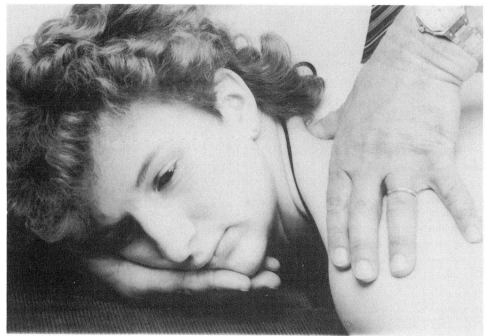

Figure 60

joints, side-bending dysfunction, and ribs that are more comfortable when elevated.' The simplicity of the methods is obvious. The shortened fibres relate to the areas where tender points are to be found, and the positioning is such as to increase the shortening already existent, whilst palpating the tender points. Ninety seconds of this is all that there is to the method. The skill required is in localizing the tender points, and identifying and duplicating the nature of the original strain or injury. (*See Figure 60.*)

Summary of Simplified Strain/ Counterstrain Technique:

Anterior cervical strains (flexion strains)
Anterior strain of C1. The tender point is found in a groove between the styloid process and angle of jaw. Treatment is by rotation of the head of the supine patient away from side of dysfunction (always maintaining pressure on Jones point). Fine tune by sidebending away from the painful side.

An alternative or second point for C1 flexion strain is ½ inch anterior to the angle of mandible. Treat by flexion and rotation approximately 45 degrees away from side of pain.

Remaining cervical anterior strain points are on or about tips of transverse processes of involved vertebrae. Treat by forward bending and rotation to remove pain from point. In general the higher the point the more rotation away from the point is needed in fine tuning. The lower the point the more flexion, and the less rotation, is required.

Posterior cervical strains (extension strains)
These tender points are found on or about the spinous processes, and treatment is by increased extension.

Extension strain of C1 has two tender points. The first lies in the occipital groove between the occiput and posterior arch of C1. Strain related to this point is treated by extension and rotation away from the point. The forehead is then used to apply pressure to increase extension (fine tuning).

The other point lies on or just lateral to the inion, and is treated by placing the head/neck into acute flexion with the chin close to the trachea.

Other extension strains in the cervical area are treated by taking the pain out of the palpated Jones point, via extension of the head on the neck.

In a bedbound patient the patient lies on the side with the painful side uppermost, so that fine tuning can be accomplished via slight sidebending and rotation towards the side of the lesion.

Exceptions include the C3 extension strain which can be treated in either flexion or extension. C8 extension strain may also be treated in slight extension, with marked sidebending and rotation away, rather than towards, the side of strain (C8 point lies on TP of C7).

Posterior thoracic strain (extension or backwards bending strain)
These are treated in the same manner as extension strains of the cervical spine. Points are usually found or, or close to, the spinous processes, bilaterally, or on the lateral paravertebral muscle mass. The lower the strain the closer is the tender point to the TP. Direct extension (backwards bending) is the method employed with the patient sidelying, seated, supine or prone. If sidelying the arms are placed so as to avoid rotation of the spine, resting on a pillow.

For the T5 to T8 levels the arms are held slightly above head level, to increase extension.

For T9 to T12 the patient lies face upwards, the operator on the side of the lesion, grasps the hand on the side opposite the tender point with his/her caudad hand, and draws the arm towards him/herself, so that the opposite shoulder lifts by 30 to 45 degrees. In this position fine tuning is accomplished. The operator's cephalid hand is inserted under the spine to palpate the point all the while. The pull on the arm on the side opposite to the lesion causes extension and rotation in the region of the strain.

Once the tender point is noted to ease in sensitivity, or tissue alteration is felt to be adequate, the fine tuning is complete and the position is held for 90 seconds.

Extension strains of the lumbar spine are treated as follows
L1 and 2. The sensitive points for these are found over the tips of the TPs of the respective vertebrae. They may be treated with the patient prone or sidelying.

If prone, the operator stands on the side opposite the strain, grasping the leg of the side of the lesion, just above the knee, bringing it up and towards the operator in a scissor like movement.

Similarly if the patient is sidelying, with side of dysfunction uppermost, the upper leg can be extended to introduce backward bending into the region of the strain.

When this is done and the palpated tender point is less painful, or when a tissue change is noted, fine tuning is accomplished by slightly raising or lowering the leg.

The tender point for extension strain of L3 is found about 3 inches lateral to the post superior iliac spine, just below the superior iliac spine. L4 tender point lies an inch or two lateral to this following the contour of the crest.

Treatment of L3 and 4 extension strains is accomplished with patient prone, operator on side of dysfunction. The operator's knee or thigh is placed under the raised thigh of the patient to hold it in extension whilst fine tuning it accomplished via abduction and external rotation of the foot. This can also be done with the patient sidelying, dysfunction side uppermost. The operator's foot is placed on the bed behind the patient's lower leg. The upper leg is raised and the extended thigh of the upper leg is supported by the operator's thigh. Rotation of the foot and positioning of the patient's leg in a more anterior or posterior plane, always in a degree of extension, is the fine tuning mechanism.

There are three L5 tender points for extension strain. The first, known as the upper pole L5 strain, is found bilaterally between the SP of L5 and the SP of S1. This is treated as in extension strains of L1 and L2 (using scissor-like extension of the leg on the side of the lesion and fine tuning by variations in position).

The middle pole L5 point is found in the superior sulcus of the sacrum and relates to strain which is treated with the patient lying on the unaffected side. The lower arm of the patient is extended over the edge of the bed and hangs toward the floor. The operator stands in front of and facing the patient. The knee of the upper leg (affected side) is flexed and rests on the operator's thigh or abdomen. The fine tuning of the area is achieved by slight movement which takes the flexed leg caudad or cephalid, or which elevates or depresses it.

The lower pole of L5 extension strain lies on the body of the sacrum, centrally. Treatment is via the same position and method as in L1 and L2 and upper pole L5.

Flexion strains of the thoracic region
In a rotation strain of the midthoracic region it is possible for there to coexist extension and flexion strains, say flexion (anterior) strain on the left and extension (posterior) strain on the right.

T1 anterior strain is located on the superior surface of the manubrium on the midline. T2 to 6 lie on the sternum approximately ½ to ¾ of an inch apart.

Anterior T7 point lies close to the midline, bilaterally under the xyphoid. Other anterior T7 points are found on the costal margin close to the xyphoid.

T8 to T11 anterior dysfunction produces points which lie in the abdominal wall, approximately 1 inch lateral to the midline.

A horizontal line ½ inch below the umbilicus locates the 10th thoracic anterior strain Jones point.

1 and 3 inches above T10 lie T9 and T8 respectively. 1½ inches below T10 is T11; and T12 lies on the crest of the ilium at the midaxillary line.

Treatment for anterior strains T1 to T6 involves the head of the supine patient being flexed to the chest whilst the Jones point is contacted as a monitor of adequate ease.

Fine tuning is by slight rotation of the chin towards or away from the side of dysfunction. The head may be supported in flexion by the operator's thigh for the necessary 90 seconds of release time.

For lower thoracic flexion strains a pillow is placed under the supine patient's buttocks, allowing the lower spine to fall into flexion. The patient's knees are flexed and supported by the operator (hand or thigh for support) who stands at waist level facing the patient and palpating the tender point. Fine tuning is by movement into sidebending and/or rotation using the patient's legs as a lever (T8).

T9 to T12 flexion strains involve the same position (buttocks on pillow, the patient's flexed knees supported by the operator's thigh (operator's foot on bed). The operator is standing on the side of the strain and, having crossed the patient's ankles, fine tuning is by movement which introduces slight sidebending, or which slightly alters the degree of flexion.

The point is constantly monitored.

T12 treatment requires more sidebending than other thoracic strains.

(Jones' method for dealing with flexion strain of the upper thoracics in non-bedbound patients involves the patient seated on a couch and leaning back onto the operator's chest/abdomen so that forced flexion of the upper body may be achieved. A variety of arm positions are used to involve particular segments.)

Anterior lumbar strains (flexion or bending strains)
Gross positioning is as for thoracic strains, anteriorly.

L1 has two tender points: One is at the tip of the anterior superior iliac spine and the other on the medial surface of the ilium just medial to ASIS.

2nd lumbar anterior strain is found lateral to the anterior-inferior iliac spine. L3 is hard to find but lies ½ inch below a line connecting L1 and L2 points. L4 point is found at the insertion of the inguinal ligament on the ilium. L5 points are on the body of the pubes, just to the side of the symphesis. Treatment is as for thoracic flexion strains except that the knees are placed together (ankles crossed in thoracic strain treatment position).

In bilateral strains both sides must be treated. L3 and 4 require greater sidebending in fine tuning.

Rib dysfunction
Depressed rib strains produce points of tenderness at the anterior axillary line.

Elevated ribs have tender points at the angle of the ribs posteriorly. The scapula requires distraction or lifting to allow for palpation of these, in those ribs lying under it. This is done by the arm of the affected side of the patient being pulled across the chest, or the shoulder being raised by a pillow with the patient supine. The operator stands on the side of the disorder, and palpation of the tender point once identified is continuous, as positional change is engineered.

The patient's knees should be in a flexed position for attention to elevated ribs, and then be allowed to move to the side of the dysfunction. Fine tuning for elevated ribs is accomplished by raising the arm or shoulder cephalid, in effect exaggerating the positional deformity. The head is turned towards the affected side to further fine tune and release the stress in the palpated tissues.

For treatment of depressed ribs, the patient is supine, knees flexed and falling to one side or the other, whichever produces better release in the tissues being palpated at the anterior axillary line. The operator is on the side of dysfunction, palpating the tender point whilst drawing the patient's arm, on the side of dysfunction, caudad until release is noted. In some cases the other arm is elevated, and even has traction applied to enhance release of tender point discomfort.

Interspace dysfunction of the ribs
Tender points for strains of these tissues lie between the insertions of the contiguous ribs into the cartilages of the sternum. Ribs are noted to be overapproximated, and the pain noted in the tender points is very strong on palpation.

The more recent the strain the more painful the points, oedema and induration will be palpable.

In chronic conditions pressure on the tissues will produce a reactivation of the extreme tenderness noted in more recent strains. These strains are found in costochondritis, the persistent pain noted in cardiac patients. They are implicated in respiratory restriction and their release assists in normalization.

Treatment is by placing the patient supine, contacting the tender point. The operator is on the side of dysfunction with his/her caudad hand providing contact on the point. The cephalid hand cradles the patient's head/neck and flexes this and draws it towards the side of dysfunction at an angle of approximately 45 degrees towards the foot of the bed.

If fine tuning is adequate the pain on palpation will ease after some 30 seconds and the position should be further maintained for the full 90 second period.

NOTE: Despite the extreme gentleness of the methods involved in strain/ counterstrain there is, in about a third of patients, a reaction in which soreness, fatigue, etc. may be noted just as in more strenuous therapeutic measures.

Chapter 11

On Energy

A variety of systems and methods have concepts of energy which differ from the normally accepted concept of this phenomenon. Energy lost or wasted by the maintenance of unnecessary muscular and fascial tension is easily demonstrable. That such a situation is undesirable is also clear for, if maintained, such a drain on energy can lead to local and general fatigue of pathological significance, as well as creating a 'feedback' by which psychic tensions are reinforced. This self-maintenance of tension states makes the recognition of the somatico-psychic aspect of pathology causation as important as that which attaches to the psychosomatic component.

Energy interference has been theorized by a number of individuals and systems. Some of these will be briefly considered since, if their theories are valid, in whole or part, then the significance to a method such as NMT is obvious. In releasing neuro-muscular contraction and tensions much more may be taking place than is realized.

Varma,[1] who gave Stanley Lief the original idea for NMT stated his views, which were derived from traditional Ayuvedic philosophy, as follows:

Vibration is the manifestation and movement of life—it is life itself. The source of all vibration is the universal force known as the *prana*, of which the most tangible manifestations are the ultra-sensitive currents of the atmosphere.

The average number of vibrations for man is 360 per second, the proportion being much higher in the head than in the feet. Thus, varying degress of high frequency and low frequency can be recorded throughout the body from the top of the head to the tips of the fingers and the toes.

These currents provide the body with varying degrees of heat in order to regulate the density of its fluid content.

We have discovered that our bodies pick up two kinds of currents at two points: the ultra-sensitive currents at the pineal gland; and the sensitive currents at the nerve fibres below the cranium.

The ultra-sensitive vibrations, starting from the pineal gland in the middle of the encephalus, pursue a circular route, passing through back and front (spinal cord and sternum), to the middle of the body. This produces a kind of circuit with two poles, the pineal gland and the cocygeal plexus. Between these two poles, the currents flow downwards to stimulate the different organs, and upwards to inform the brain of heat or cold, pain or oversensitivity. The stoppage of circulation in any part, irritation or other pathological phenomena such as indigestion, stiffness of joints and all the ailments of a disordered nervous system—every form of abnormal condition is communicated to the brain by the returning flow of sensitive currents.

If adhesions of muscular fibres occur in the region of the atlas, this current cannot pass easily, and the body suffers from the deficiency. In cases of very obstructive adhesions it is cut off, just as in the case of a 'blown' electric fuse, and the body dies.

On either side of the spinal column, from the atlas to the coccyx, we find sympathetic nerve-ganglia, which are protected by muscular fibres. These ganglia act as electric batteries which are charged with the descending current and which distribute this current to the right and left to the various organs.

Special mention may well be made of the sensitivity current which is to be found in the first of the four layers of the skin. If the latter is in normal condition, the nervous current passes freely through the nerve fibres, but if the skin becomes attached to the underlying muscle, the current cannot pass, the part loses its sensibility and is said to be paralysed.

It may be stated as a general rule that all illnesses are caused through some kind of disorder in the flow of nervous current. Such disorders are generally caused by adhesions of the muscular fibres. These adhesions may arise suddenly through an accident (such as crushing by a heavy object) or gradually, through constant exercise of a single part of the body, or through exposure to draughts or damp, causing the skin to adhere to the muscles. Such adhesions, though slight at first, obstruct the passage of the nervous current; the adhesion consequently becomes more obstinate, until, finally the passage of the nervous current becomes completely blocked, the tissues fail to be reproduced, and the organ in question loses its suppleness.

Albert Abrams M.D. the father of the 'Black Box', and either a genius or a lunatic, depending upon the entrenched viewpoint from which his ideas are examined, states his views as follows:[2]

Everything in nature is in a state of perpetual motion and the latter is continually changing from one velocity to another.

The power to change the state of motion of a body is *energy*. The total energy contained in matter depends on the extent to which it can be changed. Energy is the universal commodity on which all life depends.

All forms of energy, whether derived from heat, electricity, magnetism or gravitation are interconvertible and represent practically different varieties of motion. Energy, like matter, can neither be created nor destroyed. The first principle of energetics is, all physical phenomena (vital or chemical), are forms of motion. All these forms are susceptible to or change into one another, and in all the transformations the quantity of mechanical work represented by different modes of motions remains invariable. Atomic energy, like matter, in accordance with the Law of the Conservation of Energy, is indestructible and uncreatable. Energy is differentiated as *potential and kinetic*.

Our present conception of matter presumes a cyclic or vibratory motion of electrons and it continues as potential energy until transformed into actual energy by some exciting energy from without.

Every living being is a transformer of energy converting the environmental energy into mechanical motion, heat and nervous energy.

Investigations of all ages have espoused the theory of *human radiations*.

To some the organism in compared to a Voltaic battery which emits something akin to electricity.

The hagiologist conciliates the reality of radiations by referring to the auras in ancient pictures around the heads and bodies of Christ and the saints. The phenomena of light in materialization have been witnessed and accepted by notable scientists as spiritual phenomena. Of superstition, it has been said, that it is true psychology with the wrong dress.

The writer is convinced that the phenomena are realities independent of disembodied spirits and can be referred to the manifestations of human energy. Disocculting the occult will be possible when one attains a better understanding of the activities of living cells and when the biologist knows the laws that govern cell growth with the accuracy of the scientist knowing his laws. Every individual, it is maintained, is enveloped in a radiance (aura) invisible to the carnal eye and only perceived by the soul accustomed to it. Perception of the aura is the supposed prerogative of clairvoyance but Kilner has shown that any one can observe the 'atmosphere' surrounding the human body by aids of chemical screens, notably one containing a solution of dicyanin which, by partially paralyzing the retinal rods and cones causes visibility of the aura in a darkened room.

Philosophism, the refuge of the scientifically destitute, can never substitute objectivity in scientific research.

There are more false facts than theories and the true scientist does not hesitate to preside at a birth of a theory and officiate at its burial on the morrow. Energy liberated by the organism appears in mechanical, thermal and electrical form.

The human generates electricity statically by muscular movement.

The body may be likened to a collection of storage cells, which are liable to become highly charged, or to have their charge altered by any direct or passing current, or exciting influence. Electromotive force continues even when the body is absolutely motionless, hence the theory of chemical generation of nerve force. Electricity in the body must be constantly discharged, otherwise the electrical pressure would become umbearable. The skin, the body insulator, is not of uniformly high resistance. Sign, electromotive force and current vary with the individual. Whereas the generation of electricity in the body may be constant, its dissipation cannot be so by reason of the varying conditions of external conductivity.

Abrams went into the field of radionic diagnosis and treatment and his contribution to physical therapy included the recognition of reflex areas for diagnostic purposes and spondylotherapy, the percussion of the spinal centres, to create a vibratory response on the part of the body. The author cannot resist the temptation to quote one more paragraph from Abrams book:

> *Why does the physician fail to recognize disease in its incipiency?* Owing to the arbitary domination of the cell theory, he awaits cellular alterations which are *effects*. Disease in its incipiency is only a physiological disturbance. Just as the barometer portends a storm so may these cellular alterations be anticipated and checked. The phenomena of disease are not inert but dynamic. Thus the actions of the body should be regarded as processes and not as structures and, if the microscope is utilized as a criterion of disease when cell changes have ensued, the patient is eligible for the morgue and not the hospital.

Not, it would seem, the words of a lunatic! The concept of an energy discharge from areas of lowered skin resistance and of an 'aura' surrounding the body finds its echoes in modern electro-acupuncture and Kirlian photography.

Dr Randolph Stone has elaborated upon these ideas and has evolved a system of soft tissue and bony manipulation which is designed to restore energy balance. He has called this Polarity Therapy. he states:[3]

Polarity Therapy

In this atomic age of science we realize that matter itself is but a mass of spinning energy particles which appear as solid substances. In reality, they exist as such only because of a constant flow of energy currents between all parts and portions. As soon as that circuit is interrupted, changes begin to appear which, in the human body, are interpreted as pain or disease. The interrupted current cannot reach the core to flow through and out again. In the meantime, the opposing currents pile up energy particles at the point of interruption and act as blocks in the areas where they occur. This pressure of energy particles in any of the five fields of matter registers as intense pain or obstruction of normal energy flow, called disease.

To give an idea of his therapeutic methods the following is illustrative: [4]

Correlate the function of the vital centres through the re-establishment of polarity in the parasympathetic and sympathetic nervous systems by *Perineal and Polarity* contacts and techniques.

Rule. No relaxation of the voluntary nervous system and muscles can occur as long as the involuntary musles are locked and tense. *No bony correction should be forced.* Merely telling the patient to relax, is useless.

Have the patient lie on the left side on a soft table, with the head on a pillow, knees drawn up. The operator sits on a stool, facing the back of the patient. Trace the path of vital forces in their *bipolar* action, from the neck to the perineum.

Check the neck for tenderness and spastic muscles; with the left hand contact the sorest spot, and either inhibit or stimulate firmly (whichever happens to be indicated) over the lamina.

With the first or second finger of the right hand, find the most tender spot in the perineum, on the same side of the neck lesion. Use a finger cot on the finger of this hand, or work through thin clothing, such as a gown or underwear. Take care *never to enter an orifice when giving this treatment*, because the nerve endings we are balancing now are on the surface.

If the pulse is fast, the upper cervical area—or any sore spot over the occipital space—is lightly and slowly stimulated by a double contact, rotary movement; this applies to neck contact in general. Because this is a vagus area, you are balancing the pulse with the two nervous systems. Most pulses are fast because of habitual tension and over-strenuous, hurried living. In these cases, the ropy neck muscles can be slowly manipulated while the Perineal Contact is held.

If the pulse is slow, inhibit the tender neck areas, and further check the carotid pulse of each side of normalization each time after the two contacts are held, until the pulse is improved.

If the pulse is normal, the rule for general treatment applies:

First, inhibit the most tender area gently, then more firmly. This is the principle of 'Yin' inhibition, or drawing off energy.

Second, use heavy pressure or stimulation on the less tender area or constricted area; namely, the principle of 'Yang', to tonify.

Make firm contact with the most tender perineal spot found. The neck and the perineum are contacted *simultaneously.* Regardless of pulse, the perineal contact is made with *one finger*, and is an *upward lift* (toward the head or neck contact, on the same side). This lift is increased as relaxation allows it. If the perineum is flaccid and relaxed, then it needs tone and stimulative contacts, by repeated *upward* impacts on the contact.

Any sharp, pin-sticking sensation here, like a finger nail or knife point is due to crystallized deposits or other products of chemistry, which were carried along by the energy currents in the short-circuiting effect. It is the action of a local cataphoresis. A few inhibitions will cause this to be re-absorbed by the circulation, and carried away, as the short-circuiting is stopped and energy flows in regular paths again. When nerve relaxation occurs the spinal muscles also relax, and previous occipital and dorsal findings will have changed.

The work of Stone incorporates both the Chinese Yin/Yang concept and the Hindu *prana* concept.

Yin and Yang

In Taoist thinking all phenomena are activated by the movement of energy, the opposite poles of which are known as Yin and Yang. The interaction between these two forces is seen in human terms in, for example, the spirallic formation of the embryo and the relationship between various structures and functions. Yin and Yang are seen to operate via the medium of dynamic energy called *chi*. Harmonious flow of this energy is thought to be the prime requirement for health. In such a state the organism vibrates in harmony with its environment. The restoration of this balance is the aim of Oriental medicine in general and acupuncture in particular. Yin and Yang may be thought of as low frequency and high frequency waves respectively. There is said to be a fluctuation of the energy potential in the various body 'meridians' at different times of the day. Thus, each meridian or channel of energy has a period of maximum potential and therefore a period at which time treatment would be more likely to be of benefit. This may sound far fetched but the reader should consider the recent American findings that medication has an optimum time for its effective consumption by the individual. Different body systems have their optimum periods of activity. The study of this phenomenon by orthodox science is called chrono-biology.

Acupuncture points may be located by the measurement of the electrical potential of the skin surface. They will be found in areas of low resistance, and these areas will also be demonstrated (in Kirlian photography for example) as areas of high energy discharge. In active pathological conditions or when dysfunction has occurred these areas will also be sensitive to pressure. The relevance of soft tissue techniques becomes apparent when we realize that pressure on acupuncture points is often just as effective as needling or electrical stimulation. It is also relevant to our study to realize that all these acupuncture points lie within the muscles and fascia and many of them are identical with reflexes discovered by others and which are amenable to techniques used in NMT treatment.

The Aura

Kirlian photography is a technique using high-voltage photography. The developed plates show a luminescence or pattern of electrical discharge emanating from the entire body surface. Various interpretations have been made as to the significance of this electrical 'aura'. From the viewpoint of this study the importance is that it verifies as fact the existence of some sort of electro-magnetic discharge on the part of the body which is influenced by the state of health of the individual and by therapy, of whatever sort.

The influence may not always be to the benefit of the body and the patterns of discharge will vary accordingly. The verification of acupuncture points as areas of greater discharge is also significant, especially as these areas can be shown to become more or less active in different pathological states, and further that they can be seen to be more or less sensitive to pressure at the same times. In attempting to reach an understanding of the acupuncture phenomenon I have quoted from the work of Speransky, in my book *The Acupuncture Treatment of Pain*.[5]

> In his study of the nature of disease, Speransky explained how, after years of research, he became convinced that, in studying the processes of diseases, the traditional subdivision of the nervous system into central, peripheral, sympathetic etc. had no justification. He showed in many experiments that, from any point in the nervous system, it was possible to bring into action nerve mechanisms, the functioning of which terminated at the periphery, producing changes of a bio-physico-chemical character.
>
> He developed the thesis that any nerve point, not excluding peripheral nerve structures, could become the originator of neuro-dystrophic processes serving as the temporary or permanent nerve centre of these processes, and pointed out that whenever a procedure affected the nervous aspect of any phenomenon, the resultant changes were not only in the nerve portion concerned, but in the whole intricate complex. Also apparent from his work was the fact that irritation of any points of the nervous system could evoke changes, not only in the adjacent parts, but also in remote regions of the organism.
>
> Finally, he stated that it became evident that the usefulness of operating on the nervous system was often due to the very act of interference itself and not to its form, whilst harm depended on its form and was associated with excessive trauma. I find in these thoughts of Speransky's the justification for my views on acupuncture and, in a large part, the explanation for the acupuncture phenomenon.

Rolfing   A system of physical therapy that incorporates a concept of energy being 'locked' in the body in states of disease and being released by therapy is that developed by Ida Rolf. 'Rolfing' recognizes a total mind/body interaction and sees this reflected in the muscuoskeletal component of the body where a degree of shielding or armouring takes place to protect the individual from emotional discomforts, as well as from the conscious experience of inner hurts, that accumulate throughout life. A further concept of Rolfing is that gravity not only upholds man but that it 'feeds' him. It sees therapy as designed to release energies locked up in the armour or defence mechanism and to balance (posturally) the individual so that the forces of gravity can act and support him.

The importance of energy locked into the musculoskeletal tissues was demonstrated by Eeman.[6] His work, which was similar in direction to that of Abrams and Stone, clearly showed that without neuro-muscular relaxation there could not be mento-emotional relaxation. This observation can now be demonstrated by measuring brain wave patterns in varying stages of physical relaxation.

Cooper[7] echoes Rolf's ideas and adds some additional thoughts of some significance. He points out that osteopathic practitioners have observed and recorded the extent to which all degenerative changes in the body are reflected in the superficial fascia. Any degree of degeneration changes the nature of fascia. As this elastic envelope is stretched, manipulative mechanical energy is added to it and fascial colloid softens to become more gel-like and less solid. He states:

> It is an accepted fact that life happens only where there is protoplasm behaving colloidally. In living structures the colloids are extremely sensitive, with enormous possibilities with regard to stability and reversibility of phase. One of the characteristics of life is periodicity or rhythmicity, in other words, fluctuation between predominance of sol and gel phases.
>
> In an organism living in health, the complex totality of manifold colloidal structures behaves with appropriate periodicity and rhythm between certain phase limits. Any phase

of any of the colloidal systems which goes beyond the appropriate limit or fails to reach the limit within the proper time will affect the health of the organism as a whole. Likewise any factor, intrinsic or extrinsic, capable of altering colloidal behaviour will have a marked effect one way or another on the welfare of the organism. Physical colloidal states so paired with nervous, mental, and other characteristics and illnesses are connected with colloidal disturbances.

He goes on to point out that colloids may be influenced by five factors, i.e. physical (e.g. heat), biological (e.g. bacteria), chemical (e.g. drugs). psychic (e.g. practitioner's intention; emotion) and mechanical (e.g. pressure or friction).

Taylor[8] points out that:

It is the law of the physical universe that every system, if left to itself, changes spontaneously either slowly or rapidly in such a way as to approach a definite final state of rest or equilibrium. Likewise, it is also a law of the universe that, once this state of rest or equilibrium has been reached, no reverse change or moving away from equilibrium can be brought about without the application of some form of energy. This is the thermodynamic concept and is simply stated: a system and its surroundings are in equilibrium in such a way that any change in the energy of the system will result in a change in the energy of its surroundings.

Lawson-Wood has written widely on energy in relation to health and he states in regard to colloidal states:[9]

All life is found in the colloidal form; and there are many forms of 'gel' which have been in that state of 'gel' for a very long time and are unlikely to do other than continue the slow ageing process but which are nevertheless reversible if energy of the right kind can be applied.

Cooper and Lawson-Wood insist on the importance of operators visualizing his intention and the desired end-result of the manipulative or soft tissue treatment. This they maintain will have an effect on the colloidal state. Becker[10] makes the important additional comment on the value of the patient's consciousness being incorporated into the therapy programme in whatever dysfunction there might be. He gives the following example:

To illustrate the matter of changing the programme an individual has installed to resist a postural imbalance due to anatomical inequality in the lower extremeties: Since the programme was established to maintain body balance on an uneven base, it is obvious that simply placing a lift under the short leg will increase the problem because the programme is automatic. The muscle pulls that served to maintain balance on an uneven base will be inappropriate under the new circumstances and will create further imbalance unless the individual is trained to reprogramme the computer (i.e. his mind). So the physician explains to the patient how the new balance will affect her actions, uses whatever methods he prefers to equalize muscle tensions and fascial pulls and correct or release any impairments in articular motion, teaches the patient to cancel the old programmes by consciously releasing the muscles each time before she starts a new action and gives her some controlled exercises which call into play new standards or proprioceptive data which now will define the normal, acceptable and tolerate limits.

Becker goes on to comment on residual patterns of soft tissue stress following a traumatic incident, namely, a whiplash injury.

Here the problem is complicated by the fact that the body has been subjected to forces that entered it in a direction that crosses the normal direction of movement. Such forces tend to produce a wave-like movement within the fluid cells of the body, and the inertia of the body, which is trying to continue whatever programmes are in action at the time, causes a counterwave directed toward the point of impact. The resultant of these two sets of force vectors produces a standing wave, or ridge of energy, a kind of built-in distortion, around which the defensive programmes are installed. If the physician attempts to remove this distortion, the body activates the protective mechanisms or programmes unless the physician first dissipates this ridge of energy by appropriate manipulative means. In other words, the energy of impact and the counter-energy of resistance must be permitted to pass through each other rather than opposing one another, and then the programmes in the CNS computer which were designed to operate around this built-in distortion must be cancelled and new ones established to include the new energy.

Energy means different things to different people. Simple stress patterns locked into the soft tissues as a result of trauma or postural or emotional factors will reduce the energy potentials of the individual. Release will encourage normalization and will reduce the drain on vital energy. That is the simplistic view and if that is all that is involved it is of great value.

If, however, there do exist more subtle energy transactions which soft tissue dysfunction can interrupt then the value of the restoration of balance in this regard will be of immense value. The reader must solve the riddle to his own satisfaction. The quest for greater knowledge in this field will lead to many strange abstruse byways of human research and endeavour. That something akin to an energy field surrounds the body is not really the question. What is to be clearly established is that the existence of this has relevance to the field of health in general and manipulative therapy in particular.

[1] Varma, Dewanchand, *The Human Machine and Its Forces*, (Health For All Publishing Co., 1930).
[2] Abrams, Dr Albert, *New Concepts in Diagnosis and Treatment*, (Physico-clinical Co., San Francisco, 1922).
[3] Stone, Randolph, *Polarity Therapy*, (privately published, 1954).
[4] Stone, Randolph, *The New Energy Concept*, (privately published, 1948).
[5] Chaitow, Leon, *The Acupuncture Treatment of Pain*, (Thorsons, 1976).
[6] Eeman, L., *Co-operative Healing*, (Frederick Muller, 1947).
[7] Cooper, Gerald J., *Journal of the American Osteopathic Association*, Vol. 78, pp. 336-73 (January, 1979).
[8] Taylor, R. B., 'Bio-energetics of Man', *Academy of Applied Osteopathy Yearbook*, 1958, P. 91.
[9] Lawson-Wood, D. and J., *Progressive Vitality and Dynamic Posture*, (Health Science Press, 1978).
[10] Becker, Alan R., 'Parameters of Resistance', *Journal of the American Osteopathic Association* (September, 1973), p. 39.

Bibliography

Barlow, W., 'Anxiety and Muscle Tension Pain,' *British Journal of Clinical Practice,* Vol. 3, No. 5.

Becker, Alan R., 'Parameters of Resistance', *Journal of the American Osteopathic Association* (Sept. 1973), p. 39.

Blashy, M., 'Manipulation of the Neuromuscular Unit via the Periphery of the CNS', *Southern Medical Journal* (Aug. 1961).

Boadella, David, 'The Language of the Body in Bio-energetic Therapy', *Journal of the Research Society for Natural Therapeutics* (1978).

Cathie, Dr A., 'Selected Writings,' *Academy of Applied Osteopathy Yearbook* (1974).

Chaitow, Leon, 'An Introduction to Chapman's Reflexes', *British Naturopathic Journal* (Spring 1965).

——*The Acupuncture Treatment of Pain* (Thorsons Publishers Limited, Wellingborough, Northants, 1976).

Cooper, Gerald J., 'Considerations on Fascia in Diagnosis and Treatment', *Journ. of Amer. Ost. Assoc.,* Vol. 78 (Jan. 1979), pp 336-73.

Cyriax, J., *Textbook of Orthopaedic Medicine,* Vols 1 and 2 (Balliere).

Dittrich, R. J., 'Somatic Pain and Autonomic Concomitants', *American Journal of Surgery* (1954).

Ebner, M., *Connective Tissue Massage* (Churchill Livingstone, 1962).*

Erlinghauser, R. F., 'Circulation of CSF through Connective Tissue', *Academy of Applied Osteopathy Yearbook* (1959).

Fielder and Pyott, *The Science and Art of Manipulative Surgery* (American Institute of Manipulative Surgery Inc., 1955).

Grieve, Gregory, *Mobilization of the Spine,* (Churchill Livingstone, 1984).

Gustein, R., 'The Role of Abdominal Fibrositis in Functional Indigestion', *Mississippi Valley Medical Journal,* 66 (1944), p. 114.

—— 'A Review of Myodysneuria (Fibrositis),' *American Practitioner and Digest of Treatments,* Vol. 6, No. 4.

—— 'The Role Craniocervical Myodysneuria in Functional Ocular Disorders', *American Practitioner and Digest of Treatments* (Nov. 1956).

* Now available in a revised edition from Krieger Publishing Co., Inc., U.S.A.

Hagbarth, K., 'Excitatory and Inhibitory Skin Areas for Flexor and Extensor Motoneurons', *Acta Physiologia Scandinavia* (1952).

Jacobson, E., 'Principles Underlying Coronary Heart Disease', *Cardiologia* (1956), ppl 16-83.

Jones, L. H., 'Foot Treatment Without Hand Trauma', *Journ. Amer. Ost. Assoc.* (July, 1963).

—— *Strain and Counterstrain*, (American Academy of Osteopathy, 1981).

Korr, I., 'Spinal Cord as Organiser of Disease Process', *Academy of Applied Osteopathy Yearbook* (1976).

Lawson-Wood, D. and Lawson-Wood, J., *Progressive Vitality and Dynamic Posture* (Health Science Press, 1978).

Lewit, Karel, *Manipulative Therapy in Rehabilitation of the Motor System* (Butterworth, 1985).

Little, K. E., 'Toward More Effective Manipulative Management of Chronic Myofascial Strain and Stress Syndromes', *Journal of the Academy of Applied Osteopathy,* Vol. 68 (March, 1969).

Mennel, J., 'The Therapeutic Use of Cold', *Journ. Amer. Ost. Assoc.,* Vol. 74 (Aug. 1975).

Patterson, M., 'Model Mechanism for Spinal Segmental Facilitation', *Academy of Applied Osteopathy Yearbook* (1976).

Postgraduate Institute of Osteopathic Medicine and Surgery, *The Physiological Basis of Osteopathic Medicine* (New York, 1970).

Reich, Wilhelm, *Character Analysis* (Vision Press).

Rolf, Ida, 'Structural Dynamics', *Academy of Applied Osteopathy Yearbook* (1962).

Selye, H., *The Stress of Life* (McGraw Hill, 1956).

Stoddard, A., *Manual of Osteopathic Practice* (Hutchinson, 1969).

Taylor, R. B., 'Bioenergetics of Man', *Academy of Applied Osteopathy Yearbook* (1958).

Travell, J., 'Ethyl Chloride Spray for Painful Muscle Spasm', *Arch. Phys. Med. Rehabl.,* 33 (May, 1952), pp. 291-8.

—— 'Symposium on Mechanism and Management of Pain Syndromes', *Proc. Rudolph Virchow Medical Society* (1957).

Travell, J., and Bigelow, N., 'Role of Somatic Trigger Areas in Patterns of Hysteria', *Psychosomatic Medicine,* Vol. 9, No. 6.

Webber, T. D., 'Diagnosis and Modification of Headache and Shoulder, Arm, Hand Syndromes', *Journ. Amer. Ost. Assoc.,* Vol. 72 (March, 1973).

Youngs, B., 'NMT of Lower Thorax and Low Back', *British Naturopathic Journal,* Vol. 5, No. 11.

—— 'Physiological Background of N.M. Technique', *British Naturopathic Journal,* Vol. 5, No. 6.

Index

Note: **Bold** entries refer to tables and illustrations.

Abdominal Reflex Areas,
  Mackenzie's, 89, **90,** 189-90
Abdominal Technique
  Basic, 187-93, **190**
  General, 196-7
  Specific release, 142-7, **144,
   146**
Abrams MD, Albert, 258, 262,
  264
Acromio-clavicular (AC)
  dysfunction, 219-20, **220**
acupressure, 178, 183, 246, 247
acupuncture points, 9, 56,
  62-73, 93, 142
  see also Ah Shi points
Acupuncture Treatment of Pain
  (Chaitow, L.), 262
aerophagia, 104-5
Ah Shi points, 45, 66, 142, 178,
  247
  see also: acupressure;
   acupuncture points
akebane points, 70, **71**
  see also acupuncture points
alarm points, 67-70, **68**
  see also acupuncture
Alexander Technique, 104, 197
anaesthetic injection, 43, 48, 77
annulospiral fibres, **26,** 27
Applied Kinesiology, 62, 63,
  131, 132
  technique, 141
Arbuckle DO, Beryl, 162
  *Selected Writings of Beryl
   Arbuckle,* 56
aura, 259, 261-2
autonomic nervous system,
  23-4, 48, 52, 63

Barlow, Dr Wilfred, 18, 39,
  101, 104
Beal DO, Myron, 48, 47, 50
Becker, Alan R., 263, 264
Bennett, Dr Terence, 10, 57
Bennett's Neurovascular Reflex

Points, 48, 57-62, **60-1,** 72,
  126, 189
Blashey, Dr M., 51, 73
'bloodless surgery', 142, 143
Bosey MD, Jean, 72
Botek MD, Stephen, 64
Bourbillon, J., *Spinal
  Manipulation,* 206
breathing, 103, 105, 205, 209,
  225
Buzzell DO, Keith, 25, 27

Cathie, Dr A., 21, 22, 39
central nervous system, 25-8, 42
Chaitow, Boris, 12, 32-3, 124,
  142, 171, 186
Chapman's neurolymphatic
  reflex points, 9, 38, 44, 45,
  48, 93-4, 178, 189, 246
  definition of, 54
  location of, **163-72**
  mechanism of, 54
  and research evidence, 55-7
  and vibratory treatment, 126
chemical structure of tissue,
  34-5
chi, 70, 261
chiropractics, 10, 11, 18, 37
clinical use of NMT, 195-200
CNS, 25-8, 42
collagen, 22, 31, 34-5, 212-13
colloid, 262-3
Connective Tissue Massage
  (CTM), 23-5, 52-4
Cooper, Gerald, 262, 263, 264
CTM, 23-5, 52-4
Cyriax, J., 22, 23, 39

diagnostic and therapeutic role
  of soft tissues *see* soft tissues
diagnostic methods, 75-96
Dittrich, R. J., 47, 73
Dominant Eye Assessment, 95
drugs, 30

Ebner, Maria, 23-4, 39, 85, 96
Eeman, L., 20, 39, 262, 263
effleurage (stroking), 24, 36-7,
  149
elbow
  technique, 128, **129**
  use of, 128, 154
electro-acupuncture, 70, 72-3,
  259
emotions, 19, 97-119
end-organs, 25-7
energy, 20, 201, 257-64
  aura, the, 261-2
  Polarity Therapy, 259-61
  Rolfing, 262-4
  Yin and Yang, 261
Ernst MD, Monique, 64
etiology, 94-5
Evans, J., 47, 73
exercise, 36, 115, 161, 197
exercises, 116-18
eye positions, 205, 225

facilitation, theory of, 28-30
fascia, functions of, 16, 21-2
fatigue, 31, 100, 257
fibrositis, 22-3, 76
Fielder, 189, 193
Fielder's reflex areas, **188**
finger techniques, 123-4, **123**
fingers, use of, 33, 37, 76, 92,
  123-4, 125, 126, 128-9, 130,
  133, 137, 143-4, 145, 146,
  149, 177, 179, 180, 186, 190,
  191
fingertips, use of, 176, 179, 184,
  191, 192
Flower Spray fibre, **26,** 27
fluids, displacement of, 37, 127
friction, 37, 149
Freyette, Harrison, 133
Fuchs, Julian, 51
functional techniques, gentle,
  11, 28, 36

gamma motor system, 30

GAS, 16-17, 35, 79
gastro-intestinal dysfunction, 43, 44
Gelb, Harold, *Clinical Management of Head, Neck and TMJ Pain and Dysfunction*, 137
General Adaptation Syndrome (GAS), 16-17, 35, 99
Goldthwait, *Essentials of Body Mechanics*, 100
Golgi tendon organs, 25, **26,** 27, 37, 64, 141, 208
Goodheart, Dr George, 63-4, 141, 178
Goodridge DO, John, 204, 216, 220-1, 225, 226
gravity, 105, 156, 159, 206, 216, 262
Grieve, G., 31, 32, 36, 39, 204
Grieve's Psoas method, 136-7
Gunn, G. Chan, 64
Gutstein, R., 21, 39, 42-4, 73, 178, 189, 193

hands, use of, 37, 128-9, 143, 145, 147, 149, 156, 158
Hartman, Laurie, 24, 210-11
Heiling DO, David, 204
holistic approach, 12-13, 105, 195, 196
homoeostatic mechanisms, 17, 71, 102
Hoover, Harold, 247
hormones, 35
HSZ, 38, 57, 89-91, 93, 125-6
Human Machine and Its Forces, The (Varma), 32
Hyperalgesic Skin Zones (HSZ), 38, 57, 89-91, 93, 125-6
hypertonia, 98, 99
hyperventilation, 104
hypotonia, 98, 99

Iliotibial Band Techniques, 156-9, **158, 159**
Induration Technique, 75, 137
infiltration method, 196
intercostal treatment, 190-1
intrinsic muscles (Stabilizers), 98
irritation, 66, 67
Isaacson, 98, 99
isokinetic contraction, 203, 211, 213, 214, 230
isolytic contraction, 158, 159, 203, 212-13, 221, 229, 230
isometric contraction, 158, 159, 201, 203, 204, 205, 207, 208, 210, 216, 226, 229
isometrics, 36, 38, 136, 141, 154, 155-6
isotonic contraction, 36, 201, 203, 204, 207, 208, 210, 221, 230

concentric, 201, 203, 212, 214, 228, 230
eccentric, 201, 203, 212, 213, 221, 230

Jandra, Vladimir, 207
Jokl, Peter, 30, 31, 32, 36, 39
Jones, Dr Lawrence, 28, 29, 36, 38, 45, 66, 141
and development of technique, 241
and low back pain, 100, 119
Strain-Counterstrain, 246, 250
Jones' Technique, 241, 247-50
Jones' Tender Points, 189, 206

Kirlain photography, 259, 261
Koizumi, Kiyomi, 89
Korr, 25, 27, 28, 29, 30, 32, 248

LAS, 16-17, 35, 99
Latey DO, Philip, 101, 102
Muscular Manifesto, 101, 103
Lawson-Wood, D., 263, 264
Lewit, Karel, 36, 38, 39, 91
and HSZ, 126
Manipulative Theory, in Rehabilitation of the Motor Systems, 37, 45
and MET methods, 204-6
and Piriformis technique, 155-6
and Psoas technique, 132, 136
and TMJ problems, 141
Lief DO, Peter, 33, 34, 76
Lief, Stanley, 11-12, 32-4, 124, 142, 171, 175-86
lifting skin folds, 91-2, **91**
Local Adaptation Syndrome (LAS), 16-17, 35, 99
low back pain, 30-1, 100-1, 251
and MET, 226-8, **227**
lubricant, use of, 124, 138, 149, 174, 190
Lymphatic Pump Method, 1, 162, **162**
Method 2, 163, **163**

McConnel DO, Carl, 11, 105
McKenzie, Sir James, 10, 24, 89, 189
manipulation, 11, 18, 37-9, 115, 196, 197
theory, changes in, 20
Mann, Felix, 47, 65
massage, 10, 23-5, 36, 37-9, 52-4, 208
techniques, 147-50
Mennell, Dr J., 24, 42, 43, 73, 160
MET
Acromio-clavicular (AC) ·
dysfunction, 219-20, **220**

and antagonists, 203, 207, 210, 215
application of, 217
and barrier, 209, 210, 213, 215, 218-19
and cervical problems, 217-18, 219
development of technique, 208-9
exercise for beginners, 220-1
and extensors of wrist, 222-5, **223**
and eye movements, 205, 225
and force used, 205, 210, 212, 216
and Iliotibial band problems, 157-9
lengthening shortened muscles, 221
and localization of forces, 207-8, 209-10
and Long Biceps Tendon, 225
low back dysfunction, 31, 226-8, **227**
lumbosacral ligament pain, 225
operator-direct method, 204, 213, 218, 229
patient-direct method, 213, 229
patient-indirect method, 204, 210
and PIR, 213, 225
and piriformis problems, 154-6, **155**
and preparation of joints, 210-11
and Psoas spasm, 136-7
reduction of fibrotic change, 212-13
reporting stations, 28
spasm release, 213-15
sternomastoid treatment, 222, **222**
strengthening joint complexes, 211-12
strengthening weak muscles, 221
and terminology, 201, 203, 204
and TMJ treatment, 138, 141
torticollis, 215-16, **215**
treatment, 119, 127, 128
and trigger points, 42, 73, 203
use of, 30, 38, 207
variations summary, 229-30
and whiplash, 218-19
Mitchell, F. L., 127, 208
Endocrine Interpretation of Chapman's Reflexes, An, 161
morphology of points, 72

Moule DO, Terry G., 198-9
Muscle Energy Technique, *see* MET
muscle spindles, **26,** 27, 30, 37
muscle testing, 105-118
muscle weakness, 31, 106, 107, 108, 109, 110
muscles, role of, 241
   types of, 31, 35-7
musculo-skeletal system, 10-11, 15, 20
myodysneuria, 21, 43, 44, 189
myofascial
   needling, 64
   tender points, 242-7
   trigger points, 9, 36, 38, 41, **78-84**

Neurolymphatic Reflexes (Chapman's, 10, 93-4, 127, 161-72, **172-72**
neuro-muscular lesion, causes of, 33-4
Neuro-Muscular Technique, *see* NMT
Neurosis, effects of, 19
neurovascular points, 10
Nimmo, Raymond, 9-10, 24, 39, 55
NMT
   aims of, 195, 196
   application of, 34, 171, 196, 197
   assessment, 50
   and athletic injury, 198-9
   Basic Abdominal Technique, 187-193
   Basic Spinal Technique, 173-85
   benefits of, 77, 195-6, 199
   and Bennett's points, 62
   and Chapman's reflexes,55
   in clinical use, 195-200
   and Connective Tissue Massage, 23, 24
   continuity of contact, 179-80
   development of, 32-4
   diagnostic and therapeutic role of, 11, 12, 28, 50, 171, 177, 195
   general treatment approach, 178-9
   low back pain, 31
   and manipulation, 10, 38-9, 197
   and pain control, 64
   and postural problems, 115
   and psychotherapy, 197
   and reporting stations, 28
   role of, 38-9
   techniques, 121-71
   and theatrical performers, 199-200
   tissues involved with, 34-5

treatment, 77, 119, 128, 196-7
   and trigger areas, 41-4, 73, 177-8
   and zones of soft tissues, 89
nutrition, 22, 33, 44, 197, 213

operator
   position of, 121, 128, 133, 136-7, 143, 145, 147, 154, 156, 175, 176, **180,** 181, **182,** 184, **184, 185,** 186
   privileged position of, 150
   skills of, 171-2
orthokinetic fields, 51
osteopaths, 10, 12, 18, 20, 37, 262
over-treatment, 126, 160-1, 162, 184, 192

Page, Dr Leon, 99, 119
pain
   low back, 30-1, 100-1
   patterns, 41, 47, 77, **78-84**
   referred, 15, 38, 41, 42, 48, 65, 77, **78-84,** 126, 177
   reflex, 47-8
   source of, 18-19
   as symptom of dysfunction, 38
   threshold, 64
   types of, 15
palpation, 44, 49-50, 57, 75-7
pathways, 24, 29, 52, 77, 190
Patterson, Professor Michael, 28, 32, 39
Pauling, Linus, 22, 39
pelvic diaphragm, relaxing, 103-4
pelvic tilt, 107, 108, 109-10
Periosteal Pain Points (PPP), 38, **45-6**
petrissage, 147-9
physiotherapists, 12, 18, 37
pinch (squeeze), 181
pinch-roll technique, 126
PIR, *see* post-isometric relaxation
Piriformis Muscle Technique, 150-6, **152, 153, 155, 157**
Polarity Therapy, 259-61
positioning, spontaneous release by, 29-30
post-isometric relaxation (PIR), 38, 202, 213, 218, 219, 221, 225, 227, 228
posture, 18, 97, 101, 115
   and emotions, 97-119
   fascia, 99-100
   homoeostasis, 18
   muscles, 36, 98
   and stress, 9, 31
   and tension, 18
pressure, 20, 21, 37, 41, 126-8
proprioceptive adjustment

(Applied Kinesiology), **131,** 132
proprioceptive neuromuscular facilitation (PNF), 202
Psoas, 132-3, **132,** 133-7, **134, 135**
pulsation, 57, 71, 126

Rabagliatti, Dr, *Initis*, 32, 34
reciprocal inhibition, 36, 202-3, 210, 215, 221, 226
record-keeping, 174-5
re-education, 18, 115, 118, 197
referred pain, 15, 38, 48, 77, **78-84,** 177
   point of, 65
   and pressure, 126
   and trigger areas, 41, 42
reflex
   activity, 38, 93
   areas and somatic dysfunction, 41-73
   grouping of, 161-72, **163-72**
   pain, 47-8
   pathways, 24, 190
   points, 44-5
   relaxation, 37
   role of, 42
   systems, 9
   tendon, 27
Reich, Wilhelm, 19, 39, 104
relaxation, 30, 104, 105, 197, 205
release techniques
   specific, 193
   spontaneous, 141-2
reporting stations, 25-8, **26**
respiration, *see* breathing
resting length, full, 42, 127, 128, 203
Rolf, Ida, 20, 39, 206, 262
Rolfing, 20-1, 104, 115, 206, 236, 262-4

segments, spinal, 49, 50, 52
   facilitated, 28-9
Serizawe MD, Katsusuke, 62-3
Selye, Hans, 16-17, 35, 39, 66, 99
Sherrington's Law, 154, 207
skills
   of diagnostic assessment, 99
   of operator, 207-8, 214, 216, 242, 247
   plapatory, 57
skin
   changes, 75
   distraction, 91, 92-4
   elasticity, 125
   folds, lifting, 91-2, **91**
   reflex zones, 89-91
   rolling, 52-3, 91
   and muscles, 51, **51**
   see also HSZ

soft-tissues, diagnostic and
   therapeutic manipulation, 10,
   38-9, 197
   role of, 11, 12, 28, 50, 171,
     177, 195
   see also: NMT; Somatic
     dysfunction; zones of
     altered tissues
somatic dysfunction
   and reflex areas, 41-73
   and soft-tissue component,
     15-39
Speransky, 66-7
   *Basis for the Theory of
     Medicine, A*, 94, 262
spinal cord, 25, 28-9, 32
Spinal NMT Technique, Basic,
   173-86
spindle, muscle, **26,** 27, 30, 132,
   141, 248-9
Splenic or Liver Pump
   techniques, 147
Spondylotherapy, 130, **130,** 259
springing, 150, 218
sternomastoid contraction, 222,
   222
Stiles DO, Edward, 95, 208-9
Stiles' piriformis technique, 156,
   157
Still, Andrew Taylor, 9
Stoddard, Dr Alan, 23, 39, 137
Stone, Dr Randolph, 245, 262,
   264
Strain-counterstrain, 241-51
   and abdominal reflex areas,
     189
   CNS, 248-9
   concept of, 231-2, 248-9
   location of tender points, 233
   methods, 66
   mobile points, 232
   muscle spindles, 248-9
   myofascial tender points,
     242-7
   normalization mechanics,
     248-9
   pain relief, 246
   panic reaction 241, 242
   position of joint, 247, 248
   and reporting stations, 28
   technique, 142, 242, 247-50
   tender areas, 242
   treatment, 250-2, **250, 251**
   trigger points, 73
   value of, 246-7
Stress
   bands, 99, 246-7
   effects of, 17, 41

effects on tissues, 16-17
   emotional, 19
   and homoeostasis, 102
   and hormones, 35
   occupational, 18, 31
   and points, 66
   postural, 9
   reduction and CMT, 53
   responses, 18
   and spinal pathways, 29
stretching, 20, 36-7
   and strengthening exercises,
     116-118
stroking (effleurage), 24, 36-7,
   149
structure and function
   relationship, 97-9
symptoms
   of dysfunction, 10-11, 28
   of emotional involvement,
     102

Takeshige, Chifuyu, 64
Taylor, R. B., 19, 20, 39, 250,
   263
techniques, *see* under individual
   names
Tieriche-Leube, H., 85, 96
Tempero-mandibular Joint
   (TMJ)
   dysfunction techniques,
     137-41, 139, 140
Tender Point Technique, 241-4
tender points, 28, 36, 38, 45, 66
   spots, 189
tenderness, 76
tendon reflex, 27
tension bands, 99, 100
terminology, 15, 201, 203, 204
tests (muscle), 95, 105-118
therapeutic role of soft-tissues,
   see soft-tissues
Thie, John, 57
thumb
   technique, 121-3, **122**
   tip, use of, 190
   as treating instrument, 171,
     175, 176-7, 179, 180, 183,
     184, 186
   use of, 37, 121-3, 124, 126,
     128-9, 142, 144, 145, 147,
     149, 154, 157, 158, 190,
     191, 192
Tissue Release Technique, 128-9
tissues involved in NMT, 34-5
TMJ techniques, 137-41, **139,
140**
torticollis, 215-16, **215**

Travell, Dr Janet, 24, 41, 42,
   44, 73, 85, 160
treatment
   CTM, 24-5
   of emotional involvement,
     103-4
   pattern, 118-19
   programme, 36-7, 115-16
   of tigger areas, 43
   see also: NMT; MET; Strain-
     counterstrain
trigger areas, 21, 41-2, 43
trigger points, 21, 32
   and acupuncture, 64-6, 67, 70,
     72
   defined, 44
   and electro-acupuncture, 72-3
   and MET, 203
   and nerves, 22
   and pain patterns, 77
   symptoms from, 72-3
   treatment of, 41-2, 126-8
   and vapo-coolant technique,
     160-1
Tsubo, 62, 178, 183, 247

Ulett, George, 64
umbilicus, 192-3

Vannerson, James, 55, 127
vapo-coolant spray, 160-1, 196
Varma, Dewandchand, 32-3,
   257, 264
vasomotor dysfunction, 43
vibration, 37, 126, 257-8
viscera, 189
viscerosomatic reflexes, 48-50
visualization, 174
vitamin C, 22, 213

weight transfer, 175, 177, 180,
   191
whiplash and MET, 218-19
Williams MD, Paul, *Lumbosacral Spine, The*, 201
wrist extensors, 222-5, **223**

x-rays, 133, 218

Yin and Yang, 260, 261
yoga, 136
Youngs, Brian, 34, 39, 76, 89,
   96

zones of altered soft-tissue,
   85-9, **85-8**
   see also HSZ